D1591922

Introduction to Diagnostic Sonography

Introduction to Diagnostic Sonography

Arthur C. Fleischer, M.D.
Coordinator of Ultrasound Educational Programs
Section of Diagnostic Ultrasound
Department of Radiology and Radiological Sciences
Vanderbilt University School of Medicine
Nashville, Tennessee

A. Everette James, Jr., Sc.M., J.D., M.D.
Professor and Chairman
Department of Radiology and Radiological Sciences
Chief, Section of Diagnostic Ultrasound
Vanderbilt University School of Medicine
Nashville, Tennessee

A WILEY MEDICAL PUBLICATION
JOHN WILEY & SONS
New York · Chichester · Brisbane · Toronto

Library of Congress Cataloging in Publication Data:

Fleischer, Arthur C

  Introduction to diagnostic sonography.

  (A Wiley medical publication)
  Includes index.
  1. Diagnosis, Ultrasonic. I. James, Alton
Everette, 1938–   joint author. II. Title.
RC78.7.U4F53   616.07'54   79-19065
ISBN 0-471-05473-9

Printed in the United States of America

10 9 8 7 6 5 4 3 2 1

To our families and all those who encourage creativity

Preface

In order to attain proficiency in a particular clinical discipline, a comprehensive study of the principles applied in its daily practice must be understood. Accordingly, this book is designed for all those who wish to familiarize themselves both with the techniques of performing sonographic examinations and with the diagnostic principles employed in their interpretation. Concise discussions and illustrative case material are presented in a manner similar to that used in Felson's *Fundamentals of Chest Roentgenology*, Lalli's *Tailored Urogram*, Peterson and Kieffer's *Introduction to Neuroradiology*, and White's *Fundamentals of Vascular Radiology*. It is hoped that this book will prove effective in explaining the fundamental concepts that underlie the daily practice of diagnostic ultrasound.

To the specialty trainee, medical student, and clinician, this book provides an overview of the present applications of diagnostic sonography, with some insight regarding future developments. Clinical applications are discussed in sufficient detail to enable the primary physician or imaging consultant to employ sonography appropriately in the evaluation of certain clinical entities. The biomedical engineering principles involved in ultrasound are discussed only as they pertain to creating images of clinically useful quality.

The text is meant to be concise but complete. Each chapter begins with a discussion of the indications for sonographic studies to evaluate a particular group of clinical disorders. The technical factors that influence image quality are then mentioned as they pertain to delineation and recognition of normal anatomical structures and to the abnormalities in question. The sonographic features of common disorders are stressed and the less common entities discussed only as they significantly relate to the differential diagnosis of a particular entity. When possible, important diagnostic principles are summarized in tables. "State of the art" images were obtained whenever possible and are employed to illustrate the diagnostic entities. Areas of interest on the sonograms are indicated with only a few arrows so that the original features of the image are preserved. At the end of each chapter, a selected list of references is included for those who desire further information on a particular topic.

Arthur C. Fleischer
A. Everette James, Jr.

Acknowledgments

The authors would like to express their gratitude to many people who contributed to the composition of this book. First is Raymond L. Powis, Ph.D., whose assistance in composing the first chapter is gratefully acknowledged. The authors express their thanks to Annie M. Lindsey, R.T., R.D.M.S., and Carol Cherry, R.T., who performed many of the sonographic examinations used in this book. A debt of gratitude is owed to Betty Burnside, Sally Oliver, Sandy Strohl, Angela Sullivan, and Lynn Fleischer for their assistance in preparing the manuscript in its various editions. John Bobbitt provided expert photographic support. The artwork performed by Mary Cooley Walker and David Christia, M.D., also added greatly to the book.

The authors also acknowledge colleagues who, through their suggestions and criticism, had an important influence on the content of each chapter. These include Frank H. Boehm, M.D., for his criticism of Chapter 2; Conrad Julian, M.D., for his comments on Chapter 3; Tom Jones, M.D., for his assistance with Chapter 4; M. Louis Weinstein, M.D., for his criticism of Chapters 4 and 5; Richard M. Heller, M.D., and Sandra G. Kirchner, M.D., for their comments concerning Chapter 6; and Rosemarie Robertson, M.D., for her criticisms and illustrations for Chapter 7. Many people were kind enough to supply images of cases that the authors did not have in their teaching collection. These are acknowledged in the legends of the figures.

Finally, the authors express their sincere appreciation to their clinical and radiological colleagues whose interaction provided daily clinical input concerning the patients who were examined in our clinic.

Contents

1
Basic Principles*

*With the assistance of Raymond L. Powis, Ph.D.

HISTORICAL PERSPECTIVE

The use of reflected ultrasonic waves to create visual images of structures within the body (sonography) is a well-recognized clinical imaging technique that is now being widely accepted in medical practice. As a result of improved image quality, physicians are beginning to understand better the information obtained by sonography and to make important management decisions based on ultrasonic evaluation. This, however, has not always been the case. In the past, ultrasonic imaging techniques were poorly understood and the results were often ambiguous. There was a period of skepticism before the images were recognized as clinically valuable. Now, not only are the clinical applications of sonography recognized, but its role in present-day diagnostic evaluation has become established.

Sonography or ultrasound, as it is usually termed, has several fundamental virtues that make it an appealing diagnostic imaging modality. It is noninvasive and does not require injection of potentially toxic contrast material. Diagnostic sonography does not appear to cause significant biological harm to either the patient or the sonographer (1). (For simplicity, "sonographer" will refer to the person performing the examination, whereas "sonologist" will refer to the physician interpreting the sonogram.) The scanning equipment requires a smaller resource allocation by comparison with other valuable types of imaging devices. Thus, ultrasound is a very acceptable method of examing the body for evaluation of anatomy and pathophysiology.

Despite these virtues, ultrasound has only recently commanded widespread interest and acceptance in the medical community and the general public. Because of this increased interest, some inquisitive patients and physicians continue to ask, "Just how does this machine work?" or "Just how new is this imaging method?" To assist in answering these questions, our preliminary discussion will examine the development of ultrasonic imaging as it progressed from an engineering curiosity to its present status as a clinically relevant, diagnostic modality.

Human beings are comparative newcomers to the field of echolocation. A number of aquatic and flying animals such as porpoises and bats use ultrasound of various frequencies to locate and identify objects in the water and air (Fig 1-1). These animals echolocate by emitting bursts of ultrasound into their environment and detecting the echoes that are reflected from certain objects. This process is referred to as echolocation.

In the late 1700s, the Italian scientist Spallanzani observed that flying bats used high-frequency sound waves to navigate inside dark caves. Scientists later learned that the sound frequencies used by bats extended far beyond what human beings could hear. Similarly, marine biologists have learned that porpoises

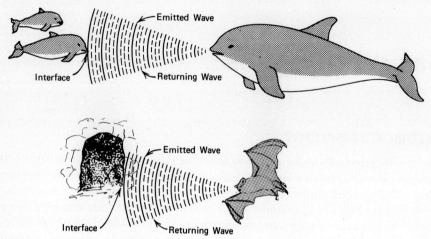

Figure 1-1. Fellow sonologists. Porpoises and bats locate objects in their surroundings by sending ultrasound waves into their environment and sensing returning echoes. The same principles are used in diagnostic sonography.

use an audible and an above-audible set of sounds to locate and characterize objects under water.

Unlike the bat and the porpoise, human beings do not have a biological source of ultrasound; therefore, until a physical source of ultrasound could be developed, it could not be investigated or used practically. The discovery of the piezoelectric effect of certain crystal substances by Pierre Curie made possible use of ultrasound by humans. Piezoelectric crystals are at the heart of all present diagnostic ultrasound systems because they produce and detect ultrasonic fields.

The piezoelectric or pressure-electric effect discovered by Pierre Curie can be observed in a limited group of crystalline materials. When pressure is applied, a small voltage is generated across the crystal, and the effect can be detected and measured. Conversely, when an electric field is applied to a piezoelectric crystal, the crystal changes shape. If the electric field is quickly removed, the crystal returns to its resting state in an oscillating manner, generating pressure waves into the surrounding medium. Because crystals will physically vibrate when struck, the piezoelectric effect can be used to "strike" a crystal into physical vibration. Since the frequency of vibration is determined by the physical size of the crystal, crystals could be ground to sizes that permitted vibrations at ultrasonic frequencies. Thus, the piezoelectric crystals (called transducers) are the basis for generation and detection of ultrasound waves in medical sonography today (Fig. 1-2).

In the early 1900s, the first device using the piezoelectric effect for echolocation was devised by the French engineer Paul Langeuvin. Langeuvin perceived that high-frequency sound waves traveled better in water than air, indicating that echolocation with ultrasound would be more easily achieved under water than in air. From this work came the modern SONAR instrument, named for *S*ound *Na*vigation and *R*anging, used to detect submarines and ocean floors in the ocean's depths during World War II and right up to today.

After World War II, the German scientists began to use ultrasound in a therapeutic mode for cancer therapy and diathermy. The application stemmed from the thermal effects of high-intensity ultrasound on biological tissues. Ultrasonic therapy was so far ahead of the diagnostics that the majority of the members of the American Institute of Ultrasound in Medicine (AIUM), which was formed in 1955, were physical therapists interested in the use of ultrasound in physical rehabilitation.

But by the late 1950s, interest in the diagnostic applications of ultrasound was growing, and several pioneers such as Drs. Howry, Holmes, Reid, and Wilds were building prototype scanners. Many of these early instruments approached our current level of technology and produced images quite comparable to those produced by present-day devices. With feasibility shown, several new applications of ultrasound rapidly evolved. In the late 1950s, Dr. Ian Donald in Scotland and others began to apply ultrasound to image the fetus. Since the fetus is suspended in a "sea of amniotic fluid," it presents an almost ideal situation for ultrasonic examination. At nearly the same time, Drs. Edler and Hertz in Sweden were devising an ultrasonic instrument that could follow the motion of heart valves; this was the beginning of the new field of echocardiography.

As the successful applications of ultrasound grew, so did the supporting technology. One of the major improvements in ultrasonic imaging occurred with the advent of gray scale image processing, first introduced by George Kossoff in the late 1960s. This technique allowed display of a range of echo amplitudes as various shades of gray rather than dots of set intensity. The information contained in a sonographic image improved markedly with this technical advance, and the utility of sonographic imaging expanded with it; the flow of technological improvements has continued. Commercial instruments are being upgraded as new ways of acquiring, storing, and evaluating data are incorporated into existing designs. Gray scale displays of wider range, new ways of storing image data, and scanning techniques that form real-time images are provided by the instrumentation now commercially available. They are signposts of things to come in an

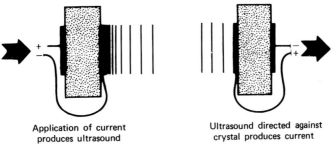

Application of current   Ultrasound directed against
produces ultrasound   crystal produces current

Figure 1-2. The piezoelectric effect. When an electrical voltage is applied to a piezoelectric crystal, it deforms the lattice structure. When the electrical supply is terminated, the crystal vibrates, producing compression and relaxation of the surrounding medium, resulting in the formation of compression waves. Conversely, when pressure waves in the medium impinge upon the piezoelectric crystal, compressions and rarefactions from the pressure wave are converted to small oscillating voltages that can be amplified and displayed.

image modality that holds an astounding potential for improving the overall quality of life through noninvasive recognition of many diseases.

Like certain other forms of medical imaging, diagnostic ultrasound requires a firm knowledge of the principles employed in the the technique. This knowledge is essential not only in interpreting the results but also in recording a representation of diagnostic quality initially. The effort devoted to understanding and mastering the basic physical principles and concepts of ultrasound is appropriate because diagnostic ultrasound provides the user with constant accessibility to biomedical engineering and physics in action. After this short introduction, the basic biophysical principles behind diagnostic sonography will be considered.

BIOPHYSICAL PRINCIPLES

Ultrasound is a longitudinal pressure wave composed of a set of compressions and rarefactions in the material carrying the wave, occurring at a frequency above human hearing (above 18,000 cycles per second or hertz) (Fig. 1-3). Diagnostic ultrasound operates over a frequency range of 1 megahertz (MHz) to 25 MHz (a hertz being 1 cycle per second and a MHz 1 million cycles per second). The compressions and rarefactions are formed by the movement of molecules in the material in which the ultrasound is propagated. Because of this, just how well ultrasound is transmitted through a material depends heavily upon the physical properties of the medium, such as density and elasticity (Fig. 1-4). Despite the form of the ultrasound wave, it conforms to a set of physical laws that govern all waves. Thus, they can be reflected, refracted, focused, and scattered, which are processes that also occur with light energy (Fig. 1-5).

Unlike light, however, ultrasound requires a medium to transport the wave form. One of the factors determining how well ultrasound can travel through a material is the density (ρ) (Fig. 1-4) (Table 1-1). Materials with molecules close together transmit ultrasound best, and the velocity of ultrasound propagation

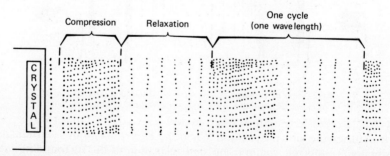

Figure 1-3. Ultrasonic waves. Ultrasonic waves consist of periodic compression and rarefaction of the surrounding medium produced by the piezoelectric crystal. One complete cycle includes the compression and relaxation phase of the wave. By definition, the frequency of an ultrasonic wave is greater than that of an audible acoustical wave, which is 18,000 cycles/sec.

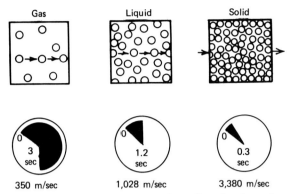

Figure 1-4. Relative ultrasonic velocities through media of various densities. The velocity of ultrasound through a medium depends on density. The more dense a structure, the faster the ultrasonic wave is propagated through the medium. The relative velocities of ultrasound through 1 kilometer volume of gas, liquid, and solids are shown. The greatest velocity is achieved as ultrasound passes through a solid structure. (Adapted from [4].)

is comparatively fast. If the molecules in the transmitting medium are farther apart, not only is propagation slower, but also the ability to couple the required movement from one part of the medium to the next is decreased. As a result, materials like water and metals transmit ultrasound well, but materials like air and gases do not. In addition, although certain substances such as bone are dense, they do not transmit ultrasound energy well because of the large amount of energy lost at their highly reflective interface. These relationships between ultrasound and the transmitting medium are useful guides to understanding how ultrasound can be potentially used. Tissues and cavities containing air do not transmit ultrasound well, and tissues such as bone and calcified lesions will

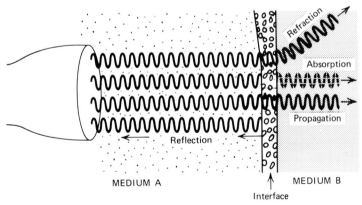

Figure 1-5. Interactions of ultrasound as it passes through two different media. When the ultrasound beam is emitted perpendicular or "normal" to the interface between mediums *A* and *B*, reflection of a part of the beam occurs. The remainder of the incident beam will be propagated through the medium. The major portion of the wave will be absorbed, resulting in heat production. When the ultrasonic beam encounters a curved surface, refraction or bending of the incident beam will occur.

Table 1-1. Velocity of Ultrasound Through Various Materials (2)

Material	Velocity (m/sec)
Nonbiologic	
Air	331
Pure Water	1,430
Sea water	1,510
Plastic	2,500
Metal	5,000
Biologic	
Fat	1,450
Vitreous humor of eye	1,520
Human soft tissue, mean value	1,540
Brain	1,541
Liver	1,549
Kidney	1,561
Spleen	1,566
Blood	1,570
Muscle	1,585
Lens of eye	1,620
Skull	4,080

decrease the amount of energy that can pass through them. Some velocities of propagation through various materials are listed in Table 1-1. From this table, it is evident that the velocity of propagation is nearly the same for most biological tissues, averaging approximately 1,540 meters/second. Because of this nearly constant velocity, a relationship between wavelength and frequency emerges, which is described by the following equation:

$$C = F\lambda$$

where C is the velocity of propagation, F is the frequency in hertz, and λ is the wavelength in the same units as the velocity length component. From the equation, one can see that as frequency increases, the wavelength decreases. We will subsequently consider how wavelength contributes to the resolution of the ultrasonic system.

Material density and the propagation velocity through any given material contribute to form another component of the ultrasound-material interaction, namely acoustical impedance, symbolized by Z. The word impedance implies some sort of resistance to propagation of acoustical waves. What is being impeded is the formation of compressions and rarefactions that form the longitudinal wave. Dense materials with a high propagation velocity have a high acoustical impedance because the molecules are already close together; therefore, compressing them further is difficult, requiring a great amount of additional energy. The acoustical impedance, then, is related to the compressibility of a material,

Table 1-2. Representative Values of Acoustical Impedance of Various Biological Materials (2)

Material	Acoustical Impedance (Z) ($\times 10^5$ gm/cm²s)
Air	0.0001
Fat	1.4
Water	1.5
Kidney	1.6
Muscle	1.7
Lens of eye	1.8
Bone	8.0

and is equal to the product of the material density, ρ, and the propagation velocity C, that is:

$$Z = \rho\, C.$$

Impedance makes all ultrasonic imaging possible, as will be subsequently discussed. Some characteristic values of acoustical impedance of certain materials are listed in Table 1-2.

As the ultrasound field propagates into the body, it passes through different tissues and interacts with the various types in varied ways (Fig. 1-5) (Table 1-3).

Table 1-3. Interactions of Ultrasound

Physical	
Absorption	Produces heat
Reflection	At echogenic interfaces
Refraction	Dependent upon angle of incident beam to interface and change in velocity at boundary between materials
Propagation	Dependent upon acoustical impedance of the material
Biologic	
Thermal effects	Insignificant with pulsed ultrasound; probably dissipated by vascularity of tissue
Cavitation	Unimportant at frequencies and intensities used for diagnosis
Microstreaming	Primarily responsible for cell membrane effect

First, the longitudinal waves of ultrasound must be passed from one region of space to another; that is, they must be propagated. When the ultrasound energy passes through an interface where the acoustical impedance changes, a very important second type of interaction takes place, namely reflection (Table 1-4). If the energy incident to that interface is not perpendicular to the interface, the ultrasound beam is bent, forming a third sort of interaction, called refraction. And as the ultrasound field passes through the various tissues within the body, energy is lost from the beam. This energy loss is called attenuation; that is the fourth major type of interaction. Most of the energy removed from the ultrasound beam appears in the form of heat. However, the amount of heat that is transferred to the medium is small, ranging from 0.25° to 0.5°C at diagnostic intensities. Since each of these interactions affects the image quality and thereby its diagnostic content, each process will be considered further.

Propagation, as pointed out earlier, involves the ability to transmit ultrasonic energy through biological tissues. But in ordinary usage, propagation takes on a more general meaning. The primary meaning of this term is the ability to transmit the ultrasound through a material by the coupling of energy from one region to the next. Conceptually linked with the propagation process is attenuation; that is, processes that remove energy from the ultrasonic beam. When a material is said to propagate ultrasound well, the statement includes the concept not only that mechanical energy is coupled well from molecule to molecule but also that energy is not rapidly lost from the propagated ultrasound beam. On the other hand, the process of energy loss is correctly called attenuation. Since it is difficult to determine just how well energy is coupled in a material, the term propagation is often used although attenuation is really meant. Although close in meaning, propagation and attenuation should be clearly separated conceptually, because, technically, they describe two different processes.

As the ultrasound propagates through a nonhomogeneous medium such as the human body, the ultrasonic beam crosses interfaces where the acoustical impedance sharply changes. At such an interface, a portion of the incident ultrasonic energy is reflected (Fig. 1-6). Just how much energy happens to be reflected depends on the reflectivity of the interface, expressed as the reflectivity

Table 1-4. Magnitude of Reflection at Various Interfaces (2)

Interface	Percent Reflection (%)
Blood-brain	0.3
Blood-kidney	0.7
Water-brain	3.2
Blood-fat	7.9
Muscle-fat	10.0
Muscle-bone	64.6
Brain-skull bone	66.1
Water-skull bone	68.4
Air-any soft tissue	100.0

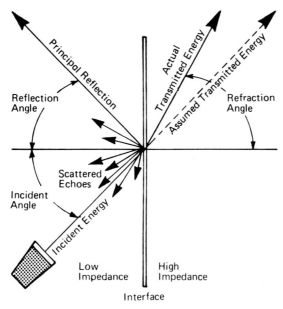

Figure 1-6. Reflection, scatter, and refraction. This diagram illustrates the three inter-actions of the incident beam that may occur at an interface between media of low and high impedance. A portion of the beam that is directed nearly perpendicular to the surface is reflected. The remainder of the beam is either scattered or propagated. By moving the transducer, the portion of the beam that is scattered can be detected. When the beam encounters a curved surface, the beam can be bent or refracted. Beam refraction alters the expected course of the incident beam and may result in faulty registration of echoes distal to a curved surface. Beam refraction may also occur when a beam traverses substances of markedly dissimilar acoustical impedance. Beam refraction frequently oc-curs when imaging intrathoracic structures distal to the diaphragm. (Courtesy of Raymond Powis, Ph.D., Unirad Corp., Denver, Co.)

coefficient, R, which is a function of the relation of the two acoustical impedances. R is expressed by the equation:

$$R = \frac{Z_1 - Z_2}{Z_1 + Z_2}$$

where Z_1 is the acoustical impedance in material 1 and Z_2 is the acoustical imped-ance in material 2. Since these changes in acoustical impedance occur at organ interfaces and structural boundaries within organs, the echoes can be used to create an image representing the organs and their internal structures. Most of the tissue characterization echoes, however, come from a slightly different process called scattering. These echoes can be viewed as reflections from sites of acoustical impedance changes at structures much smaller than the acoustical wavelength. For example, the wavelength for a 2.25-MHz sound beam is 0.68 mm, making the scattering sites that are detected within an organ less than 0.68 mm. Because the sites are small and project the reflected energy in many directions, scattering sites produce much smaller amplitude echoes than large interfaces. To distin-guish between the two mechanisms, reflection from large interfaces is called

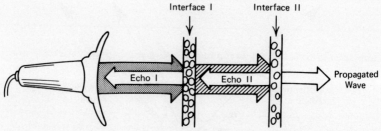

Figure 1-7. Echo production and detection. Because the acoustical impedance of the first medium is different from that of the second, not all of the incident energy is propagated into the second medium. When the incident beam is nearly perpendicular to the interface, some of the energy is reflected as an echo that can be detected by the transducer. By measuring the time interval between the initial ultrasound pulse and the echo, the distance between the interface and the transducer can be measured.

specular reflection and reflection that occurs at small interfaces is termed scattered reflection. It is these subtle changes in acoustical impedance at organ boundaries and interiors that allow diagnostic ultrasonic image formation.

At boundaries of interfaces with an acoustical impedance change, the velocity of propagation also often changes, permitting the process called refraction to occur (Fig. 1-6). This bending of the sound beam is sufficiently similar to the bending of light at an interface that the same equation may be used to describe both. This equation is an expression of Snell's law and relates the angle of incidence with the angle of refraction as a function of the two velocities of propagation. The equation is:

$$\frac{C_1}{C_2} = \frac{\sin_i}{\sin_r}$$

where i is the angle of incidence, r is the angle of refraction, and C_1 and C_2 are the velocities of propagation in materials designated 1 and 2. Refraction is important in diagnostic ultrasound as a source of artifacts and in the engineering of acoustical lenses. According to the equation, the angle of refraction approaches zero as the angle of incidence approaches zero. Stated differently, the effects of refraction are negligible when the ultrasound beam axis is perpendicular to the reflecting surface. The refraction that occurs when the incident beam is not perpendicular to an interface is one of the reasons the transducer is placed as perpendicular as possible to the organ of interest (Fig. 1-8). Thus, the wave sent from the transducer has the greatest opportunity to be reflected directly back and to record most accurately the location and strength of the wave form energy change.

As ultrasonic energy is propagated through the body, undergoing reflection and refraction, the beam loses energy. The major form of energy loss is the production of heat. The longitudinal wave is a mechanical one that requires in its formation the organized motion of molecules. Heat, on the other hand, is also mechanical motion of molecules, but disorganized and random. The conversion of ultrasound to heat, then, is rather direct; from organized to disorganized molecular motion. The amount of heat produced within a medium as ultrasound is passed through it depends on several factors, including the elasticity of the medium and the frequency and intensity of the ultrasonic beam. At the frequencies and intensities used for diagnosis, the temperature increment is small, ranging from 0.25° to 0.5°C in excised organs. The effects of this heat increment are lessened by the cooling effect of an intact vascular system.

Energy is lost from the incident beam with each reflection from a boundary between an organ as well as the scattering that occurs within the soft tissue structure. Energy can also be lost when the tissue acts in a very nonelastic way. And all these losses are frequency-dependent, increasing as the frequency increases. Various measurements of biological tissue show that a nearly uniform rate of tissue attenuation occurs through most biological materials. This attenuation is approximately 1 decibel per centimeter per MHz, where the dB or decibel is defined as:

$$dB = 10 \log_{10} \frac{I_1}{I_2}$$

and I_1 and I_2 are the sound intensities being compared. Thus, a 3.5-MHz ultrasonic field will be attenuated about 3.5 dB for every centimeter of tissue traversed. This number, however, should be considered only a gross approximation since the attenuation within any given tissue can demonstrate great variance. Because tissue attenuation significantly influences diagnostic imaging, ultrasonic scanning devices are designed to compensate for attenuation. Adjusting the machine properly for this compensation is a large part of the "art" in diagnostic ultrasound and will be considered in detail in the instrumentation section.

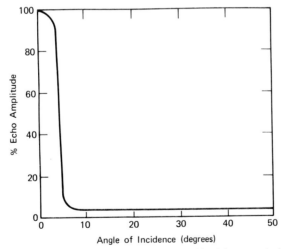

Figure 1-8. Echo amplitude as a function of angle of incidence relative to an interface. Because the interface acts like a mirror, moving the transducer slightly off normal with respect to the interface, this causes the echo to be reflected away from the transducer, decreasing the likelihood of recording the echo. This concept has practical significance, for if the transducer surface is greater than 5 degrees off normal from the interface, it is unlikely that the returning echo will be recorded. (Adapted with permission from Goldberg [2].)

Although the organization of an ultrasound scanning device is yet to be discussed, several practical rules for the use of ultrasound can be gathered from the physical principles thus far elaborated. For example, the poor transmission of ultrasound in air explains why a coupling gel is used to transfer ultrasound from the transducer housing and into the body. Further, the poor transmission through gases also explains the artifacts from bowel loops that contain gas, and why transmission of ultrasound through lung is very difficult. In addition, since the transducer is both the producer and detector of ultrasonic waves, a reflection from an interface cannot be detected unless the echo passes through the transducer. The highest amplitude echo will be detected, then, when the transducer is perpendicular to the interface being imaged. As shown in Figure 1-8, the echo amplitude diminishes precipitously when the transducer is off normal by as little as 5 degrees. Thus, transducer position relative to the interface being imaged is a very important factor of image information and quality.

With these physical principles as a data base, the physics underlying the echo-ranging process and instrumentation can be discussed.

PRINCIPLES OF ECHO-LOCATION

Producing a sonographic image depends upon the ability of the scanning device to depict correctly the position and magnitude of echoes returning from interfaces within the body. The first assumption made for an echoranging system is that the velocity of propagation is constant. For biological systems, a velocity of 1,540 meters/second is the value chosen, since it approximates velocities through most soft tissue structures of the body. Since the propagation velocity is assumed to be constant, distance can be measured by measuring the time required for a burst of ultrasonic energy to leave the transducer and return, technically defined as the time of flight. For most diagnostic ultrasound systems, the means of measuring time is the horizontal sweep of an electron beam of a cathode ray tube (CRT). The sweep on the CRT must begin when the burst of ultrasound leaves the transducer; therefore, the pulser that strikes the crystal and the sweep generator on the CRT are synchronized. A master system clock performs this synchronization. In addition, the system must have a receiver that amplifies and processes the returning echoes so that they can be presented on the CRT. All the basic elements of an echoranging system are included. The arrangement is shown in Figure 1-9.

With an average tissue propagation velocity of 1,540 m/sec, it takes only 6.5×10^{-6} sec for ultrasound to traverse 1 cm of tissue. This value is initially used to adjust the sweep speed on the CRT trace. The time required for any echo to arrive from a reflective interface is determined by the time required to reach the interface and return to the transducer. Thus, 1 cm of range on the CRT will be approximately 13×10^{-6} sec long. Therefore, by making a centimeter range on the CRT 13 μsec long, the range of an interface can be read directly from a CRT screen. Representative range values can be set up on the screen by having a small electronic indicator (pip) appear every 13 μsec along the trace. The use of these numbers will become clearer after we discuss the echoranging process.

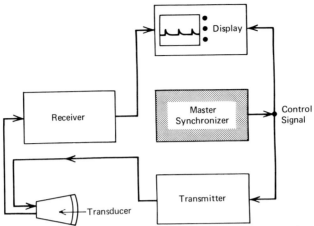

Figure 1-9. Basic organization of an echo-ranging unit. Master synchronizer transmits simultaneous impulses to the transmitter and the display module. The receiver detects the relation of the impulses from the transducer to the initial transmitted pulse, which in turn is sensed by the display module.

For illustration, consider a target 10 cm from the transducer (Fig. 1-10). It will require approximately 65 μsec for the ultrasound burst to leave the transducer and reach the interface. But for the transducer to signify the presence of an interface, it must receive an echo, and that echo will not be received for another 65 μsec during the return trip, or a total elapsed time of 130 μsec. For this reason, the time representing 1 cm on the CRT is twice as long as in the

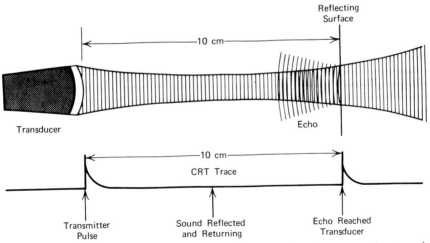

Figure 1-10. Echo ranging. By coordinating the electronic pulse sent to the transducer with an electronic sweep on the cathode ray tube (CRT) and moving the trace at a known fraction of tissue propagation velocity, the distance of an interface can be directly measured off the CRT. Each 13 μsec of trace movement will represent 1 cm of tissue. In this example, an interface 10 cm distal to the transducer required 260 μsec for "the time of flight" which corresponds to that distance. (Adapted with permission from Powis [5].)

tissues. The operational cycle of a diagnostic imaging device is simply to generate a pulse of ultrasound and prepare to receive (listen) for the echoes. In most current instruments, this cycle is repeated about 1,000 times every second to produce a flicker-free image on the CRT. The frequency of this pulse-listen cycle is called the pulse repetition rate (PRR). In summary, the position of interfaces within the body can be determined by measuring the time interval between the initiation of a pulse from the transducer and the return of an echo to the surface of the transducer.

INSTRUMENTATION

Obtaining consistent images of diagnostic quality depends greatly upon the function of the equipment and how well one understands the physical principles of the instrumentation and how each component of the system influences image quality. This discussion will begin with the interface between the patient and machine, the transducer, and continue through those features of a typical scanning device that are important determinants of image quality (Fig. 1-11).

Transducers

As previously stated, the transducer is the central feature of ultrasound imaging systems because it is both the producer and the detector of the ultrasound waves (Fig. 1-12). The transducer is situated at the interface between the patient and

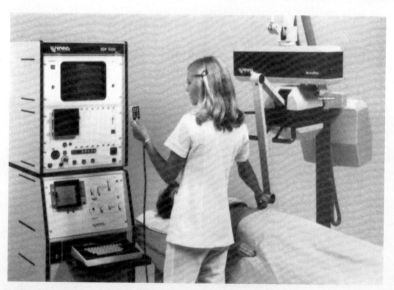

Figure 1-11. Gray scale sonographic imaging device. A sonographer is holding the transducer with the right hand while scanning the patient. The transducer is mounted on a scanning arm that can be moved in many directions. The sonographer holds the controls to the scanning arm movement in the left hand while viewing the image on the screen. Externally, the scanning console consists of two CRTs, one television (TV) monitor, and numerous switches for controlling the gain and time gain compensation (TGC). (Courtesy of Courtney Stanley, R.D.M.S., Unirad Corp., Denver, Co.)

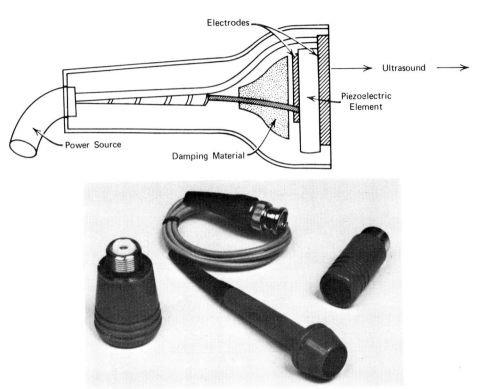

Figure 1-12. Single-element transducers. Transducers come in various shapes, sizes, and frequencies. Single-element transducers contain only a single piezoelectric crystal, whereas multielement transducers like those used for real-time scanning contain several smaller transducers. Most single-element transducers can be exchanged readily by attaching them to the main scanning arm. The top diagram shows the essential components of the transducer. In addition to the piezoelectric element and electrodes that produce ultrasound, the transducer contains a damping material that controls the amount of "ringdown." It is important to limit the "ringdown" time so that the transducer is maximally receptive to the returning echoes. (Courtesy of Dapco, Inc., Ridgefield, Conn.)

the machine, transforming mechanical to electrical energy and electrical to mechanical energy with each pulse-listen or send-record cycle. The frequency of transducer vibration is determined by the crystal thickness. When the crystal is thicker, the frequency of vibration is lower, and when the crystal is thinner, the frequency of vibration is higher. The ultrasonic field is produced by electrically deforming a piezoelectric crystal and allowing it to attain or "ring down" to its resting state. The crystal can be made of quartz but is more commonly made of materials such as lead titanate zirconate or barium titanate. The return to the resting state ("ringdown") should be made in as short a time as possible; hence, the crystal ringing is damped (like the shocks on an automobile) to decrease the number of cycles in the ringdown. An energy-absorbing material, sometimes called a damping material, is placed on the back surface of the crystal to remove vibrational energy rapidly from the crystal, effecting a rapid return to the resting state. When the compression waves of ultrasound reach the transducer as an echo, the deformation of the crystal produces a set of oscillating voltages at the resonant frequency of the crystal. These voltages are used to produce the electrical signals that represent echoes on the display. Thus, the physical energy is converted back to electrical energy.

Once a piezoelectric crystal is set into physical vibration, the ultrasound field extends outward from the crystal face with a width close to the size of the crystal diameter. If the crystal surfaces are moving uniformly, the whole crystal surface acts in unison as if it were a perfect piston. As the field progresses outward from the transducer face, it goes through a series of maximum and minimum intensity values and then begins to fall off smoothly as the field diverges, much like the light field from a flashlight. At the last maximum where the field begins to diverge is a limit or boundary of the near field, which extends from this limit back to the transducer. The area that is located distal to this boundary and where divergence of the beam occurs is called the far field. The association of these two fields is shown in Figure 1-13. The distance of this near field boundary (NFB) from the transducer face is a function of the transducer diameter and

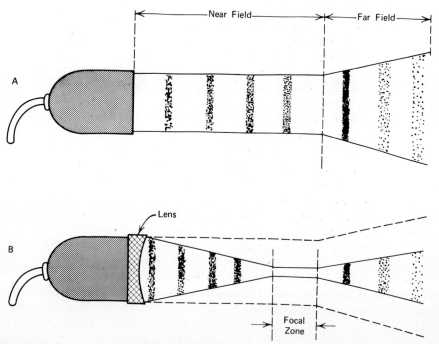

Figure 1-13. Near field and far field. The upper portion of this diagram (*A*) reveals the divergence of the incident beam that occurs in the far field. The beam appears coherent in the near field. The point at which the beam begins to diverge is termed the near field boundary. Objects that are imaged in the far field have less lateral resolution than those imaged in the near field. The lower half of this diagram (*B*) shows the beam profile emanating from an externally focused transducer. The acoustical lens is usually of curved plastic material which serves to focus the incident beam at a certain range distal to the transducer. This area is called the focal zone. The best resolution occurs within the focal zone. However, even with a focused transducer, the beam begins to diverge distal to the focal zone.

the transducer vibrating frequency. The equation for the position of the NFB is:

$$\text{NFB} = D^2/4\lambda$$

where D is the transducer diameter and λ is the wavelength of the transducer resonant frequency. This equation describes an important relationship between the transducer frequency and the transducer diameter. As the frequency decreases and λ becomes larger, the near field boundary moves closer to the transducer. This relationship between transducer size and frequency has an influential role in the overall resolution of the scanning system.

When using an ultrasound system for diagnostic imaging, two sorts of information are desired about the reflective interface: how far the interface is from the transducer, and the dimensions of the interface. An estimate of interface dimensions can be made by moving the transducer over the surface and determining when the echoes from the interface begin and cease. One should recognize that the ultrasound beam will generate echoes as long as the interface is within the sound beam from the transducer. Thus, if an attempt is made to determine the size of an interface smaller than the beam width, the measurement will produce a minimum value equal to the effective beam width. The effective beam width is dependent on where the interface is located in the field. The smallest beam width can be found in the near field; the expansion in size in the far field produces an even greater error in estimating size. Another type of error appears when two interfaces are separated by less than the beam width, for they will not be distinguished as two separate structures. Thus, the wide beam in both the near and far field begins to degrade information by making small targets appear larger than they really are and by failing to distinguish two interfaces separately if they are in too close proximity. This sort of resolution transverse to the beam axis is termed lateral resolution and is a major source of error in any ultrasonic system. The mechanisms of lateral resolution are illustrated in Figure 1-14.

A method of partially circumventing the problems introduced by beam width and the poor lateral resolution it produces is to narrow the field physically. One method to accomplish this is to decrease the transducer width. This, however, brings the near field boundary closer to the transducer and increases the rate of expansion of the far field. Narrowing the dimension of the transducer is not an effective way of narrowing the ultrasonic field size.

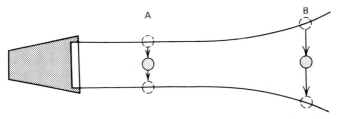

Figure 1-14. Lateral resolution. The echo of an object placed within the near field (*A*) will be better resolved than if the same object is imaged in the far field (*B*). Lateral resolution is influenced by the frequency of the ultrasound beam used, width of the transducer head, and the pulse width. (Adapted with permission from Powis [5].)

One of the earliest and partially successful ways of narrowing the ultrasound field was to use the wave properties of ultrasound and apply an acoustical lens to the transducer (Fig. 1-13B). The lens was attached to the front portion of the crystal that was placed in contact with the body surface. Certain of these lens systems are in current use, and the transducer employing this type of focusing is said to be an externally focused transducer. The lens-crystal arrangement results in conforming a beam to a particular shape as depicted in Figure 1-13B. The focusing produces a narrow region in the beam called the focal zone. Within this zone, the lateral resolution is greatly improved, as well as the delineation of targets of interest that are located outside the focal zone.

Lens changes are not the only means of focusing an ultrasonic beam. Figure 1-15 demonstrates two other means: bending the crystal and using an ultrasonic mirror. Such techniques are effective because of the wave properties of ultrasound. By bending a wave front with a mirror or by bending the crystal surface, succeeding wave fronts may also be bent, causing the beam to converge on a focal point. The physical law governing this process is called Huygen's principle. The transducers that are focused by bending the crystal are termed internally focused and are now the most frequently used devices for obtaining focused ultrasonic beams. Despite these extensive efforts to produce focusing, the resulting beams have finite widths, and problems created by poor lateral resolution continue to be significant.

In an attempt to improve the lateral resolution, it is assumed that the near field boundary has an influential role in this process. Focusing can occur within the bounds of the near field; therefore, by choosing the correct ratio between the transducer size and frequency, the near field boundary can be located far enough from the transducer to place the focal zone in an appropriate region of interest within the body. An incorrectly chosen ratio will cause the focal zone

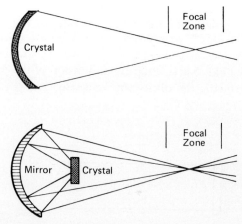

Figure 1-15. Internal and mirror focusing. The ultrasound beam may be focused by curving the transducer so that a focal zone is produced. This type of transducer is said to be "internally focused." An alternative method of focusing the beam is by the mirror technique. In this method, the beam is aimed toward a curved mirror that shapes the beam to converge at a certain focal zone. (Courtesy of Raymond Powis, Ph.D.)

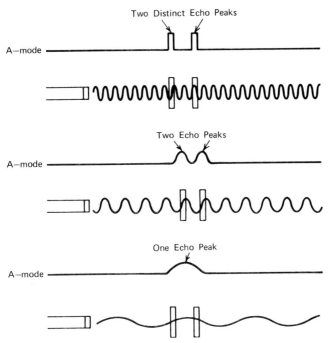

Figure 1-16. Axial resolution. Axial or depth resolution depends primarily on the wavelength of the ultrasound beam. At a high-frequency or short wavelength, two objects can be easily distinguished, whereas with longer wavelengths, the objects appear as a single echo. In order for two objects to be resolved, they must be at least a wavelength apart. For the usual diagnostic devices, the wavelength used is approximately 0.5 to 1 mm. (Adapted with permission [2].)

to lie too close to the transducer, making it difficult to obtain the best lateral resolution. As a consequence, most of the transducers used in abdominal scanning are larger than those used for echocardiography because the heart is closer to the transducer than the liver or kidneys. Also, the liver is a "solid" organ that we often need to examine internally. To move it farther from the transducer, the focal zone is often placed close to the near field boundary. A simple calculation of transducer diameter and frequency will allow one to determine the expected length and distance of the focal zone for any transducer. Many of the current transducers have focal zones labeled, not by number or quantitative form, but by general terms such as near, medium, and far focus. The near field boundary equation thus becomes quite useful in finding the focal zone limit. Since the focal zone provides the best lateral resolution, transducer selection should be based on location of the focal zone and the anticipated dimensions of the region to be studied, with the purpose of making these properties commensurate.

Besides determining the range of an interface and measuring its dimensions, one can place interfaces very close together along the beam axis. The closest position of two interfaces that can still be imaged as two is described as the axial resolution of the system (Fig. 1-16). Axial resolution is directly a function of the pulse width or wavelength and frequency. The axial resolution improves as the frequency is increased or as the wavelength decreases.

Controlling pulse width is the damping process in the transducer. If the pulses are too long, they crowd together echoes from sequential interfaces, making it difficult to determine whether one or two interfaces are present. Even with very heavy damping on the crystal, a finite time is required to begin and stop the vibration of the crystal. As a consequence, about five or six cycles of vibration are needed to start and stop the crystal, regardless of the frequency used. This independence of ringdown and frequency means that transducers of higher frequency can be chosen to improve the axial resolution. Moving to higher frequencies also means improved lateral resolution, because the focusing process is also better at higher frequencies. However, using a transducer of higher frequency also means a decrease in penetration, since the tissue absorbs more of the beam energy. One then has the problem of choosing the correct transducer frequency for a particular examination, balancing the requirements of lateral and axial resolution against the decreased penetration of higher frequencies (Table 1-5). Sometimes, one does not have a choice if the equipment has a poor frequency response that limits what frequencies can be used with the machine. Many of the manufacturers, however, are designing machines with wide frequency responses that give the user a wider choice of transducer frequencies (Table 1-6). The selection guidelines for particular transducer frequencies and focal zones will be discussed in each chapter as the techniques for evaluation of a particular organ system are considered.

Consideration of all these methods of circumventing the inherent limitations of transducers leads the present discussion to transducer design. A schematic transducer with its various components is shown in Figure 1-12. The crystal is located inside a housing with a backing material to absorb energy. Attached to the crystal are wires that conduct electrical energy to excite the crystal and to conduct electrical signals produced by the effect of the returning echoes on the transducer crystal back to the amplifiers in the scanning device. The crystal may be bent or a lens may be placed in front of the crystal to focus the ultrasonic energy into a focal zone. Some transducer manufacturers are now placing a matching layer of material in front of the crystal to achieve better coupling of the ultrasonic energy from the crystal into the tissue and from the tissue back into the crystal. These coupling layers of material are ground to one-quarter

Table 1-5. Important Factors That Influence Resolution

RESOLUTION depends upon ultrasonic FREQUENCY, which is indirectly proportional to wavelength and beam width.
  The greater the FREQUENCY used, the shorter the WAVELENGTH, the better the depth and lateral RESOLUTION
  The higher the FREQUENCY, the more collimated the BEAM WIDTH and the better the lateral RESOLUTION
The amount of PENETRATION of the incident beam depends directly upon FREQUENCY and DIAMETER of the transducer.
  The higher the FREQUENCY, the less the amount of tissue PENETRATION
  The WIDER the transducer head, the GREATER the PENETRATION
FOCUSED transducers provide the best RESOLUTION within a certain range that is at a specified distance away from the transducer.

Table 1-6. Transducers and Their Clinical Applications

Type of Ultrasonic Imaging	Transducer Type	Common Uses
Static	2.25-MHz, 19-mm diameter with long focus (10–15 cm)	Echocardiography, gravid patients, obese patients
	3.5-MHz, 19-mm diameter with medium to long focus (7–10 cm)	Abdominal organs, pediatric patients
	5.0-MHz, 6-mm transducer with short internal focus (3–5 cm)	Thyroid, superficial organs
	10-MHz with 1–2 cm focus	Eye, thyroid, parathyroid, superficial vessels
Real time	Linear array	Obstetrics, biopsy, aspiration
	Phased array	Cardiac imaging, survey of region of interest
	Mechanical sector	Cardiac imaging, abdominal survey
	Rotating transducer	Alternative to above
Aspiration	2.25-MHz with central lumen	Renal cyst aspiration, amniocentesis, thoracocentesis
Doppler	Continuous wave or pulsed dual sending and receiving transducers	Evaluation of blood flow, detection of fetal heart tones

wavelength thickness; therefore, the transducers are called "quarterwave" transducers. This technology makes coupling or transfer of energy into and out of the crystal more efficient without changing the efficiency of the crystal. Thus, for the same pulsing voltage applied to the crystal, quarterwave transducers theoretically provide higher energy output into the tissues.

Although transducers used in B-scanning and echocardiography initially may seem complicated, they are simple in comparison with the transducers used for real-time imaging (Fig. 1-17). The design purpose and basic principles of real-time imaging devices, however, are well within the understanding of the interested reader. These transducers are specialized for either an electrical or mechanical scan that occurs so rapidly that, as the interfaces change in the composite ultrasound field, these interfaces can be followed on the display. The effectiveness of real-time imaging can best be appreciated in viewing and evaluating a dynamic organ that has a characteristic motion, such as the heart. Echocardiography is only one field in which real-time imaging has applications. Rapid abdominal scanning, instantaneous structure location, visualization of vessel wall movement

Figure 1-17. REAL-TIME SCANNING DEVICES

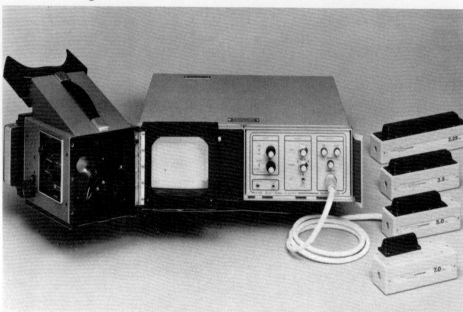

Figure 1-17A. Real-time sonographic scanning device and linear array transducers. Real-time scanning devices are usually smaller than static gray scale scanning devices and thus may be portable. Types of real-time transducers are described in the text. (Courtesy of Dwight White, R.D.M.S., A.D.R. Corp., Tempe, Ariz.)

and other physiological anatomical motion, as well as obstetrical scanning, are other current applications of real-time scanning.

Transducers used for real-time scanning can be divided into four major categories:

1. Mechanical scanners, in which the transducer is physically moved by a motor and mechanical linkage arrangement
2. Mechanical scanners, in which several transducers are mounted in a cylinder and rapidly rotated (rotating head transducers)
3. Phased arrays, in which a focused beam is synthesized from several small, unfocused transducers and, with the same technique, steered in a sector scan
4. The linear array, in which a beam is synthesized from array components and scanned down the array (Fig. 1-17)

None of these real-time techniques is ideal for all applications. Alternatives and compromises are made, balancing such considerations as cost of the device, resolution, image display format, convenience of the study, and size and configuration of the field of view. For example, phased arrays allow excellent lateral and axial resolution of the techniques. They are, however, the most expensive because of the computer control required to synthesize the beam, steer it, and slide the focal zone to maintain a nearly constant lateral resolution over the whole field. In addition, all the sector scanners, mechanical and electrical, have a limited

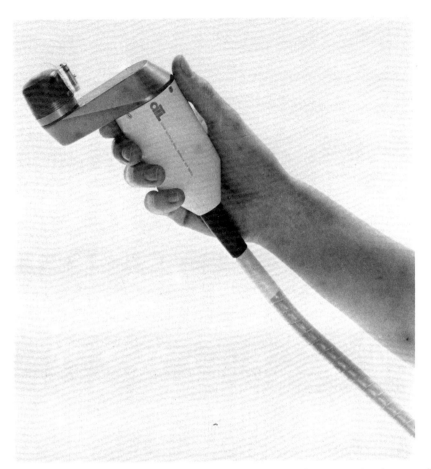

Figure 1-17B. Rotating head transducer. This real-time transducer contains three smaller transducers which rotate within the housing. The small size and curved surface of the transducer facilitates imaging between ribs. (Courtesy of Janet E. Kloock, A.T.L. Corp., Bellevue, Wa.)

field of view when compared with the linear array. Linear array transducers, because of the large transducer housing, are difficult to maneuver between ribs and under subcostal regions. For these areas of the body, a real-time transducer with a small, curved head, such as a mechanical sector of phased array transducer, can be used. Real-time capabilities are incorporated into many standard B-scanners, providing the user with a versatile approach to imaging.

A question that frequently arises is "will real-time scanning replace B-scanning?" At present the two techniques appear to be more complementary than competitive. The first obstacle to real-time scanning replacing B-scanning is the distortion inherent in both sector scanners and linear arrays that limits the accurcy of depicting internal structure. Such distortion is not present on single-element B-scanners. Another concern would be the limited gray scale presentation that is at present inherent in real-time displays. This may eventually be overcome, but the image distortion is inherent in the current technology. Recognition of the

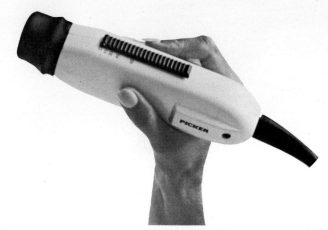

Figure 1-17C. Mechanical sector real-time transducer. A motor within the transducer housing sectors the transducer. A phased-array real-time transducer has a similar appearance. Both are used in cardiac evaluation and abdominal survey. (Courtesy of Thurmond Clardy, Picker Corp., Northford, Conn.)

problem with distortion and resolution has focused attention on improving image accuracy and real-time systems, with the promise that they may soon approach the B-scanner in image quality. Finally, it is thought that in the near future, real-time imaging will be as much a part of abdominal scanning as fluoroscopy is of radiographic examination of the gastrointestinal tract.

Scanning Arm

In a B-scanner, the transducer is attached to a scanning arm that confines the motion of the transducer to a single plane. Within the plane, the position of the transducer is located and recorded by potentiometers or other encoders that follow the joint positions on the arm. The output from these sensors, which is converted to a set of control voltages that position the event (trace) representing the sound beam axis on the CRT display, is used to calculate the transducer position. An accurate trace position depends on the accuracy of the potentiometers; and a significant part of any quality assurance program is to measure the alignment or registration of the arm translators. Arms that are out of alignment produce artifacts that cannot be easily detected by simply viewing the images. After some experience, one can often detect anomalies in the image quality, such as an abnormally wide outline of the body, that suggest incorrect function of arm registration. The presence of a misalignment can be easily documented by scanning one of the standard phantoms that are commercially available, such as one recommended by the American Institute of Ultrasound in Medicine (AIUM).

Basic Instrument Organization

The transducer produces and detects ultrasonic energy, and the arm informs the machine where in the scanning plane the transducer is located. The echoes that reach (are reflected to) the transducer are converted to an electrical burst of radio frequency oscillations that must be converted to a signal to be displayed and synthesized into an image. This function is performed by the organization of electrical components of the scanner. The general organization of a typical B-scanner is shown schematically in Figure 1-18. Following the signal stream not only will provide a description of how the ultrasonic echoes are converted to a signal for display but will allow determination of which machine adjustments are critical in order to obtain images of diagnostic quality.

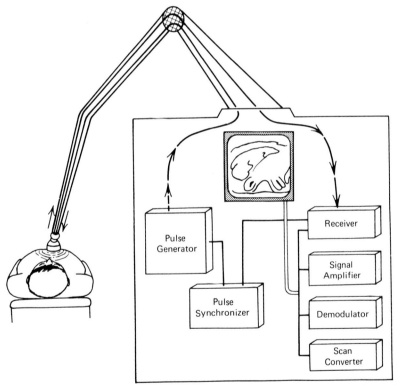

Figure 1-18. Components of a B-scanner. The pulse generator initiates the pulse that is sent to the transducer for production of an ultrasonic wave. The pulse synchronizer coordinates the generation of pulses with the particular instrument's processing capabilities. When an echo is detected by the transducer, the signal is sent through a series of electronic circuits that include a receiver, signal amplifier, demodulator, and scan converter. After the impulse is processed by the circuits, a visible image is produced. (The text contains more detailed discussion of the components of a B-scanner.)

When the echoes reach the transducer, the crystal converts the series of compression waves into a set of oscillating voltages with a frequency approximating the resonant frequency of the transducer. This places the frequency in the radio frequency (rf) spectrum; hence, the first amplifiers are radio frequency or rf amplifiers. Once amplified, the rf signal is sent to the demodulator, which rectifies and filters the rf, leaving just the envelope of the rf pulse. This signal, called a video signal, is amplified and sent to the display. The video signal is used to modulate the brightness of the spot on the cathode ray tube that represents the original echo from the interface. Display of the echoes as dots on the CRT is called a B-mode (B = brightness) display, and since the transducer is scanned over the body, the system is called a B-scanner or B-mode scanner. The image can be displayed either as a gray-scale image, in which the dots are varied in intensity according to the signal level, or as a bi-stable image, in which the dots are all presented at the same intensity regardless of signal level. On the display, the position of the trace is determined by the information of arm position that is transmitted to the X and Y axes of the display.

The gain of the B-scanner is determined by the gain in the rf amplifiers and the video amplifiers. Because we are attempting to image echoes from both close and distant targets and have their intensity reflect the characteristics of the interface and not the distance, this is a difficult problem. Often the more distant targets need to be seen, but when the gain is increased enough to image them, the echoes close to the transducer become too large and saturate (overwhelm) the amplifiers, distorting the image by causing false signal dropout and amplifier blocking. When the gain is reduced to optimize visualization of the close targets in immediate proximity to the transducer, the more distant targets may not be seen at all. What is needed is a variable gain that is low for the close echoes and high for the more distant echoes. This problem is addressed by a circuit known as time gain compensation or TGC. This circuit generates a curve that is shaped by front panel controls and adjusted by the operator while performing the study. The curve is retraced on each pulse-listen cycle and is adjusted to match the attenuation of the tissue.

The effect of the TGC is explained and illustrated in Figure 1-19. The goal of the operator is to increase the system gain at the same rate as the tissue is attenuating the ultrasonic energy. Thus, the first part of the TGC curve is a ramp function. The TGC increases rapidly with distance. It is over this region that attenuation is compensated. When the TGC is set properly, interfaces with the same reflectivity within the region that the ramp is increasing will have similar signal levels. This gain makes signal representation according to strength of the reflection and not distance from the transducer. Once the ramp or compensation is complete, the signals will once more decrease according to the tissue attenuation. This process of compensation is frequently called swept gain or depth gain compensation. The curve used to control the rf amplifiers in Figure 1-19 could just as well have been used to control the gain in the video amplifier.

Starting the TGC curve is the master pulse generator, which is the housekeeper for the system. The pulse to the transducer and the sweep on the CRT trace must also be synchronized; hence, they are also under the control of the master generator.

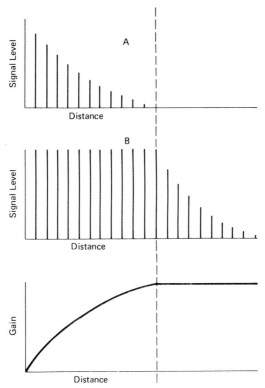

Figure 1-19. Time-compensated gain. Without a time-compensated gain curve, the echoes that are produced in the near field would limit the amount of the beam propagated into deeper structures. The time-compensated gain is displayed on the A-mode trace on a separate CRT. With time-compensated gain, far field echoes are enhanced and near field echoes de-emphasized since the beam is not substantially attenuated by the echoes produced in the near field. (Adapted from Powis [5].)

These are the essential elements of any B-scanning system. Although the elements of the different types of units may reach various levels of sophistication, their role in the overall operation of the system remains the same. The end product is the image shown on the display.

Just how data is displayed is important and is determined by the instrumentation. Should the echoes be displayed inappropriately, the image quality may suffer or can be misleading. One of the oldest and still valuable means of display is the A-mode display. In this technique, the trace moves over a CRT screen and is displaced along the Y axis when an echo appears. The displacement is proportional to the echo amplitude; thus, this display gives echo range and amplitude information. Echo range and amplitude information can be useful on a B-scanner, and nearly all the current scanners have an A-mode display. The echo amplitude and position information is used to adjust the system TGC and often assists in identifying moving echoes. The A-mode display does not store data; therefore, attempting to form a two-dimensional image from the A-mode would require a huge image memory. The A-mode display simply shows what echoes happen to be appearing in the ultrasonic field in which the direction the transducer is pointing at that particular time.

If the trace is made in the same way as in the A-mode but the beam is turned on and off by the presence or absence of an echo, a B-mode display is formed. Further, the trace on the CRT can be moved over the screen following the position of the transducer. If the CRT has a memory, then a scan over the body will generate an image composed of all the echo dots formed in the B-mode trace. This is the standard display for the B-scanner. Early displays used storage CRTs and variable persistence CRTs to store the echo signals received during a scan, but these displays had serious limitations and it was not until fabrication of present-day scan converters that good gray scale imaging became possible. These scan converters deserve special attention and will be treated in a separate subsection of this chapter.

Modes of Display

The electrical impulses from returning echoes can be displayed in three major modes: A-mode (A stands for amplitude of a signal peak, which represents the strength of the echo); B-mode (B as we have previously discussed refers to brightness of a CRT dot, which represents the strength of an echo); TM- and RT-mode (TM refers to time-motion or dynamic imaging display of a B-mode trace; RT is used to denote real time) (Fig. 1-20). Each mode has its particular advantages and disadvantages for various applications.

Figure 1-20. MODES OF DISPLAY

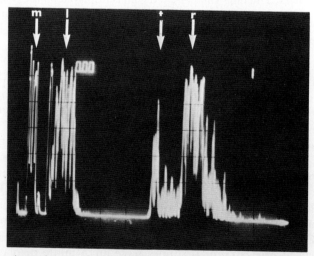

Figure 1-20A. A-mode. A stands for amplitude. This A-mode tracing was obtained with the transducer placed on an eyelid and directed into the eye. The "main bang" (m) or initial pulse appears as a peak on the CRT trace. The height of the peak corresponds to the amplitude of the echo. Echo peaks are recorded within the eye arising from the lens (l) and retina (r). A group of echoes is present proximal to the retina representing an ocular tumor (t).

The A-mode displays echoes by representing the amplitude of the echo as the height of a signal peak. In the past, A-mode scanning was used for an evaluation of patients with cranial trauma by examining for a shift in midline intracranial structures due to such disorders as a subdural or epidural hematoma. This technique employs placing a transducer above the ear on the thinnest portion of the temporal bone and directing the beam toward midline structures (falx cerebri, septum pellucidum). In general, displacement of midline structures such as the falx cerebri and septum pellucidum becomes clinically significant when they are shifted more than 3.0 mm. Because of the dependence on operator skill and lack of specificity of this method compared to computerized tomography (CT) scanning, the clinical importance of A-mode echoencephalography has diminished. At present, the most useful roles for A-mode displays are in adjusting TGC curves and evaluation of cystic lesions and in aspiration and biopsy procedures. In the latter application, the range of an area for aspiration or biopsy, as well as the location of the needle, can be assessed. These particular procedures will be described in more detail in Chapter 5.

A-mode displays are limited in their utility, however, because of the small sampling volume and lack of anatomical landmarks in establishing exactly where the ultrasound beam is directed. As stated, an important use of A-mode is to verify the relative amplitude of echoes seen on a B-scan. The high-amplitude distal echoes characteristic of cystic masses are easily shown on an A-mode tracing (Fig. 5-10). In addition, no echoes will be seen between the proximal and distal walls of a cyst, even at high-gain settings. Solid masses, however, demonstrate numerous fine echoes within the outlines of the mass, echoes that can be enhanced by increasing the system gain.

B-mode imaging electronically displays the amplitude of an echo as the brightness of a spot of light on a CRT. From the point of view of sitting on top of an A-mode pattern looking down, the spots can be thought to represent the peaks of the A-mode echoes. A B-mode scan is constructed by passing the transducer over the body and storing the returning echoes on a storage display as the data points are acquired (Fig. 1-20B).

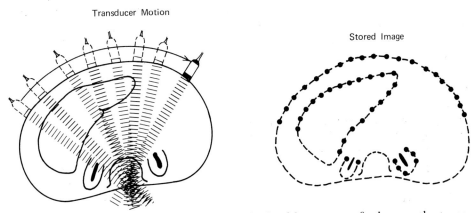

Figure 1-20B. B-mode. B-mode images are obtained by storage of echoes as the transducer is moved over a body area. (This is considered in detail in the text.)

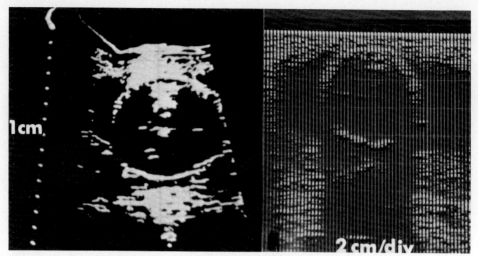

Figure 1-20C. Real time. The real-time image of a fetal biparietal diameter (*right*) is compared to a bi-stable B-mode image obtained through the same plane (*left*). The individual lines that are frequently apparent result from the ultrasound emissions from each transducer element.

B-mode images can be obtained either in a bi-stable scan, where the boundaries of a mass are easily delineated, or in gray scale, where the subtle differences in internal soft tissue interfaces can be demonstrated by their different shades of gray. In general, gray scale imaging affords display of soft tissue interfaces, whereas bi-stable processing is characterized by enhanced delineation of mass borders. Either display can be set up for either a white-on-black or a black-on-white image. As will be subsequently discussed, studies of physiologic and cognitive perception appear to demonstrate that a white-on-black image seems best for evaluating the outline of organs, whereas black-on-white appears to be preferred for detecting subtle differences in gray scale shades (5).

Another type of B-mode display is real-time, dynamic imaging, which is particularly suited for evaluation of moving structures. Real-time sonographic imaging is similar to fluoroscopy in that images are shown on a CRT format and the dynamics of echo sources can be observed. Real-time imaging employs a transducer consisting of several smaller transducers or a single one that moves along a prescribed tract and is able to perform a set of rapid B-scans so quickly that the dynamics of the echo sources can be followed. Real-time sonographic imaging can be used to survey areas of interest quickly, follow a vessel to its origin, localize an organ, or provide a rapid scan of different body regions. This last application can also be performed using the survey mode available in newer digital systems. Generally, real-time systems provide a fast and effective method of examining the body, but also have inherent limitations on the field of view, depending on which transducer is used.

TM-mode is the method used currently for most echocardiography (Fig. 1-20D). In this display format, a B-mode trace is moved as a function of time to show the dynamics of tissue interfaces. Echoes emanating from ventricular, valvular, and pericardial interfaces can be displayed and their motion

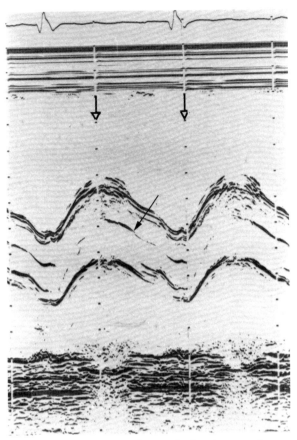

Figure 1-20D. TM mode. TM- or M-mode stands for time-motion mode. The motion of the echo sources toward and away from the transducer with respect to time is depicted. Centimeter markers (*open arrow*) are displayed each second. This image was obtained when the transducer was directed toward the aortic valve. The central linear echo represents the movement of the echo arising from the closed aortic leaflets (*arrow*).

studied (Chapter 7). Real-time cardiac scanning is an additional method for evaluating the motion of heart structures as well as valvular disorders. In this method, a single hand-held phased array or mechanical sector transducer is placed at specific sites that allow dynamic delineation of the heart and its internal configuration.

The Doppler technique is most often used to examine moving structures and blood flow. All the Doppler units use the Doppler principle, which is best described as an apparent change in frequency of a sound source in motion, such as a train whistle as it approaches and passes a stationary listener (Fig. 1-21). Doppler instruments contain separate sending and receiving transducers that can detect a change in frequency of the reflected pulse resulting from motion of the reflecting target. This principle is used to detect diminished or altered flow in vessels, fetal heart motion, or blood flow to a major abdominal organ. Newer systems are equipped with both static and Doppler scanning devices, which assist in detecting not only anatomical derangements but also abnormalities

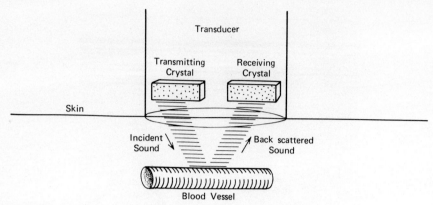

Figure 1-21. Diagram of Doppler instrument. A Doppler instrument contains a transmitting and a receiving crystal that senses change in the frequency of the incident beam as it encounters a moving target. In this case, the flow of blood within the vessel would change the frequency of the emitted ultrasound beam and be detected at the receiving crystal. By quantifying the change of frequency that occurs, the incident velocity of blood flow can be estimated.

in flow. By coupling pulse-echo techniques with Doppler techniques, both anatomical and flow information can be obtained.

Scan Converter Displays

Few innovations have changed diagnostic ultrasound as much as gray scale imaging. In large measure, this is a result of applying scan converter technology to ultrasound. The instrumentation has changed once more with the newly introduced digital scan converters. Understanding the digital scan converter, however, requires understanding the older analog scan converter. Knowing both may have some advantages since several manufacturers still produce both types of instruments, thereby providing the physician or other user with options to suit particular clinical requirements.

A schematic of the analog scan converter is shown in Figure 1-22. The scan converter tube is constructed much like a cathode ray tube. An electron beam is formed, focused, and moved just like a standard CRT. The target for the electron beam is a dielectric matrix, which provides the memory for the system. The image is stored on the dielectric matrix as a charge distribution over the surface. The energy of the electrons in the electron beam is kept low enough for more electrons to be stored on the dielectric than are removed. The number of stored electrons is determined by the electron beam current, which is a function of the echo signal level. In effect, the echo signal levels modulate the electron beam current, controlling the amount of stored charge representing an echo. Again, this is how the intensity of a single data point in the final image is related to that particular original event.

Once the charge is stored, the same electron beam is then used to read the image. This is accomplished by moving the beam over the charge distribution

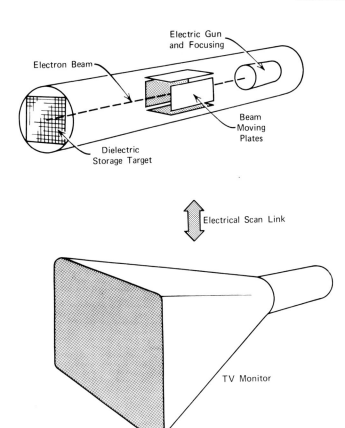

Figure 1-22. Scan converters. In the scan converter, the memory required to store the images is provided by a matrix of insulating cells on which electrons are stored. In an analog scan converter, the image is stored as a charge distribution that must be "read" by an electron beam and mapped onto a TV monitor screen. By allowing the charge density of the stored image to control the reading beam curve, a signal is generated that regulates the beam current to the TV monitor. Analog scan converters provide excellent gray scale images but are dependent on operating factors that may reduce reliability. The digital scan converter is positioned at the same point in the signal stream as the analog scan converter. This circuit converts the analog signal levels to a set of binary numbers. Once the signal is converted to binary numbers, the numbers are stored into a computer-like memory. The image is stored, not as a set of charges, as in the analog system, but as a set of binary numbers. (Courtesy of Raymond Powis, Ph.D.)

in a standard TV raster scan. As the beam moves over the charge, the beam current will change according to the charge that is present where the beam is pointing. These charges are used to control the beam current in a TV monitor linked to the scan converter raster scan. In this manner, the image is stored on the dielectric matrix as a distributed charge and mapped onto the screen of the TV monitor. The scan converter derives its name from the conversion of the scanning rate of the arm that holds the transducer into a standard TV scanning rate.

Now that the image is stored on the dielectric matrix, some of the problems fundamental to this image-storing technique become evident. For example, if the dielectric target does not have a uniform temperature, the ability to store charges will not be uniform and neither will the gray scale display. Thus, differences in gray tone on the image would not represent differences in interfaces in tissue but a technical artifact. In addition, approximately 10 pulse-listen cycles are required for the charge on the dielectric to reach equilibrium with the electron beam; hence, the transducer scanning speed can affect image storage. This means that it is possible for the user to move the transducer too fast over the surface of the patient.

The scan converter reads the stored image with the same electron beam used to make that image. Thus, the stored electrons can interact with the electron beam; that is, reading them results in electrons being removed from the memory. In this instance the image will slowly degrade simply from electron beam reading of the image. Because of these relationships, the analog scan converter is noted to be temperature- and voltage-sensitive. Despite these sensitivities, analog scan conversion still provides one of the most successful means of storing and obtaining gray scale images.

Although the digital scan converter makes an ultrasound system more quantitative or "digital," functionally the instrumentation proximal to the scan converter is basically the same as in an analog system. Therefore, all the potential problems with transducers, scanning arms, TGC, rf amplifiers and others, still exist as part of the system. Only the means of storing the image is different from that in analog systems. The digital scan converter is positioned at the same point in the signal stream of the entire system as the analog converter. The interface between the analog and digital segments of the instrument is the analog-to-digital converter (ADC). This circuit converts the analog signal levels to a set of binary numbers. The value of this number depends upon the signal level and the number of bits (value or data points) possible in the binary system. A five-bit system can assume 2^5 or 32 values. A four-bit system can assume 2^4, or 16, values. Since each of these values can represent a gray scale level on the TV monitor, the two systems are said to be a 32 and 16 gray level system, respectively. Once the signal data are converted to binary numbers, the numbers are stored as numbers (specific data points) in a computer-like memory. The position of the data within the memory depends upon the scan arm position to which the transducer is affixed and along which trace the echo appeared. Handling this position assignment is an addressing program stored on a specialized electrical component called a PROM (programmable read-only memory) (Fig. 1-23). The image, in contrast with the analog system, is stored, not as a set of charges, but as a set of binary numbers. These numbers have none of the properties of stored charges; hence, many of the problems that are inherent in converters will not be present.

"Reading out" of the digital memory is a process of reading memory contents, address by address, as if a raster scan were performed over the image. Digital memory reading out is more uniform than with the analog scan converter. This process is also handled by a PROM, which adjusts the reading to be compatible with a standard TV format. All the processes of the analog scan converter are carried out, but completely in a digital format.

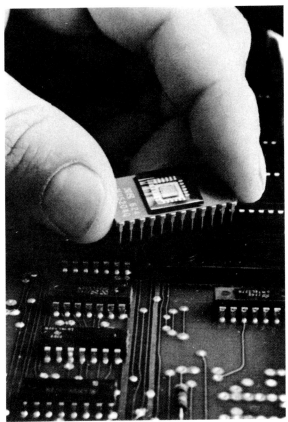

Figure 1-23. Programmable read-only memory circuit (PROM). This miniaturized electric circuit is an essential part of all digital scan converters. It is necessary for the retrieval and assignment of the proper location of an echo that is stored in a digital format. (Courtesy of Norman Goldman, Picker Corp., Northford, Conn.)

Gray Scale Displays

Fundamental to the display of gray scale images is the presentation of a CRT dot in proportion to the signal level. Thus, the dot representing an echo is changed in intensity as the echo amplitude is changed. The question then arises, how does one know what the signal level happens to be? Estimating absolute signal levels by estimating absolute intensity levels visually is very difficult. In part, this problem originates with the eye, which is not an intensity sensor but a contrast sensor (5). Therefore, the ability to perceive a particular echo will always be referenced to adjacent signal levels and to the background intensity level.

Since the eye is a contrast sensor, the eye requires some type of reference with which to make contrast comparisons. This reference is usually the background level of light or adjacent portions of the visual field on the ultrasound image. The ability to see small changes in intensity for both a portion of the visual field against a background and between two adjacent fields against a common background is determined by the background illumination. This relationship is referred to as Weber's law and basically states that the relative sensitivity of the eye increases as the intensity of the background level increases until a constant ratio of change to background illumination is reached. At this point, the ratio is independent of the background illumination. The optimal relation between change in light intensity to background illumination at which the eye can act as the best contrast discriminator can be easily reached in the bright display from a TV monitor. This ratio is usually somewhere between 0.01 to 0.001. This means that given the proper conditions, the human eye can detect somewhere between 100 and 1,000 gray levels. The limiting factor in the total data transfer from the television or CRT monitor to the eye may be the limitations of the monitor and which type of protocol (pre- or postprocessing) is being used to integrate the image.

Some signal compression occurs in any ultrasound instrument as the echoes reaching the transducer are converted to electrical signals that are in turn shaped for presentation on the display. Signals from the transducer may be spread over a range of values of 10,000 to 1. The internal operations of the machine on these signals tends to compress the signal range to about 100 to 1, a 40-dB dynamic range. Because most displays cannot appropriately respond to this large signal range, the signals are often further compressed to about 50 to 1 or less. Simply, the strongest and weakest signals must be spread between the display range of the recorder. The limits of the recording format are usually from pure white to black, with the intervening values represented by shades of gray.

One of the most successful means of displaying gray scale levels, as we have stated, is by the analog scan converter. This display system uses a dielectric matrix to store the image as a charge distribution. But within the storage and reading processes are the mechanisms that will degrade the image. As a result, the analog scan converter has inherent instabilities and some lack of reproducibility over long-term usage. Many of these undesirable characteristics may be overcome with digital scan converters.

The digital scan converter has generated a new set of considerations for the user. For example, many of the new scan converters display 32 shades of gray. Can the human eye detect 32 shades of gray? The answer is yes, but this ability is controlled by the physiology referred to briefly earlier in this discussion. Because the eye tends to contrast-enhance the sharp boundaries of echoes presented on a digital scan converter, the images on a digital format appear "grainy" and more "contrasty" than images obtained from analog systems (Figs. 1-24A,B). Indeed, these images appear quite digital in that individual pixels (picture elements) can be seen when the image is magnified. They make up a mosaic pattern that becomes smoother when viewed at minification factors of 3 or 4 to 1. Esthetic quality is partly the issue in the controversy over analog and digital images. Analog images appear "smooth" and do not show the regions of sharp contrast perceived in the digital image. This image, in which the transition of shades of gray is not so abrupt, is more familiar and esthetically pleasing to many users. The manufacturers, sensitive to this reaction, have attempted to make the digital images appear more analog-like and less digital. The idea is make the image as smooth as possible without losing image information. With most digital scan converters, attempts to smooth out the image do not appear to have

Figure 1-24. ANALOG VS. DIGITAL IMAGES

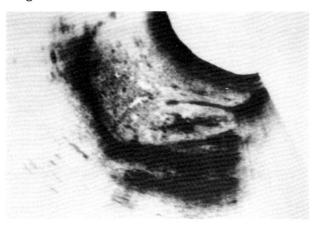

Figure 1-24A. Analog versus digital images. This longitudinal scan taken 6 cm to right of midline shows an analog image of the liver and right kidney. Note the homogeneous texture of the liver.

significantly compromised the image data content for most present day clinical purposes.

In the finished product displayed by either format, gray scale provides the visual texture of a B-scan image. This texture is used to provide information concerning the soft tissue within and around normal structures and soft tissue masses. The diagnostic usefulness of gray scale imaging is difficult to quantify, but its introduction to ultrasound has drastically enhanced recognition of subtle

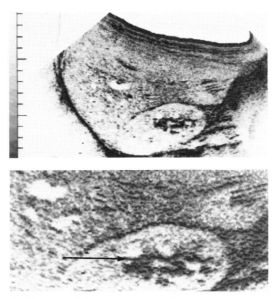

Figure 1-24B. A digital image of the same patient demonstrates an equally grainy texture of the liver resulting from the digital image. In general, a difference in texture between analog and digital images is not apparent when an image of less than 3:1 minification is used. However, the individual pixel elements are readily detected when a digital image is magnified (*arrow in bottom image*). (Courtesy of Thomas Kirkham, Xonics Corp., Des Plaines, Ill.)

changes in tissue texture associated with pathological conditions. It has certainly increased the clinical usefulness and acceptance of diagnostic sonography.

Estimating tissue qualities through gray scale images introduces another factor for consideration in recording the image. Should the image represent echoes as black dots on a white background or the reverse, referred to as a black-on-white or a white-on-black format? This has also been a subject of controversy. Many authorities on diagnostic sonography somehow believed they had to make a choice and use the same format on every study; consequently, using this logic, one type of display had to be proved superior. If one considers the data objectively, it appears that the physiology of the eye determines which format to use to achieve a certain result and when to use it.

At the outset, the eye does not detect white-on-black in the same manner as black-on-white. Single cell measurements, experimental creation of optical illusions, and Weber's law show the eye is more sensitive to changes in intensity when data are shown on a black-on-white image. Conversely, the eye contrast enhances and makes larger (an illusion) white-on-black images. Thus, to use the best gray scale sensing ability of the eye to estimate tissue texture, a black-on-white image would be favored. However, to examine organ boundaries and linear structures, one would prefer a white-on-black image. The decision of which format to use is also a function of personal preference of the physician and what sort of photographic record (Polaroid or hard-copy) is available.

PRINCIPLES OF SONOGRAPHIC INTERPRETATION

Since ultrasound is still relatively new in its general application to clinical medicine, this imaging modality lacks some of the technical standardization of more established diagnostic methods. Clinically useful (good) images are obtained empirically in many instances. Certain techniques can be performed, however, in attempts to optimize scan quality. Many of these maneuvers are acquired through direct clinical experience. However, understanding the fundamental principles will greatly expedite this process.

Before a patient is scanned, one should always be aware of the reason for the study and any additional pertinent clinical data. The examination should be monitored by a physician so that questions asked prior to the examination are answered as completely as possible. Each sonographic examination should be tailored to the clinical questions posed by the overall clinical assessment of the patient.

As to the value of confirming a radiographic abnormality in two projections, one must be able to visualize the region of interest by synthesizing the ultrasound appearance on both longitudinal and transverse planes. Sonographic imaging has the flexibility to image an abnormality in many degrees of obliquity. This versatility should be fully exploited by delineating an observation or abnormality in at least two scanning planes. Because an imaging procedure that employs tomography displays only a limited region of the body, a diagnostic modality such as ultrasound, with its limited field of view, is not an ideal screening procedure. Because of its noninvasive and nontoxic qualities, however, sonography remains an excellent technique for initial evaluation of many pathological disorders.

The images used in this text are oriented using the convention accepted for both ultrasound and CT images. The patient's head is to the reader's left of the display for longitudinal scans and the patient's right is to the reader's left for transverse scans. On longitudinal scans, the xiphoid, umbilicus, and symphysis pubis are indicated by a vertical line created by lifting the transducer off the patient's abdomen while making the scan (writing). A marker system composed of a series of dots 1 cm apart is included in most scans to provide accurate estimate of distance.

Specific criteria for evaluating soft tissue masses have been established (6). These include the size and location of a mass, its overall sonographic qualities, internal consistency, shape, attenuating properties, and integrity of surrounding soft tissue interfaces (Table 1-7). The introduction of gray scale sonography has offered improved depiction of these features and, in particular, the portrayal of the internal consistency and borders of a mass.

Table 1-7. Criteria for Sonographic Characterization of Soft Tissue Masses

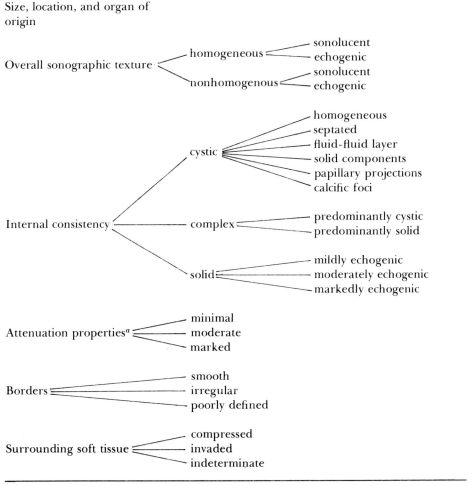

Size, location, and organ of origin

Overall sonographic texture
- homogeneous
  - sonolucent
  - echogenic
- nonhomogenous
  - sonolucent
  - echogenic

Internal consistency
- cystic
  - homogeneous
  - septated
  - fluid-fluid layer
  - solid components
  - papillary projections
  - calcific foci
- complex
  - predominantly cystic
  - predominantly solid
- solid
  - mildly echogenic
  - moderately echogenic
  - markedly echogenic

Attenuation properties[a]
- minimal
- moderate
- marked

Borders
- smooth
- irregular
- poorly defined

Surrounding soft tissue
- compressed
- invaded
- indeterminate

[a]Linear scans only.

Using the criteria listed in Table 1-7, one can separate soft tissue masses into cystic, complex, and solid categories. Cystic masses exhibit the following sonographic properties:

1. An echo-free center, even at high instrument gain settings
2. A smooth, well-defined wall
3. An increased amplitude of echoes beginning at the posterior wall and proceeding distally (acoustical enhancement) (Fig. 1-25A)

On the other hand, solid masses usually exhibit the following sonographic patterns:

1. Internal echoes that increase with an increase in instrument gain settings
2. Irregular, often poorly defined walls and margins
3. Low-amplitude echoes posterior to the mass due to increased acoustical attenuation by the soft tissue of the mass (shadowing) (Fig. 1-25C)

A complex mass is generally regarded as a lesion that contains both sonolucent and echogenic areas on the image which originate from both fluid and soft tissue components within the mass (Table 1-8) (Fig. 1-25B).

In general, the relative echogenicity of a soft tissue mass appears to be related to a variety of constituents, including the collagen content, interstitial components, vascularity, and degree and type of tissue degeneration (7,8,9). This observation is demonstrated by the relatively high echogenicity of uterine leiomyomas when compared with lymphomas. Leiomyomas, because they consist of smooth muscle and collagen, often appear as echogenic masses, whereas the lymphomas are commonly sonolucent because they contain little connective tissue and maintain a high degree of internal homogeneity in acoustical impedance. The complex appearance of most hemangiomas probably arises from the many internal interfaces of the numerous vessels within these masses. Masses that

Figure 1-25. MAJOR SONOGRAPHIC CATEGORIES OF MASSES

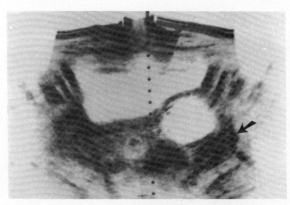

Figure 1-25A. Cystic mass (transverse, 4 cm above symphysis pubis). This left adnexal mass appears as a well-defined, spherical, sonolucent (echo-free) mass that exhibits distal acoustical enhancement (*arrow*). The major sonographic features of a cystic mass are seen.

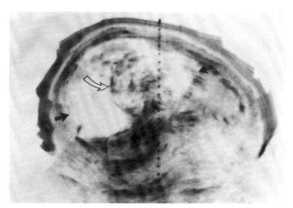

Figure 1-25B. Complex mass (transverse, 10 cm above symphysis pubis). This mass (*solid arrows*) contains both sonolucent and echogenic (echo-producing) components (*open arrow*). Complex masses usually contain both fluid and soft tissue (solid) contents and frequently represent either cystic masses with solid internal components or solid masses with internal cystic degeneration.

contain large amounts of fat often appear echogenic, probably because of the relatively inelastic properties of fat (10).

The amplitude of echoes distal to a mass can be used to evaluate the ultrasonic attenuation properties of that mass. Masses that have little or no attenuation will produce high-level echoes distal to the mass. The ultrasound transmission is said to be excellent. Conversely, solid masses that have a large amount of ultrasonic attenuation will markedly decrease the amplitude of echoes distal to that mass. Assessing these transmission properties requires linear, single-pass scans over the mass. The hydration of the tissue and degree of vascularization of a mass will alter acoustical properties, changing not only the propagation properties but also the acoustical impedance changes at boundaries within the mass. Masses that are well perfused present less acoustical impedance than masses that have only a limited vascular supply. This general observation applies up until the mass becomes so necrotic that its center is liquid; then it may appear as a cystic structure.

The sonographic texture of an organ depends, for the most part, upon the internal arrangement of the tissue. For example, the high collagen content of the portal triad and supporting elements of the liver parenchyma create a sono-

Table 1-8. Sonographic Characterization of Soft Tissue Masses

	Cystic	*Complex*	*Solid*
Internal texture	Sonolucent	Mixed	Echogenic
Attentuation[a]	None to minimal	Moderate	Moderate to marked
Shape	Spherical	Variable	Variable
Borders	Smooth, well-defined	Variable	Variable

[a]Linear scans only.

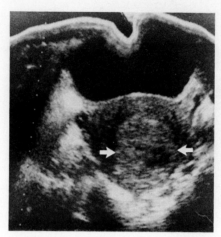

Figure 1-25C. Solid mass (transverse scan, 4 cm above symphysis pubis; white-on-black image, white = echoes). This mass contains many internal echoes, which implies its solid consistency. In contrast to cystic masses, solid masses appear more echogenic when imaged with higher gain settings.

graphic pattern for the liver different from that of the renal cortex. Tissues relatively devoid of interstitial components such as the central neutral tissue are minimally echogenic, and appear as a homogeneous texture. Inhomogeneous patterns within an organ are frequently encountered in masses that are undergoing a cystic internal degeneration, which often results in a complex echo pattern. Masses such as a dermoid cyst that contains fluid, fatty, and calcific components also emanate a complex pattern.

The wall of a mass should be carefully evaluated, as well as the soft tissues interface that surrounds it. Cystic masses with thick walls may represent either an inflammatory or neoplastic process within the wall of a cyst. Occasionally, thickened walls are seen with a cystic mass that has twisted about a pedicle. This is thought to be vascular congestion of the cyst wall. Pathological thickening of a cyst wall is illustrated by clear cell carcinoma depicted in Figure 3-2E which was located in the thickened posterior wall of an endometrioma. Thickening of a cyst wall can have the same ultrasound appearance as cellular debris that has layered out along the dependent wall of the cyst. This entity can be distinguished from a truly thickened wall by scanning the patient while placed in different positions to detect any gravity dependence of the apparent wall material. This point will be subsequently emphasized.

The regularity of the soft tissue borders that surround a mass should be examined closely by scanning the mass in at least two planes. Since cysts usually enlarge by fluid accumulation in their center, they tend to enlarge in a concentric fashion, and cause regular compression of surrounding soft tissue. This type of enlargement is reflected by a well-defined, smooth border. Infiltrative tumors, on the other hand, usually display irregular borders that often indicate tumor invasion into the surrounding soft tissues. Even though the sonographic findings may indicate a benign mass, current ultrasonic techniques cannot visualize the tissue histology well enough to differentiate benign from malignant masses accurately. Microscopic examination of tissue samples is frequently the only method by which such a judgment can be made.

If all three of the sonographic criteria used to define a cystic mass cannot be definitely established, an alternative characterization should be strongly considered. Although not normally required to make a diagnosis of a cyst, the A-mode trace can assist in substantiating the B-mode findings. The walls of the cyst defined should appear as a distinct echo peak with an echo-free interior.

As stated earlier, diagnostic information can also be obtained from echoes distal to the interface of interest. For example, most gallbladder calculi exhibit high reflection and complete attenuation of the incident beam at their interface. This situation produces a complete or "clean" shadow, as opposed to shadows secondary to a partially gas-filled bowel which reveal a mottled appearance. The gas and mucus contained within collapsed bowel scatter the incident beam, resulting in an incomplete, mottled, or so-called "dirty" shadow. Shadowing distal to a calcified structure of highly reflective area may be more apparent when the area is scanned using a transducer of higher frequency. This concept of the different types of shadowing will become much clearer with additional illustration and specific clinical examples forthcoming in other chapters of this book.

One must be able to distinguish erroneous or artifactual echoes from true echoes and patterns created by lesions representing a pathologic condition from those due to unusual appearances of normal structures or faulty use of the instrumentation. The most commonly encountered artifact in abdominal and pelvic scanning is caused by reverberation. Reverberations are caused by a series of rapid reflections from a strong interface that sets up a series of spurious echo arrangements. This artifact can be recognized by its regular spacing of echoes and diminishing strength as the artifact proceeds distally through the image. Such artifacts can usually be diminished by decreasing the gain in the region of the artifact. Reverberation artifacts are frequently created at echogenic interfaces such as gas-filled bowel (Fig. 1-26). Reverberations are also seen at the anterior surface of a fluid-filled bladder resulting from the high reflectivity of the bladder-urine interface.

Other artifacts that sometimes appear include the shadowing produced by a rib or calcific lesion that can obscure echoes distal to the interface. If the ultrasound beam crosses an interface with a change in propagation velocity, refraction can occur at the interface, causing another form of artifact. And large curved and highly reflective interfaces can act like acoustic mirrors, creating phantom images of structures close to the transducer that appear deep in the tissue. This type of artifact is frequently encountered when a phantom image of a hepatic mass is created on the opposite side of the diaphragm.

In addition to tissue-created artifacts, artifacts can be created by the scanning technique. For example, sector scans made with the patient breathing can cause serrated-appearing borders on what are really smooth cystic walls. Compound scanning can sometimes fill in areas with echoes to exclude anatomical information useful for diagnosis (Fig. 1-27B). This is often referred to as overwriting.

At very high gain settings or with the TGC improperly assigned, spurious echoes or "noise" within the system can be produced, filling in cysts with in-

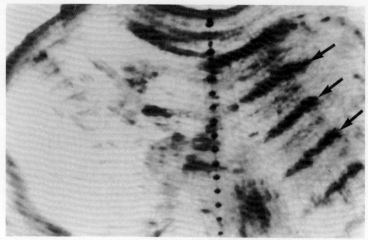

Figure 1-26. Reverberation artifact (transverse abdominal sonogram at level of the xiphoid). To the right of the image, periodic linear echogenic interfaces have a constant distance between them and diminish in intensity as they pass through the body (*arrows*). This reverberation artifact is produced by gas within the body of the stomach.

Figure 1-27. SCANNING FACTORS THAT INFLUENCE IMAGE QUALITY

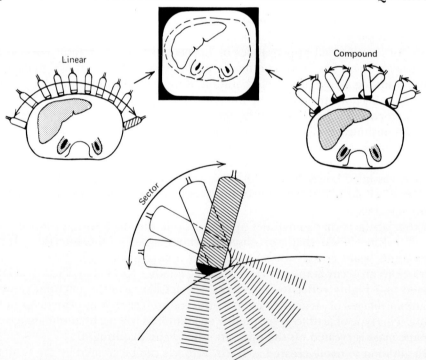

Figure 1-27A. Scanning techniques. Linear scans are performed to demonstrate the attenuation values from the various internal structures of a structure or organ. Compound scanning is used to delineate boundaries between structures that are not adequately depicted by simple linear scans. Sector scans are performed when the transducer is moved in an arc but held in the same area of the body. Sector scans should be performed in the intercostal spaces to avoid rib artifacts.

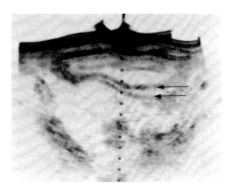

Figure 1-27B. Artifacts introduced by compound scanning (transverse view, 4 cm above symphysis pubis). The posterior wall of the bladder appears as a double line because the interface was scanned twice, with probable movement between scans (*arrows*). A compound motion of the transducer is suggested by the overlapping configuration of the path of the transducer on skin surface.

strument noise rather than actual tissue echoes (Fig. 1-28B). This can cause one to misinterpret a cystic structure as a solid one. Such an artifact is easily recognized by understanding the properties and operation of the machine and by reducing the gain to a useful and non "noise-introducing" level (Fig. 1-28A).

The reliability of measurements made on a CRT as well as portrayal of soft tissue interfaces can change as the CRT ages. Therefore, the instrument should be checked daily for proper gain and arm registration with a standard phantom. In general, ultrasonic scanners do not have any established standards for day-to-day variations in equipment. Phantoms or test objects such as those approved by the AIUM can be used to measure whether or not the arm registration is proper (Figs. 1-29A,B). A new standard phantom has been developed for

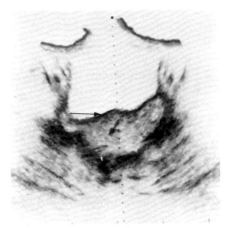

Figure 1-27C. Proper scanning (transverse view, 4 cm above symphysis pubis). The contralateral adnexa are imaged by limited sector scans on each side of the bladder. The posterior wall of the bladder is depicted as a single, continuous interface (*arrow*) rather than a double interface that was seen when a compound scanning motion was used.

Figure 1-28. TGC AND GAIN ADJUSTMENTS

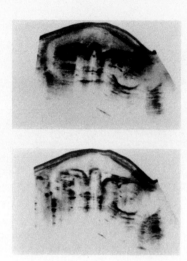

Figure 1-28A. TGC settings. Both images were obtained in the midline of a gravid uterus containing a single fetus. One image (*top*) was obtained with not enough near-field suppression, which resulted in recording spurious echoes from the placenta-fetus interface (*arrow*). When the TGC was properly adjusted, the fetal structures in the near field are better portrayed (*bottom*).

standardizing the different gray scale shades using substances of different acoustical impedance such as oil, water, and fat. With increasing need for equipment standardization, new phantoms will become commercially available, permitting users to acquire a great deal of information on the operational state of their particular scanning device (Fig. 1-29C).

If a standard phantom is available, one should begin each day by scanning the phantom to detect any drift in the scan converter or other parts of the instrument. Very often, scanning a standard-size patient's abdomen with the same transducer will detect changes in the gray scale qualities of the machine if a phantom is not available. Without an attempt to measure drift in ultrasonic devices, the user cannot determine whether the machine is in fact performing to its intended specifications. An improperly calibrated machine will make diagnostically suboptimal images. Failure to understand and properly employ the available instrumentation is probably the greatest source of clinical underutilization of diagnostic ultrasound at the present time.

BIOLOGICAL EFFECTS

Since ultrasound is a form of mechanical energy that can interact with living tissue, it is incorrect to assume that ultrasound has absolutely no biologically deleterious effect on living cells even at diagnostic levels. When discussing the biological effects of ultrasound, it is important to consider both the intensity, either in terms of spatial or time averages, and the length of exposure. At present, the quantification of ultrasonic beam intensity is imprecise. Estimates of intensity are expressed in units of watts per square centimeter (W/cm^2). These units refer

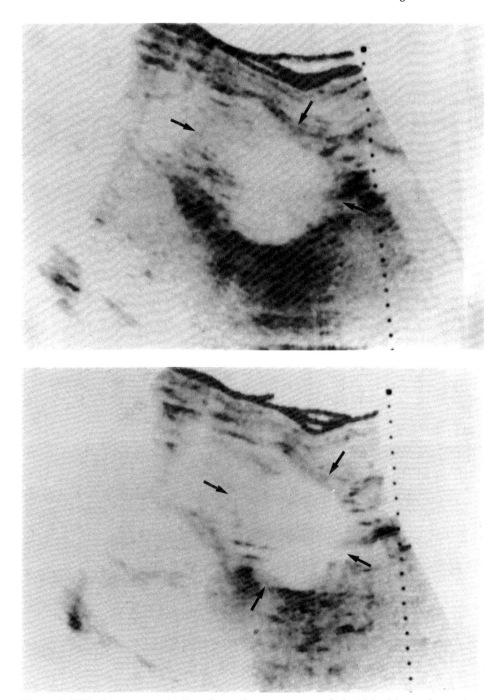

Figure 1-28B. Improper gain. Spurious echoes were recorded within this renal cyst when an excessively high gain setting was used (*top*). The echoes recorded within the cyst represented "noise" generated by the scanning system. The sonolucent features of the cyst were readily apparent when the proper gain setting was used (*bottom*). In order to establish the cystic nature of a mass, scans should be performed at low- and high-gain settings.

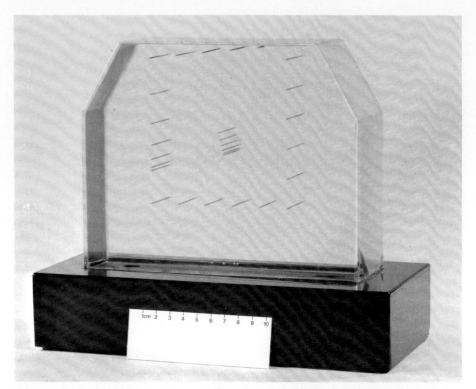

Figure 1-29A. Standard A.I.U.M. test phantom. This water-filled test phantom consists of numerous wires suspended within a plastic housing. When scanned from all sides, this type of phantom can be used to determine approximate axial and lateral resolution and alignment of the scanning system.

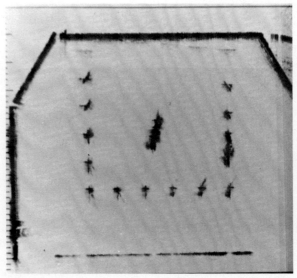

Figure 1-29B. Image of phantom. Since this scanning device was in alignment, the echoes arising from the wires intersect each other (*arrow*).

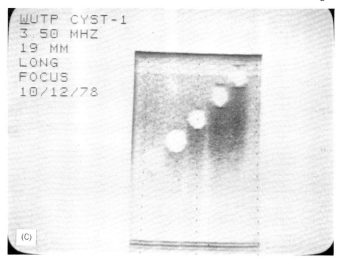

Figure 1-29C. Soft-tissue equivalent phantom. This image was obtained by moving the transducer over the top of the phantom. The gel that is contained within the phantom has a similar echogenicity to human liver. Simulated within the phantom are 2 cm "cysts." (Courtesy of Donald R. Jacobson, Radiation Measurements, Inc., Middleton, Wisc.)

to the amount of energy per unit time (watts) crossing an area of 1 square centimeter anywhere within the ultrasonic field.

Most diagnostic imaging devices are pulsed rather than continuous. The ratio of the transmission time to the total time of the pulse-listen cycle is referred to as the duty cycle and is less than 1% for most scanning devices. Thus, the instrument transmits for less than 1% of the time and listens for the rest. For most diagnostic purposes, the average intensity of ultrasound ranges from 0.002 to 0.05 W/cm², whereas therapeutic ultrasound used in diathermy ranges from 0.5 to 2.0 W/cm². Ultrasonic energy is occasionally used for ablative therapy, and here the intensities range from 50.0 to 100.0 W/cm² (Table 1-9).

Admittedly, some potentially adverse biological effects such as coagulation of blood and neurological injury have been observed in some experiments using 1,000 to 1 million times the intensity of diagnostic ultrasound (11). Despite these findings, no definite adverse biological effects have been documented for the intensities used in diagnostics. The experiments have ranged from measuring anomalies in plated cells to epidemiological studies involving thousands of patients (1). Despite this evidence, the effects remain unclear and further investigations into the implications of ultrasound will be necessary to define the biological effects unequivocally.

Table 1-9. Relative Intensities of Ultrasound Used in Medicine

Diagnostic	0.002–0.05 W/cm²	Pulsed time average
	0.5–1.0 W/cm²	Continuous wave Doppler
Diathermy	1–3 W/cm²	Continuous wave
Ablative (surgical)	50–1,000 W/cm²	Focused

The biological effects of ultrasound can be considered in three major categories. These include production of heat by absorption; cavitation, which is largely seen at lower frequencies and very high intensities; and direct effects such as microstreaming, which exerts effects on the cell membrane.

Tissue heating at diagnostic levels is so minimal that it cannot be reliably measured, and because it is so small, it is thought to be of little biological significance. In addition to the normal conduction of heat away from the region of the ultrasonic field, the vascular supply of an organ also aids in the removal of heat from the exposed region.

Cavitation involves the production of microbubbles in the carrying liquid during the relaxation phase of the ultrasonic wave. The microbubbles can come into resonance with the ultrasonic field when they reach the proper size. This phenomenon is generally not observed at the high frequencies and low intensities used in diagnostic ultrasound.

Microstreaming refers to a phenomenon in which microcurrents are produced in the liquid medium surrounding cells. Microstreaming is considered a "direct" effect because no intermediate steps exist between the agent and the effect. This phenomenon may be able to affect enzyme systems and cell permeability. Because of microstreaming, biologic effects of ultrasound appear to be centered on the cell membrane rather than the nuclear contents.

Investigations from a clinical and epidemiologic emphasis attempting to detect possible adverse effects of ultrasound have been ongoing for the last 25 years. Much more investigation appears to be needed before definitive conclusions about the biological effects of ultrasound can be reached. Of the epidemiologic studies completed, none shows any significant increase in either the total number of or any particular type of congenital anomalies in persons subjected to ultrasound in utero (12). No increase in congenital anomalies was observed in human abortuses after exposure to diagnostic ultrasound for as long as 10 hours prior to therapeutic abortion. Exposures of internal genitalia of rats at high intensities (10 to 100 W/cm²) have shown no change in reproductive capacity or genetic anomalies in the offspring (1).

Several in vitro investigations of the effects of ultrasound on living cells in tissue culture have demonstrated certain effects. Chromosomal damage due to ultrasound was reported in one study, but studies by other investigators attempting to corroborate these single findings indicated that the results may have resulted from laboratory error (10). In addition, the findings were considered inconclusive because the procedure for scoring chromosomal aberrations was both inexact and subjective. No definite chromosomal aberrations have yet been reported, even with intensities up to 8.0 W/cm² and exposure times up to 20 hours. In general, cells in culture appear to be more susceptible to damage from high-frequency ultrasound during the M-phase of the cell cycle. This is a time of mechanical separation of DNA into daughter cells, and the mechanical properties of ultrasound could interact with this process. Certain effects on colony formation, plating efficiency, and other tissue growth characteristics have been observed; the biological implications of these are as yet unknown (14).

Because of microstreaming, ultrasonic energy can exert a major biological effect on the surface membranes of cells. This has been documented by measuring effects on enzyme systems such as an ATPase attached to a membrane surface. To date, no biologically significant effects have been documented from these observed membrane effects.

At present, there appear to be no definite adverse biological effects from pulsed diagnostic ultrasound. The need for further investigation of biological effects and standardization and measurement of the dose and patient dosimetry remains. At present, the dose received by a patient in a diagnostic study can only be estimated, either by calibrating a transducer that is used to map the spatial profile of the diagnostic transducer or by using a radiation microbalance to measure the average power from a transducer. Other biological methods of analysis are being investigated as well, including the adhesion of cells in culture before and after insonation (14). Despite attempts at completely accurate and reproducible dosimetry, the exact measurements continue to await development of the proper technology. However, with the knowledge presently available, it appears that ultrasound may be used in those situations in which there is a clear clinical need with less biological risk than with most alternative imaging techniques (15).

SUMMARY

The authors feel that this chapter forms the basis for the reader's understanding of the clinical applications to follow. We hope that the reader, while considering the specific clinical uses of ultrasound which are presented in the remainder of this text, will feel free to refer back to the principles discussed in this chapter.

REFERENCES

General

1. Aximi, F., Bray, P., Marangola, J.: Ultrasonography in obstetrics and gynecology: Historical notes, basic principles, safety considerations, and clinical applications. *CRC Critical Reviews in Diagnostic Radiology* 8(2):153–166, 1976.
2. Goldberg, B., Kotler, M., Ziskin, M., Waxham, R.: *Diagnostic Uses of Ultrasound.* New York: Grune and Stratton, 1975.

Physical Principles

3. McDicken, W.: *Diagnostic Ultrasound: Principle and Use of Instruments.* New York: John Wiley and Sons, 1976.
4. Carlson, E.: Ultrasound physics for the physician: A brief review. *J. Clin. Ultrasound* 3(1):71–80, 1975.
5. Powis, R.: *Ultrasound Physics: For the Fun of It.* Denver: Unirad Corp., 1978.
6. Wells, P. N. T.: *Physical Principles of Ultrasonic Diagnosis.* New York: Academic Press, 1969.

Diagnostic Principles

7. Kossoff, G., Garrett, W., Carpenter, D., Jellins, J., Dadd, M.: Principles and classification of soft tissue masses by gray scale echography. *Ultrasound in Med. Biol.* 2:89–104, 1976.

8. Fields, S., Dunn, F.: Correlation of echographic visualization of tissue with biological composition and physiologic state. *J. Acous. Soc. Am.* 54(3):809–812, 1973.
9. Cunningham, J., Worten, W., Cunningham, N.: Gray scale echogenicity of soluble protein and protein aggregates (an *in vitro* study). *J. Clin. Ultrasound* 4(6):417–420, 1976.
10. Scheible, W., Ellenbogen, P., Leopold, G., Siso, N.: Lipomatous tumors of the kidney and adrenal: Apparent echographic specificity. *Radiology* 129:153–156, 1978.

Biological Effects

11. Baker, M., Dalrymple, G.: Biological effects of diagnostic ultrasound: A review. *Radiology* 126:479–483, 1978.
12. Freimanis, A.: The biological effects of medically applied ultrasound and their causes. *CRC Critical Reviews in Radiation Science*, 1970, pp. 639–670.
13. Hellman, L., Dufuss, G., Donald, I., Sunden, B.: Safety of diagnostic ultrasound in obstetrics. *Lancet* 1:1113–1115, 1970.
14. Siegel, E., Goddard, J., James, A., Siegel, E.: Cellular attachment as a sensitive indicator of the effects of diagnostic ultrasound exposure on human cultured cells. *Radiology* 133:175–179, 1979.
15. Nyborg, W.: *Physical Mechanisms for Biological Effects of Ultrasound*. Rockville, Md.: Bureau of Radiological Health, 1977.

2
Obstetrical
Sonography

INDICATIONS

The desire for a biologically innocuous diagnostic modality to evaluate the fetus in utero served as a major impetus for the development of sonographic imaging techniques in the early 1960s. Since the fetus is surrounded by amniotic fluid, this is an ideal circumstance to image by sonographic methods. Thus, sonography is considered a desirable modality for evaluation of the gravid patient and fetus. Extensive investigation concerning the possible adverse biological effects of ultrasound at diagnostic levels has, to date, failed to reveal any biologically significant side effects.

Sonography can be used for evaluation of the pregnant patient from 4 to 5 weeks' menstrual age (since last menstrual period) up to the time of delivery. Sonography is frequently employed to estimate gestational age, both in patients who present with a uterus "too-large-for-dates" and in those who are uncertain of the date of their last menstrual period. Sonography is also frequently performed in patients who are considered at high risk for developing complications during pregnancy and in the immediate postpartum period.

The following is a list of the obstetrical disorders or problems in which sonography has been found to be particularly useful. These conditions are listed according to frequency of request for sonographic study, which can be considered a reflection of diagnostic efficacy. For purposes of discussion, the applications of sonography in obstetrics are presented according to the stage of pregnancy in which they are particularly helpful.

A. Throughout pregnancy
   1. Confirm the presence of intrauterine pregnancy (combined with laboratory determinations)
   2. Estimate gestational duration and evaluate date-size discrepancy
   3. Confirm the presence of a multiple gestation
   4. Localize and evaluate the placenta
   5. Evaluate the amount and distribution of amniotic fluid
   6. Confirm fetal viability (combined with Doppler examination, real-time scanning)

B. First trimester
   1. Confirm suspected molar gestation
   2. Confirm suspected ectopic pregnancy
   3. Confirm suspected abortion

C. Second trimester
 1. Localize placenta prior to amniocentesis
 2. Evaluate fetal growth

D. Third trimester
 1. Confirm or exclude presence of placenta previa
 2. Evaluate congenital anomalies

E. Maternal disorders occurring during pregnancy
 1. Cholecystitis
 2. Pancreatitis
 3. Vascular aneurysms
 4. Hydronephrosis of pregnancy and urinary tract infection

F. Postpartum
 1. Evaluate retained products of conception
 2. Evaluate the extent and severity of postpartum infection such as endometritis

SCANNING TECHNIQUE

Sonographic examination of the gravid patient should be performed in a systematic manner using both longitudinal and transverse scans (4). Scans performed in oblique planes should be used when delineation of a structure is incomplete using routine longitudinal and transverse planes. Since penetration of and past the structures of the gravid uterus is necessary for adequate obstetrical sonograms, a 2.25- or 3.5-MHz transducer with medium to long internal focus is used for most obstetrical sonograms

A full-bladder technique is imperative in studying patients in the first trimester as well as in evaluating patients with possible placenta previa. Examination with the patient's bladder full is not so important in the second trimester, at which stage the gravid uterus displaces the bowel out of the pelvis. A fully distended bladder accomplishes two goals: (1) it displaces the echo-scattering bowel out of the pelvis, thus providing an "ultrasonic window" into the pelvis; and (2) the urine-filled bladder serves as a reference of sonolucency for comparison of the echogenic properties of different structures. Filling the bladder is accomplished by having the patient drink two to three glasses of water prior to examination. Catheterization of the bladder and instilling sterile saline may be necessary in patients whose oral intake is restricted.

It is because the various organs located within the pelvis are confined within a limited space defined by the osseous structures that distension of the bladder will displace out of the pelvis proper the bowel that normally lies within the pelvis (Figs. 2-1A,B). A markedly distended bladder, however, can cause spurious distortion of the uterus and its contents (5). For instance, a markedly distended bladder can compress the uterus and result in apparent flattening of the normally oval gestational sac, giving it an apparent abnormal configuration. In the later stages of pregnancy, an overdistended bladder may result in a low-lying placenta simulating a true placenta previa. This occurs as a result of dis-

Figure 2-1. NORMAL, NONGRAVID UTERUS AND OVARIES

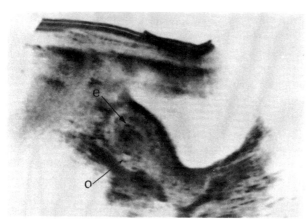

Figure 2-1A. Normal, premenstrual uterus (longitudinal scan, midline with patient's head to left of image). The uterus is a pear-shaped structure that lies immediately posterior to the distended bladder. The endometrium (e) is depicted as a linear echogenic interface in the center of the uterus. Surrounding the endometrium is a sonolucent halo probably representing hypertrophied and edematous endometrial glands. The ovary (o) appears as an elliptical structure that contains one or two small sonolucent foci probably representing unruptured follicles.

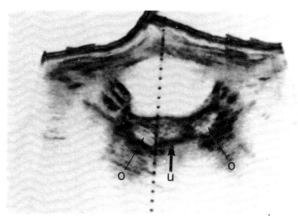

Figure 2-1B. Normal adnexa (transverse, 4 cm above symphysis pubis, patient's right to left of image). The uterus (u) appears as a central, mildly echogenic rounded structure with the ovaries on each side (o). These structures and their supporting ligaments comprise the "genital axis." Gas-filled bowel that is present behind the uterus and ovaries prohibits delineation of structures posterior to the genital axis. The oviducts are only infrequently visualized because they have a tortuous course and are below the resolution of the scanning system.

tortion of the lower uterine segment and placenta when the bladder is overdistended. In order to determine the true position of the placenta in these cases, the patient should be allowed to empty her bladder partially. A series of longitudinal and transverse scans outlining the lower uterine segment should be performed to assess any change in configuration of the placenta before and after partial voiding (5).

Real-time sonography can be used in conjunction with static gray scale scanning for rapid screening and overall evaluation of the fetal presentation and several major organs of the fetus. The fetal brain and heart should be routinely examined. The falx cerebri, thalami, and lateral ventricles within the cranium should be identified. The heart appears as a fluid-filled structure contracting rhythmically in the fetal thorax. Real-time sonography is particularly helpful as a means of locating the fetal abdomen for intrauterine transfusions (45).

SONOGRAPHIC "MILESTONES" OF NORMAL PREGNANCY

Certain features of the developing pregnancy can be used as sonographic "milestones" to establish that there is normal progression of an intrauterine pregnancy. These features are summarized in Table 2-1. A normal intrauterine pregnancy can be inferred if these features are documented at certain stages of development during the pregnancy.

Gestational Sac

As early as two to three weeks after implantation of the fertilized zygote into the endometrium (four to five weeks' menstrual age), a small oval gestational sac can be visualized using gray scale sonography (Figs. 2-2A,B). On occasion, sonography can suggest the presence of an intrauterine pregnancy before the patient is aware that she is pregnant or before routine (urine) pregnancy tests become positive.

Table 2-1. Sonographic "Milestones" in Pregnancy

4–6 weeks[a]	Gestational sac identifiable
6–8 weeks	Embryonic pole and decidua identifiable
7–12 weeks	Fetal crown-rump length measurable
8–10 weeks	Fetal "motion" identifiable by real-time scanning
8–12 weeks	Fetal heart tones audible by Doppler instrument
11–15 weeks to term	Biparietal diameter measurable
12–27 weeks	Placental growth maximal
25 weeks to term	Major fetal viscera discernable
25–35 weeks	Maximal uterine growth and "ascension" of the placenta

[a]± 2 weeks.

Figure 2-2. NORMAL FIRST TRIMESTER PREGNANCY

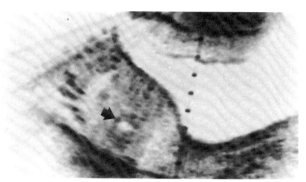

Figure 2-2A. Normal three- to four-week gestational sac (longitudinal, midline). The developing gestational sac (*arrow*) is depicted as a cystic structure within the uterine lumen. An embryonic pole is not seen at this stage of pregnancy.

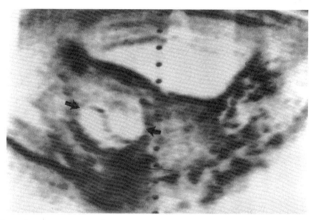

Figure 2-2B. Sonolucent corpus luteum cyst (transverse, 4 cm above symphysis pubis). There is a predominantly sonolucent right adnexal mass (*arrows*) representing a corpus luteum cyst that contains liquefied contents. These cysts occur normally during the first trimester of pregnancy and may appear echogenic or sonolucent (Fig. 2-13A), depending on their internal composition. When they contain organized hematoma, they are demonstrated as echogenic masses, whereas when the clot liquefies, they appear sonolucent. The wavy echogenic interface seen within this predominantly cystic mass probably represents a forming synechia.

The beta-subunit of human chorionic gonadotropin (HCG) is a specialized laboratory test to assess a particular portion of the HCG hormone. This test is very sensitive for the detection of functional chorionic tissue. Although the HCG beta-subunit test can be used in a quantitative manner, it may be positive only nine days after implantation.

By three to five weeks, an oval gestational sac should be apparent as a sonolucent area located within the region of the uterine fundus. A localized area of thickening along the rim of the gestational sac should also be adequately delineated; this represents the decidual tissue that will eventually form the placenta. At five to six weeks' menstrual age, an embryonic "pole" should be seen as an echogenic

57

focus within the gestational sac in the region of the chorion frondosum (Figs. 2-2C,D).

In early stages of the first trimester, the approximate duration of gestation can be estimated by measuring the diameter of the gestational sac (6) (Table 2-2). Estimations of gestational duration by gestational sac measurements should be correlated with an overall estimation of gestational age as evidenced by the size of the uterus. In general, the uterine fundus is at the level of the pelvic rim at 12 weeks and usually reaches the region of the umbilicus at approximately 20 weeks. Because the bladder displaces the uterus out of the pelvis when fully distended, the uterine size will usually be one to two weeks greater when it is estimated by ultrasound than when it is estimated by palpation on routine physical examination.

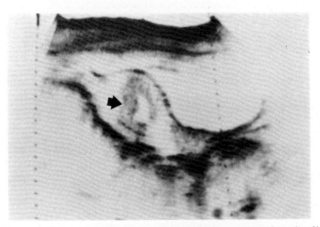

Figure 2-2C. Normal five- to six-week intrauterine pregnancy (longitudinal, midline). The developing embryonic pole appears as a focal soft tissue protuberance in the gestational sac (*arrow*).

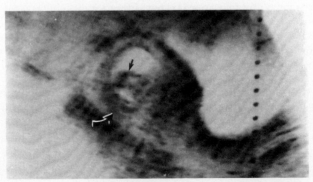

Figure 2-2D. Normal six- to eight-week pregnancy (longitudinal, midline). The embryonic pole (*arrow*) is well formed. The decidua shows a localized thickening along the posterior aspect of the gestational sac representing the developing chorion frondosum (*curved arrow*), which corresponds to tissue that will eventually form the placenta. An embryonic pole should be seen within the gestational sac after eight weeks.

Table 2-2. Estimation of Gestational Duration in the First Trimester[a]

Menstrual Age (weeks)	Gestational Sac (mm)[b] (SD ± 1 to 2 weeks)	Crown-Rump Length (mm) (SD ± 1 to 4 days)	Biparietal Diameter (mm) (SD ± 1 week)	Trunk (mm) (SD ± 1 week)
3				
4				
5	10			
6	20			
7	30	10		
8	45	17	10	
9	60	25	12	
10	70	32	14	
11		40	17	
12		55	21	18
13		65	25	21
14		80	29	24
15		100	33	28

[a]Adapted from Flamme (14).
[b]Measured by greatest diameter of gestational sac.

Occasionally, more than one gestational sac will be recognized early in pregnancy. It is not uncommon for one of the gestational sacs to fail to develop, whereas another sac develops into a normal gestation (32). The abortion of one of the sacs may or may not be clinically apparent to the patient.

From 8 to 11 weeks on, the contents of the gestational sac, such as the placenta and fetus, can be delineated. The embryonic pole appears as a localized protuberance emanating from the peripheral aspect of the gestational sac and projecting into the amniotic cavity.

Between approximately 8 and 12 weeks, a measurement called the crown-rump length of the fetus can be used to determine gestational age (7). The crown-rump length is obtained by delineating the greatest longitudinal length of the fetus. Estimates of gestational age using the crown-rump length are very accurate, having a standard deviation of ± 4 days, and can be readily obtained using real-time sonography (Figs. 2-2E, 2-3A,B).

Biparietal Diameter

Beginning at approximately 13 to 15 weeks, the fetal head can be evaluated and its biparietal diameter (BPD) measured. It is emphasized that the biparietal diameter must be obtained perpendicular to the falx cerebri. Otherwise, scans that are obtained with the transducer orientation oblique to the falx will overestimate the cranial size and will give a faulty estimation of gestational duration. Occasionally, the BPD can be difficult to obtain because of motion of the fetal head in the uterus during the examination. Because of rapid change in the position of the fetus while it is in the uterus, it may be difficult to image the biparietal diameter using a static imaging device (Fig. 2-4A). For this reason, real-time sonography can be used for rapid and accurate delineation of the biparietal diameter.

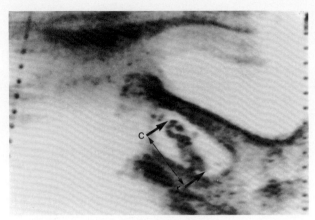

Figure 2-2E. An 11-week fetus (modified longitudinal, along the longitudinal axis of fetus). The crown-rump length is represented by the distance from c to r. In this fetus, the crown-rump length is readily identified and measures 4.0 cm, which corresponds to a gestational age of 11, ± 1 week. Crown-rump measurements are used to estimate gestational duration between 8 and 11 weeks. For proper measurement of the crown-rump length, scans should be obtained along the longitudinal axis of the fetus.

Growth of the fetal head is linear only during the second trimester of pregnancy. Between 12 and 30 weeks, the linear relation is most accurate, having a standard deviation of ± 1 week. During this phase of pregnancy, the growth of the fetal head is approximately 2 to 3 mm per week. From 32 weeks to term, the enlargement of the fetal head is nonlinear. The standard deviation during this time is approximately 2 weeks and the rate of head enlargement is about 1 mm per week (Table 2-3) (8).

Figure 2-3. NORMAL SECOND TRIMESTER PREGNANCY

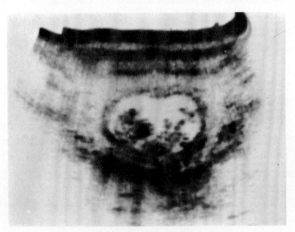

Figure 2-3A. A 12- to 13-week fetus (modified transverse view, 8 cm above symphysis pubis). The developing fetus is demonstrated with its back on the dependent portion of the amniotic cavity. The entire fetus can frequently be delineated in a single scan at this stage of development.

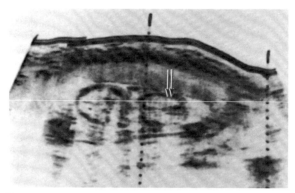

Figure 2-3B. A 20-week fetus (longitudinal, midline, the symphysis pubis and maternal umbilicus are marked by centimeter markers). The fetus is imaged from crown to rump, and the fetal head is in the uterine fundus. The bony structures of the fetus such as the ribs produce distal acoustical shadowing (*arrows*) creating a "venetian blind" effect. The placenta is anterior and homogeneous in texture. The fetal vertebral column is seen as two echogenic horizontal interfaces in the lower part of the fetal body. The falx cerebri can be identified as a central echogenic interface oriented in a horizontal manner located in the center of the fetal cranium. Centimeter markers denote the level of the umbilicus and symphysis pubis.

Figure 2-4. NORMAL THIRD TRIMESTER PREGNANCY

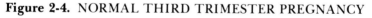

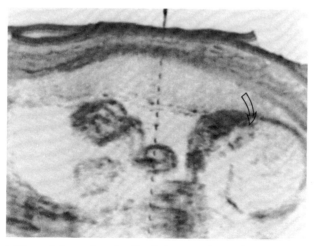

Figure 2-4A. A 30-week fetus (longitudinal, 4 cm to right of midline). Fetus has achieved enough size to make it difficult to delineate the entire fetus on a single scan. The fetus is in a cephalic presentation, and the fetal orbits can be delineated (*curved open arrow*). Fetal extremities are imaged in cross section. The placenta is anterior and has a homogeneous texture.

Table 2-3. Estimation of Gestational Age by Biparietal Diameter[a]

Biparietal Diameter (mm)	Gestational Age (to nearest half-week)
2.0	12
2.1, 2.2	12½
2.3	13
2.4, 2.5	13½
2.6	14
2.7, 2.8	14½
2.9	15
3.0	15½
3.1, 3.2	16
3.3	16½
3.4, 3.5	17
3.6	17½
3.7, 3.8	18
3.9, 4.0	18½
4.1	19
4.2, 4.3	19½
4.4	20
4.5, 4.6	20½
4.7	21
4.8, 4.9	21½
5.0	22
5.1	22½
5.2, 5.3	23
5.4, 5.5	23½
5.6	24
5.7, 5.8	24½
5.9	25
6.0	25½
6.1, 6.2	26
6.3	26½

Table 2-3. (Continued)

Biparietal Diameter (mm)	Gestational Age (to nearest half-week)
6.4 ⎫ 6.5 ⎭	27
6.6	27½
6.7 ⎫ 6.8 ⎭	28
6.9	28½
7.0 ⎫ 7.1 ⎭	29
7.2	29½
7.3 ⎫ 7.4 ⎬ 7.5 ⎭	30
7.6	30½
7.7	31
7.8	31½
7.9	32
8.0	32½
8.1	33
8.2	33½
8.3	34
8.4	34½
8.5	35
8.6	35½
8.7	36
8.8	36½
8.9	37
9.0	37½
9.1	38
9.2	38½
9.3 ⎫ 9.4 ⎭	39
9.5 ⎫ 9.6 ⎭	40
9.7 ⎫ 9.8 ⎭	41
9.9	42

^aAdapted from Chilcote and Asokan (6).

Because the fetal head can be most reliably imaged in the second trimester and the fetal growth is linear during this period, evaluation of the biparietal diameter for estimation of gestational age is optimal at midpoint in the second trimester; between 22 and 30 weeks. Gestational age and growth of the fetus may be better estimated if serial examinations are performed, preferably during the early and late second trimester (9). Percentile growth curves for the fetus in utero have been devised similar to those used for documentation of growth during the neonatal period (14).

Fetal Weight

Although the biparietal diameter can be used to estimate fetal gestational age, it is not as accurate a measure of fetal growth as serial estimates of the fetal weight. The weight of the fetus is also a more accurate measure of fetal maturation and can be estimated by measuring the abdominal circumference of the fetus at the level of the umbilical vein. The umbilical vein appears as a rounded, sonolucent structure immediately beneath the anterior abdominal wall of the fetus (Fig. 2-4B). Measurement of the fetus as it pertains to estimation of fetal growth parameters and detection of intrauterine growth retardation is discussed in detail in another subsection of this chapter.

Placenta

Sonographic imaging allows documentation of the structural and positional changes of the placenta during pregnancy. Sonography is most frequently employed to evaluate patients who present with third trimester bleeding which may be due to placenta previa. Sonography can also detect structural changes in the placenta as depicted by changes in the sonographic texture.

Early in pregnancy, the chorionic tissue that eventually forms the placenta (Fig. 2-2C) appears as a focal area of thickening on the periphery of the gestational sac. Probably due to its high degree of vascularity and numerous villous structures, the chorion frondosum is more echogenic than the surrounding myo-

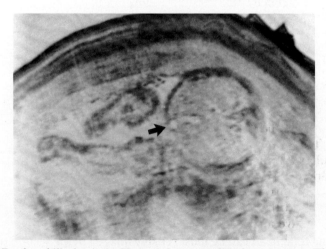

Figure 2-4B. Fetal umbilical vein in 30-week fetus (modified transverse). This sonogram was obtained through the fetal abdomen at the level of the umbilical vein. The umbilical vein appears as a tubular sonolucent structure immediately beneath the anterior abdominal wall of the fetus (*arrow*). Measurement of the fetal abdominal circumference should be made at this level. Crossed fetal legs are seen to the right of the fetal abdomen.

metrium. At this stage of pregnancy, the gestational sac appears to encompass the entire amniotic cavity and the placenta begins to cover an increasing proportion of the endometrial surface. During the latter weeks of the first trimester, the placenta may appear on ultrasound study to cover the entire endometrial surface. Since placental growth is maximal during the late first trimester and middle to early second trimester (12 to 25 weeks), the placenta usually occupies a major portion of the endometrial surface. However, the uterus experiences its greatest growth during the third trimester, the proportion of the endometrial surface occupied by the placenta diminishes to approximately two-thirds to one-half at term (3).

Although there is apparent change in the position of the placenta in relation to the internal cervical os during pregnancy, this phenomenon appears to be best explained by differential growth of the lower uterine segment during the third trimester rather than by actual change in implantation site of the placenta. The change in the location of the placenta during pregnancy has been referred to as placental "migration" (16). However, it is probably best referred to as "ascension" of the placenta or "anteriorization" or "posteriorization" (18). Since it is common for a placenta that appears to lie in the lower uterine segment during the second trimester of pregnancy to move from the lower uterine segment as the pregnancy approaches term, it is important to recognize this phenomenon and ascribe proper clinical significance to this process. It is, therefore, suggested that if a low-lying placenta is encountered in the second trimester of pregnancy, the patient should be examined one to two weeks prior to expected delivery to exclude the presence of a placenta previa. If bleeding occurs before term, a repeat obstetrical sonogram is recommended.

Besides showing change in the location of the placenta, sonography can depict textural changes in the placenta as the pregnancy approaches term. Since the placenta has such a large reserve capacity, many of these textural changes are observed without clinical expression. Focal areas of sonolucency are frequently encountered in near-term placentas. The texture pattern has been referred to as placental "mottling" (15). The sonolucent areas correspond to areas of hydropic change in the placenta resulting from a diminished number of villi combined with pooling of blood in the intervillous space. Another common textural inhomogeneity in the placenta that is encountered as pregnancy progresses is a subchorionic sonolucent band representing subchorionic fibrinoid collection (Fig. 2-12C). As the name implies, this entity can be differentiated from the sonolucent band near the basal plate of the placenta, which represents the venous drainage of the placenta, by its characteristic location beneath the chorionic plate. Calcification may be observed along the basal plate and septa. In most cases, this is a normal change in the placenta as it undergoes senescence near term. Placental infarcts usually appear as areas of relative sonolucency. Almost half of the placenta can be infarcted and its function remain normal.

The shape of the placenta may also change as term is approached. Focal bulging of the myometrium may be seen secondary to mild uterine contractions (Braxton-Hicks) and/or areas of unsoftened portion of the uterus. An "unsoftened" portion of the uterus is thought to represent the portion of the myometrium that is yet to be stretched (21, 22). A thickened portion of the uterus may have an appearance similiar to that of the placenta, although it is usually more echogenic than the myometrium (21).

Amniotic Fluid

Because an excessive or diminished amount of amniotic fluid may be a clue to suggest certain anatomical or functional anomalies of the fetus, the amount of amniotic fluid should be subjectively assessed in each pregnancy. The amount of amniotic fluid gradually increases during pregnancy, usually reaching a peak in the late third trimester. In general, the amniotic fluid should be no more than the volume occupied by the fetus and placenta. Hydramnios can also be detected by indirect signs, such as excessive thinning of the placenta. Other investigators calculate the amount of amniotic fluid by subtracting the volume occupied by the fetus and placenta from the total intrauterine volume. Standards for enlargement of the total intrauterine volume have been established by various methods (2).

At the other end of the spectrum, diminished amounts of amniotic fluid can be encountered in patients with premature rupture of membranes, fetal demise, or renal agenesis. In these cases, the fetus occupies the majority of the intrauterine volume and only small amounts of amniotic fluid can be identified. Amniocentesis may be difficult to perform in these patients because of the small amount of amniotic fluid.

Fetal Structures

In the third trimester of pregnancy, some of the major abdominal organs of the fetus can be delineated (Figs. 2-5A, B, C, D). Structures that are commonly delineated in the mature fetus include the urine-filled bladder, fluid-filled bowel,

Figure 2-5. NORMAL FETAL STRUCTURES

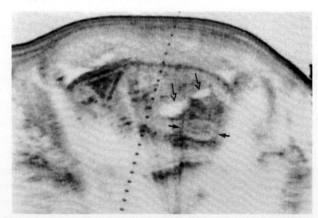

Figure 2-5A. Fetal bowel and kidney (longitudinal, midline). Since the fetus swallows amniotic fluid in utero, several of the larger segments of the fetal gastrointestinal tract, such as the stomach (*open arrows*), appear as tubular sonolucent structures. Peristaltic movement of the bowel can be demonstrated using real-time scanning. The fetal kidney is also delineated as an elliptical structure with a central echogenic interface corresponding to the renal pelvis (*solid arrows*). (Courtesy of Karen Parker, R.D.M.S., and Clifton Greer, M.D., Baptist Hospital, Nashville, Tenn.)

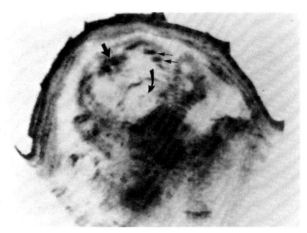

Figure 2-5B. Fetal thoracic structures (modified transverse, through fetal thorax). The vertebral body (*large arrow*) and ribs (*small arrows*) can be delineated. The fetal heart appears as a rounded, sonolucent structure (*curved arrow*) located anterior in the thorax surrounded by sonolucent, fluid-filled lungs.

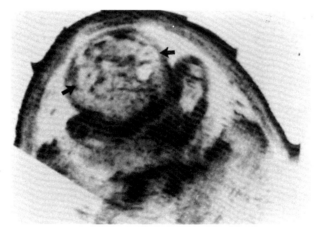

Figure 2-5C. Fetal kidneys (modified transverse, through upper abdomen of fetus). The kidneys appear as sonolucent, rounded structures that contain a central echogenic interface (*arrows*). The cystic structure anterior to the left kidney is probably the fluid-filled stomach.

heart, and kidneys. Since the fetus swallows amniotic fluid in utero, the fetal bowel appears as tubular sonolucent structures that change their configuration with peristalsis (41). Similarly, since the fetus excretes urine into the bladder from the kidneys, this structure appears as a sonolucent mass in the fetal pelvis. The external genitalia of male fetuses appear as localized convexity or outpouching from the perineum when the fetal pelvis is delineated in transverse section (Fig. 2-5D). The configuration of the scrotum can be simulated by edematous labia in a female fetus.

Real-time sonography has allowed greater visualization of the intracranial structures of the fetus. The lateral ventricles appear as slit-like intracranial struc-

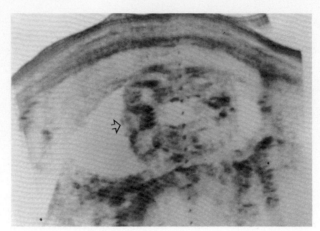

Figure 2-5D. Fetal scrotum (modified transverse, through fetal perineum). The urine-filled bladder is represented by the sonolucent structure in the fetal pelvis. The fetal scrotum appears as localized soft tissue protuberance between the legs (*open arrow*).

tures that have a characteristic configuration. The body of the lateral ventricles should measure no more than 1.2 cm, and the ratio of the hemispheric thickness to ventricular dimensions normally ranges between 0.25 to 0.34 (36).

ESTIMATION OF GESTATION DURATION

As stated previously in this chapter, sonography is a very useful modality for estimating the gestational age of a pregnancy beginning at four to five weeks' menstrual age and up to the time of delivery. Menstrual age refers to the number of weeks that have elapsed since the first day of the last menstrual period and is used synonomously with the gestational age (46). Different parameters can be employed to estimate the gestational age during the various stages of pregnancy.

Gestational Sac Size

In the first trimester, the average of the three diameters of the gestational sac can be used as a measure of gestation duration (Table 2-2). It is emphasized that estimation of the gestation duration by measurement of the gestational sac has inherently a two-week standard deviation. Averaging the three diameters of the gestational sac is preferred to using only one diameter, since the gestational sac may be flattened by an overdistended bladder (5) (Fig. 2-2B).

Crown-Rump Measurements

From 8 to 11 weeks, gestational age can be estimated from measurements of the crown-rump length of the fetus, as previously noted (Table 2-2). For estimation of the gestational age by the crown-rump length, one must obtain an image that depicts the entire length of the fetus (7) (Fig. 2-2E). The standard deviation for estimation of gestation duration by crown-rump length is estimated to be ± 1 to 4 days. Measurement of the crown-rump length can be expedited by real-time scanning.

Biparietal Diameter

After 12 to 13 weeks, the gestational duration can be accurately assessed by the biparietal diameter (BPD). Since the fetal head can be imaged readily, correlation between BPD and fetal age has been extensively documented. Estimation of gestation duration from the 13th to 15th week to term is reliable and accurate (8, 9) (Table 2-3). Beginning at 11 to 13 weeks, the fetal head can be recognized as an ovoid structure with a central linear interface in the middle representing the falx cerebri (Fig. 2-6A,B). Because enlargement of the fetal head past 32 weeks is nonlinear and associated with a greater standard deviation than in the second trimester, estimation of gestation duration by biparietal diameter measurements is most accurate when obtained at the midpoint of the second trimester. In the second trimester of pregnancy, the biparietal diameter enlarges at a rate of approximately 2 to 3 mm per week. The standard deviation of the biparietal diameter measurement after 32 weeks increases to about two weeks, whereas during the second trimester of pregnancy, it is approximately ± 1 week. It has been shown that the most accurate assessment of gestation duration is based on two or more measurements of the biparietal diameter, one at midpoint in the second trimester and one at midpoint in the third trimester (9). The growth of the BPD can be correlated with the weeks elapsed between examinations.

Figure 2-6. FETAL HEAD GROWTH

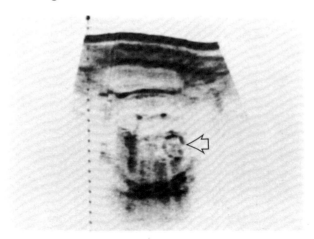

Figure 2-6A. Biparietal diameter at 12 weeks (transverse, 4 cm above symphysis pubis). The fetal head appears as a rounded structure (*open arrow*). The biparietal diameter is approximately 2 cm, which corresponds to a 12-week pregnancy. This is for practical purposes the earliest stage of pregnancy in which the biparietal diameter can be delineated with present instrumentation.

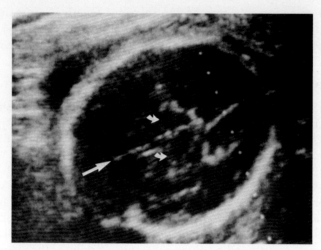

Figure 2-6B. Biparietal diameter at 34 weeks (longitudinal, midline). The fetus is in a transverse lie. The biparietal diameter of the fetus is approximately 8.3 cm, which corresponds to 34 weeks, ± 1 week. The falx cerebri appears as a central linear echogenic interface (*large arrow*) that is symmetrical with the outer tables of the skull. The thalami appear as almond-shaped structures to either side of the falx (*small arrows*). Measurements of the biparietal diameter should be determined only on those images in which the falx cerebri is symmetrical with the outer tables of the skull. Whether or not the outer tables are symmetrical with the falx can be determined by measuring with a caliper the distance from the falx to the outer table on one side and comparing it to the distance on the other side. The biparietal diameter is estimated by the distance between points taken at the center of the echogenic interfaces representing the fetal cranium.

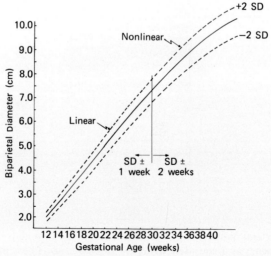

Figure 2-6C. Growth of the biparietal diameter. Enlargement of the BPD from 20 to 32 weeks is linear, with a standard deviation of one week. From approximately 32 weeks to term, the enlargement of the BPD is nonlinear and has a two-week standard deviation.

EVALUATION OF FETAL GROWTH

Sonography can be used in the assessment of the anatomic growth and maturation of the developing fetus. Fetal growth can be assessed by the increments of fetal weight and BPD and total intrauterine volume (TIUV) (2). Charts similar to that used for documentation of growth of neonates have been established for documentation of growth parameters in utero (14). A measurement of the BPD and/or fetal weight that falls below two standard deviations of the established growth curve is suggestive of intrauterine growth retardation (IUGR). In some patients, when the fetus has symmetrically retarded growth, a marked discrepancy between dates and fetal size is suggestive of intrauterine growth retardation.

In the early first trimester of pregnancy, fetal growth can be assessed by following the progression of the embryonic pole into a fusiform structure representing the developing fetus. The assessment of fetal growth assumes greater clinical importance in the second trimester, when IUGR is usually first suspected. Although the gestation duration is readily estimated by biparietal diameter, growth of the fetal head usually is not affected by intrauterine growth retardation. Fetal growth is best evaluated by serial assessment of the TIUV during the second and third trimesters.

Table 2-4. Fetal Weight as Estimated by Abdominal Circumference[a]

Abdominal Circumference (cm)	Estimated Fetal Weight (kg)
21	0.90
22	1.03
23	1.18
24	1.34
25	1.51
26	1.64
27	1.88
28	2.09
29	2.28
30	2.49
31	2.69
32	2.90
33	3.10
34	3.29
35	3.47
36	3.64
37	3.79
38	3.92
39	4.02
40	4.10

[a]Figures shown only for 50th percentile. Adapted from Sabbagha, Hughey, and Depp (9).

Fetal weight should be calculated from measurements of the fetal abdominal circumference at the level of the umbilical vein (Fig. 2-4B) (Table 2-4). The accuracy of the estimation of fetal weight by the abdominal circumference depends on the size of the fetus. For example, when the fetus weighs approximately 1 kg, the standard deviation is ± 100 gm, and when the fetus weighs 4 to 5 kg, the standard deviation is approximately 500 gm (13).

DETECTION OF MULTIPLE GESTATION

Ultrasound studies are effectively used to detect multiple gestations beginning at approximately four to six weeks' menstrual age up to term (Figs. 2-7A,B). Usually, patients in whom a multiple gestation is suspected are seen in the second trimester with a uterus too-large-for-dates. Occasionally, the patient will have a history of multiple gestations.

In some cases, more than one gestational sac will be seen early in pregnancy, but only a singleton fetus will be delivered. This is thought to be the result of subclinical abortion of one of the sacs, with retention of the other (32).

As pregnancy progresses, multiple gestations can be detected by delineating more than one fetus within the uterus (Figs. 2-7C,D). Occasionally, separate amniotic cavities can be identified by a linear echogenic interface in the center of the amniotic cavity representing the two amniotic membranes. Multiple gestations may be first suspected on a sonographic study when more than one gestational sac is delineated within the uterus. The two fetal bodies usually can be detected if one delineates their boundaries and graphically maps them on paper as a composite of the points seen on individual scans. It is often difficult to obtain a scan that demonstrates both fetal heads on the same image (47) (sometimes this is stated as being necessary to establish the diagnosis of multiple

Figure 2-7. MULTIPLE GESTATION

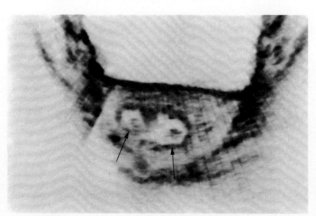

Figure 2-7A. Twin pregnancy at approximately six weeks (transverse, 2 cm above symphysis pubis). Two gestational sacs that contain embryonic poles can be delineated (*arrows*). Even though two gestational sacs are delineated in the early stages of pregnancy, it is not uncommon for this type of pregnancy to result in delivery of a single fetus. This is thought to occur as the result of spontaneous regression or abortion of one of the gestational sacs.

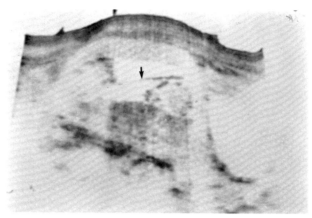

Figure 2-7B. Twin gestation at 12 weeks (longitudinal, midline). Two amniotic sacs that are separated by a common membrane (*arrow*) can be identified. Two separate placentas are delineated, as well as two fetal bodies. This implies a biovular twin pregnancy.

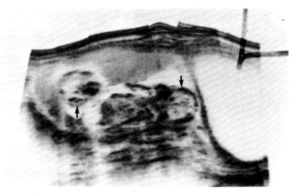

Figure 2-7C. Twin gestation at 20 weeks (longitudinal, midline). Two fetal heads can be identified (*arrows*). The fetal positions in the lower uterine segment can be delineated from crown to rump. The other fetus is in a breech presentation.

gestation). Generally, in either a singleton or multiple gestation, it is prudent to map out the location of the fetus or fetuses within the uterus so that more than one fetal body and their presentation can be indentified. Most commonly, the two fetuses in a multiple gestation will lie in a cephalic and breech presentation, although a double vertex presentation is also common. Biparietal diameters of twin gestations are slightly less than normal for singleton pregnancies. Therefore, 1 to 2 mm should be added to the BPD of a twin if a BPD chart for singleton gestation is used. A discrepancy of fetal heads greater than 4 mm suggests retardation of growth of one of the fetuses from any cause (33).

EVALUATION OF PATIENTS WITH FIRST TRIMESTER BLEEDING

When a patient presents with uterine bleeding in the first trimester of pregnancy, one must consider several diagnostic possibilities. In the majority of cases, the

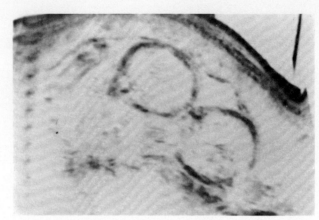

Figure 2-7D. Twin gestation at approximately 31 weeks (longitudinal, midline). Two fetal heads are delineated, both in a cephalic presentation. The biparietal diameters are within 1 mm of each other, measuring approximately 7.5 cm. Since the biparietal diameters of twins are slightly smaller than those of a single fetus, 1 to 2 mm should be added to a BPD determination of a twin if the standard BPD chart for single pregnancies is used. The biparietal diameters of twin fetuses should be within 4 mm of each other. Otherwise, growth of one of the fetuses may be retarded.

sonographic features of those entities that are associated with first trimester bleeding are distinctive enough for them to be differentiated on the basis of their appearance.

Abortion

Threatened or incomplete abortions are identified on ultrasound studies by the finding of a markedly distorted and irregular gestational sac in a uterus that is minimally enlarged. When compared to a normal gestational sac in an uncomplicated intrauterine pregnancy, the embryonic pole in patients with abortion is usually ill-defined and irregular in shape. In addition, the distorted gestational sac may be located lower than normal in the region of the lower uterine segment (Fig. 2-8B).

An excessive amount of uterine bleeding during the first trimester usually implies that progression of the pregnancy is threatened. In some cases, development of the embryonic pole is terminated, resulting in a "blighted ovum." In this condition, embryonic membranes and amniotic sac may continue to develop, although the embryonic development has ceased. The usual sonographic appearance of a blighted ovum is of a fluid-filled amniotic cavity without evidence of a normally developed embryonic pole. Usually, only a small soft tissue projection into the gestational sac representing the remaining portions of the embryonic pole can be identified (Fig. 2-8A).

Terminated development that occurs later in the first trimester is associated with uterine bleeding. This event is described as an "abortion." Incomplete abortion refers to partial expulsion of the products of conception from the uterus. Sonographically, this condition appears as a distorted, irregular gestational sac in which the fetal pole and placental structures are indistinct. Hemorrhage and blood may be seen within the uterine lumen as sonolucent areas (Fig. 2-8B).

Missed abortion implies that the patient has experienced uterine bleeding without passage of products of conception. Portions of the fetus and embryonic membranes are still within the uterus (Fig. 2-8C). As is seen with cases of incomplete abortion, missed abortions are visualized as irregular, distorted intrauterine contents. In both cases of abortion, the uterus is smaller than expected by dates. Serial examination of these patients often shows lack of development of chorionic tissue or embryonic development (30).

Figure 2-8. ABORTION

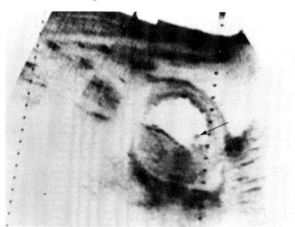

Figure 2-8A. Blighted ovum (longitudinal, midline). Only a small residium of tissue remains in the region of the embryonic pole (*arrow*). The amniotic cavity has developed normally, and there is a marked discrepancy between the size of the amniotic cavity and the size of the embryonic pole, indicating the presence of a blighted ovum.

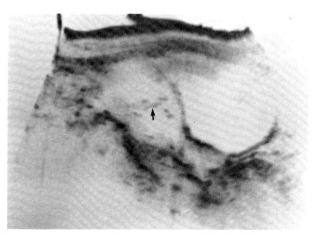

Figure 2-8B. Incomplete abortion (longitudinal, midline). Within the uterus, there is a distorted gestational sac that contains irregular internal contents representing retained products of conception (*arrow*).

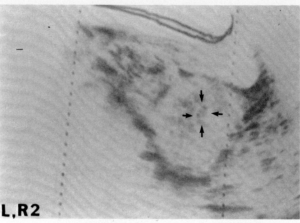

L,R2

Figure 2-8C. Missed abortion (longitudinal, 2 cm to right of midline). This patient experienced vaginal bleeding with incomplete passage of products of conception. Bleeding occurred one month prior to her ultrasound examination. Within the uterus, there is a distorted gestational sac (*arrows*). This appearance is not unlike that seen in early molar pregnancy.

Molar Gestation

Another common cause of first trimester uterine bleeding is a hydatidiform mole or molar pregnancy. Clinically, patients with this condition present in the first trimester with excessive uterine bleeding and occasionally with severe preeclampsia. The uterus in patients with a molar gestation is usually too-large-for-dates if the major portion of the molar tissue has not been expelled at time of presentation (Fig. 2-9A). Theca lutein cysts are present in approximately one-third of patients with hydatidiform moles and can be recognized sonographically as multilocular, bilateral cystic adnexal masses (31). These cysts often achieve their largest diameters when HCG production is greatest, between 12 and 22 weeks, and usually regress after removal of molar tissue (Fig. 2-9E).

The sonographic features of a molar pregnancy are often diagnostic (Figs. 2-9A,B). Numerous echoes of small, rounded vesicular tissue and/or an echo texture similar to that of a hydropic placenta are seen. The vesicular texture of the intrauterine contents emanates from the numerous hydropic chorionic villi that are characteristic of molar tissue.

Prior to the introduction of gray scale scanning, hydatidiform moles were noted to exhibit a "snowstorm" texture when scanned in high-gain and high-output settings. However, with the use of gray scale sonography, fine internal detail within these masses such as may be emanating from areas of internal hemorrhagic degeneration and products of conception that occasionally coexist with a mole can be delineated (Fig. 2-9G). The hemorrhagic degeneration that frequently occurs within these masses can be recognized as irregular areas of sonolucency within the mass (Table 2-5).

One should be aware that approximately 2% of molar gestations have an accompanying fetus and/or gestational sac. It is important to recognize this sonographically since patients with coexistent fetuses may be managed differ-

Figure 2-9. TROPHOBLASTIC DISEASE

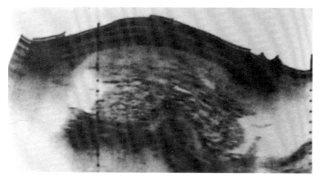

Figure 2-9A. Hydatidiform mole (longitudinal, midline). The uterus is enlarged and contains tissue that has a vesicular texture. This pattern originates from the numerous hydropic villi. There are sonolucent areas in the region of the uterine fundus that probably represent a residual portion of the fluid-filled amniotic cavity that has not been completely occupied by molar tissue.

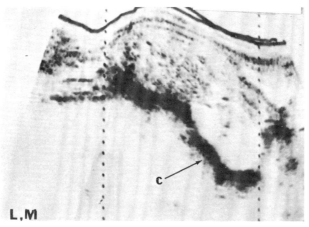

Figure 2-9B. Hydatidiform mole with theca lutein cyst (longitudinal, midline). Besides the enlarged uterus that contains tissue of a vesicular texture, a multiloculated cyst (c) is present. The cyst represents a theca lutein cyst. Such cysts are frequently bilateral and multiloculated, and are associated with hydatidiform moles in one-third of patients with a molar pregnancy.

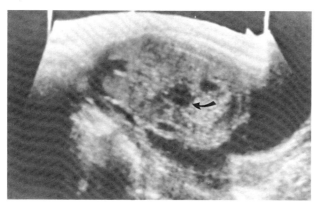

Figure 2-9C. Hydatidiform mole with internal hemorrhagic degeneration (longitudinal, midline; white-on-black image). This sonogram reveals sonolucent areas in the mole due to areas of internal hemorrhagic degeneration (*arrow*). Such areas are commonly encountered within large molar masses.

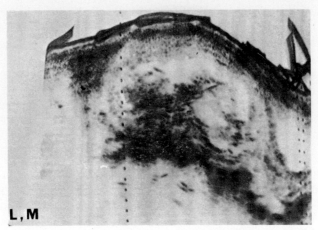

Figure 2-9D. Hydatidiform mole with marked internal degeneration (longitudinal, midline). This mole contains irregular areas of cystic and solid tissue and was distinguished from an intrauterine pregnancy because the internal contents did not simulate fetal parts or a placenta.

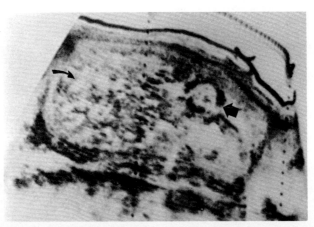

Figure 2-9E. Hydatidiform mole with coexistent 16-week fetus (longitudinal, 2 cm to left of midline). Vesicular intrauterine tissue is present (*curved arrow*) representing hydatidiform mole. A 16-week fetus is demonstrated by the ovoid structure representing the fetal head (*large arrow*). Approximately 2% of women with hydatidiform moles will have a coexistent fetus. This condition is important to recognize sonographically since these patients may be managed differently from those without a coexisting fetus.

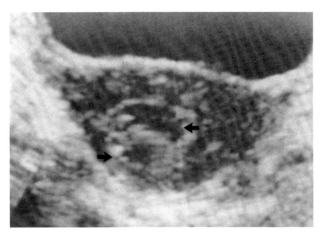

Figure 2-9F. Retained molar tissue after spontaneous expulsion (magnified view, transverse, 5 cm above symphysis pubis, white-on-black image). Within the uterus, there are rounded, sonolucent masses of various sizes representing retained molar tissue (*arrows*). This patient experienced spontaneous expulsion of a hydatidiform mole and presented with elevated levels of human chorionic gonadatropin (HCG). The clinical considerations included an early intrauterine pregnancy or retained molar tissue. The sonogram suggested the presence of retained molar tissue, indicating the need for dilatation and curettage of the uterine contents.

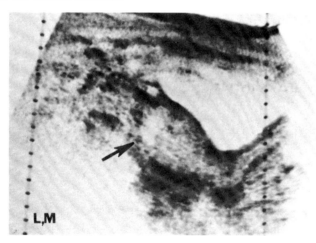

Figure 2-9G. Locally invasive recurrent trophoblastic disease (longitudinal, midline). This patient presented two months after suction curettage of molar tissue from the uterus. She had elevated HCG levels and a persistently enlarged right adnexal mass. Within the uterus, there is a sonolucent, irregular area in the region of the uterine fundus representing the infiltrative tumor and resultant hemorrhagic necrosis of the myometrium (*arrow*).

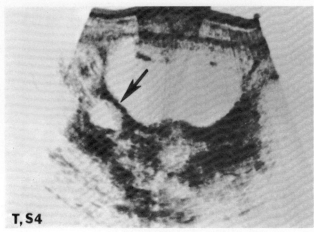

T, S4

Figure 2-9H. Persistently enlarged theca lutein cyst (transverse view, 4 cm above symphysis pubis). Same patient as in Figure 2-9G showing persistently enlarged right cystic adnexal mass representing theca lutein cyst (*arrow*). Theca lutein cysts are seen in approximately one-third of patients with benign hydatidiform mole. These cysts usually regress after adequate therapy. When they fail to regress after expulsion of a hydatidiform mole, recurrent or invasive trophoblastic disease should be considered.

ently. Distorted gestational sacs that occur with hydatidiform moles can be differentiated from areas of internal hemorrhagic degeneration, for well-formed gestational sacs will show evidence of decidual reaction and a well-defined embryonic pole. Conversely, areas of irregular internal hemorrhagic degeneration can be detected as irregular sonolucent areas without evidence of a well-defined embryonic structure (Fig. 2-9B). If the fetus is 10 weeks old or more, the fetal structures can be identified and distinguished from areas of irregular internal hemorrhagic degeneration (Fig. 2-9C).

Table 2-5. Differential Features of Hydatidiform Mole

Hydatidiform mole	Vesicular pattern of intrauterine contents
	Uterus too-large-for-dates
	One-third of cases associated with bilateral theca lutein cysts
	Approximately 2% associated with coexistent fetus
Incomplete or missed abortion	Uterine size only minimally enlarged
	Distorted outline of gestational sac
	If pregnancy test negative, helpful to include in differential diagnosis
Degenerated uterine leiomyoma	Nonhomogeneous, echogenic mass causing nodular enlargement of uterine outline

The sonographic features of invasive trophoblastic disease are much more subtle than those of hydatidiform moles. In most cases in which invasive trophoblastic disease is suspected, sonography can only be confirmatory of the clinical and laboratory findings (Fig. 2-9E) (31). However, ultrasound studies can be helpful in identifying residual molar tissue after a dilatation and curettage has been performed or spontaneous expulsion of molar products has occurred (Fig. 2-9D). Sonographic signs of invasive trophoblastic disease include irregular sonolucent areas within the myometrium that are surrounded by high-level echoes indicating hemorrhagic necrosis and invasion of the myometrium (Fig. 2-9G). Besides the laboratory findings of persistently elevated HCG levels, residual chorionic tissue function can be documented by sonographic evidence of persistently enlarged theca lutein cysts (Fig. 2-9F).

The malignant variety of invasive trophoblastic disease or choriocarcinoma can disseminate rapidly and on ultrasound may not reveal demonstrable textural abnormality of the uterus. This is illustrated by the patient seen in Figures 2-9I,J, who presented with a right hemiparesis secondary to frontal lobe metastatic lesions, delineated by computerized tomography. The overall texture of this patient's uterus was not distinctly abnormal.

Ectopic Pregnancy

Greater experience in using ultrasound to evaluate patients suspected of having an ectopic pregnancy has made it possible to establish the diagnostic value of the various sonographic features of this condition (24–28). More importantly, sonography can be helpful in the exclusion of an intrauterine pregnancy in a patient suspected of having an ectopic pregnancy.

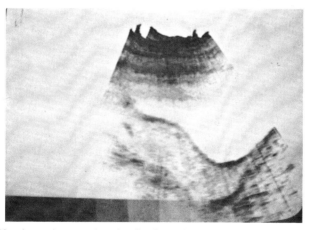

Figure 2-9I. Choriocarcinoma (longitudinal, midline). This patient presented with a right hemiparesis. The uterine texture appeared normal, although there was evidence of metastatic disease to the frontal lobes demonstrated by computerized tomography (CT). Although dissemination to other organs of the body may be already evident, invasive trophoblastic disease can produce only very subtly changes in the sonographic texture of the uterus.

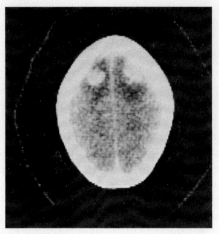

Figure 2-9J. Metastases from choriocarcinoma. This CT scan of the patient in Figure 2-9I reveals evidence of two frontal metastases from a choriocarcinoma.

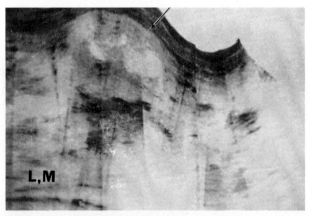

Figure 2-9K. Choriocarcinoma (longitudinal, midline). The uterus is markedly enlarged and shows sonolucent areas representing hemorrhagic degeneration (*arrow*). This patient had choriocarcinoma that revealed extensive necrosis of the myometrium. (Courtesy of Barry Goldberg, M.D.)

   Clinically, patients with ectopic pregnancies commonly present with a palpable adnexal mass, uterine bleeding, and lower abdominal pain. By using a specific laboratory test for establishing pregnancy, namely the beta-subunit of HCG, the presence of functioning chorionic tissue can be established. Because the sonographic features of ectopic pregnancy and tubo-ovarian abscess and other adnexal masses may be quite similar, one should be aware of the results of the pregnancy and beta-subunit tests before offering a diagnosis. The diagnosis of ruptured ectopic pregnancy can be inferred if unclotted blood is aspirated from the cul-de-sac. However, if blood is clotted, this may result in a negative culdocentesis, leading to the false impression of an absence of an ectopic pregnancy.
   Since the muscular layer of the oviduct becomes overdistended by the enlarging gestational sac, there is separation of the chorionic tissue from the muscular

layer, usually with resultant hemorrhage. When this occurs, the bleeding will usually be extensive enough to threaten the life of the developing embryo. Abortion of the embryo and products of conception into the uterus or more commonly out into the peritoneal cavity can occur. Most frequently, the oviduct itself ruptures, which results in intraperitoneal bleeding and cul-de-sac hematoma.

The various sonographic findings that can be observed in patients with an ectopic pregnancy are listed in Table 2-6 and illustrated in Figures 2-10A–J. They are categorized into those that are "diagnostic" and those that are "suggestive." The term "suggestive" refers to findings that are not diagnostically specific for an ectopic pregnancy by themselves but can, in combination with other findings, make the presence of an ectopic pregnancy likely. Usually more than one of the sonographic features is commonly observed in patients with an ectopic pregnancy. In general, the greater the number of sonographic findings that are diagnostic or suggestive of an ectopic pregnancy, the more reliable the diagnosis. The differential diagnosis is given in Table 2-7.

Since the false-negative rate of diagnosis of ectopic pregnancy (approximately 10%) is high, one should consider this entity in any patient of reproductive age who presents with a compatible history, positive pregnancy test (beta-subunit), and a palpable adnexal mass that suggests the presence of an ectopic pregnancy. Although ultrasound examination of ectopic pregnancy may fail to demonstrate any abnormal findings, this study is very important, since it can be used to exclude

Table 2-6. Sonographic Signs of Ectopic Pregnancy

	Unruptured	Ruptured
Diagnostic signs	1. Absence of intrauterine gestational sac 2. Complex adnexal mass representing extrauterine gestational sac or products of conception 3. Fetal motion by real-time scanning, or fetal heart tones by Doppler examination, or fetal parts emanating from extrauterine gestational sac	1. Absence of intrauterine gestational sac 2. Mixed or echogenic mass representing ruptured gestational sac and cul-de-sac hematoma 3. Fluid or organized clot in cul-de-sac
Suggestive features	4. "Enlarged" uterus with decidual proliferation	4. Free intraperitoneal fluid 5. "Enlarged" uterus with decidual proliferation 6. Deviation of uterus by complex adnexal mass

Table 2-7. Differential Diagnosis of Ectopic Pregnancy

Common	Symptoms similar to ectopic pregnancy
Hemorrhagic corpus luteum cyst (follicular and paraovarian)	May appear as echogenic if contains organized clot
	Usually sonolucent once liquefaction of clot occurs
Dermoid cyst	Usually complex, predominantly cystic mass with focus of high-level echoes corresponding to sebum and/or calcified contents
Hydro(pyo) salpinx, Tubo-ovarian abscess	Usually complex mass
	Pus and cellular debris may layer; mobile fluid-fluid layer
Uncommon	
Cystadenoma	Serous variety usually cystic; mucinous, multiloculated
Fluid-filled bowel	Tubular structure with peristaltic movement; occasionally valvulae conniventes, haustra can be seen
	Configuration change with repeat scan
Degenerated or pedunculated uterine leiomyoma	Attachment to uterus can be visualized
Endometrioma	Usually appears as multiple cystic, or mildly echogenic mass of various sizes if contains clot
	Associated with infertility
Rare	
Bicornate uterus, gravid in one horn	Nongravid horn contiguous with uterus
Solid ovarian adenocarcinoma	Complex, predominately solid pelvic mass
Intrauterine pregnancy with ectopic pregnancy	Rare (1:30,000 pregnancies)
	Increased incidence in patients taking ovulation stimulatory drugs

an intrauterine pregnancy. When the evaluation of a patient with a suspected ectopic pregnancy reveals no sonographic abnormality, the clinician should not be dissuaded from further diagnostic evaluation such as by laparoscopy. When ectopic pregnancy is demonstrated on ultrasound, one can, without delay, take steps to establish the diagnosis and proceed with treatment.

The sonographic appearance of an ectopic pregnancy depends on whether it is unruptured or whether rupture and intraperitoneal bleeding have occurred

(Fig. 2-10A–H). The most common finding in patients with ectopic pregnancy is a complex adnexal mass. The sonographer should establish that the mass is outside the uterus by performing scans that may be oblique to the transverse or longitudinal plane.

Rarely in an unruptured pregnancy, a viable fetus within an extrauterine gestational sac can be delineated. Instead, a sonographically complex tubular

Figure 2-10. ECTOPIC PREGNANCY

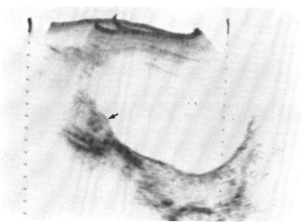

Figure 2-10A. Unruptured ectopic pregnancy (longitudinal, midline). The uterus is devoid of a gestational sac. There is a rounded, complex mass superior to the uterus (*arrow*) that probably represents the developing gestational sac and thickened muscular layers of the oviduct.

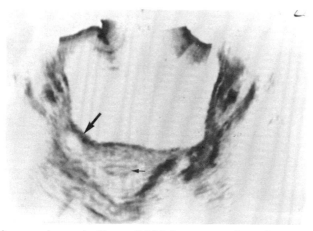

Figure 2-10B. Same patient as in Figure 2-10A (transverse, 2 cm above symphysis pubis). The endometrial lining appears echogenic (*small arrow*), and there is evidence of a small right, predominantly cystic adnexal mass that represented a corpus luteum cyst within the right ovary (*large arrow*). At surgery, this patient was found to have an unruptured left tubal ectopic pregnancy. This scan emphasizes that there may only be very subtle sonographic findings in an unruptured ectopic pregnancy. In this patient there was only endometrial thickening and suggestion of a small, complex left adnexal mass.

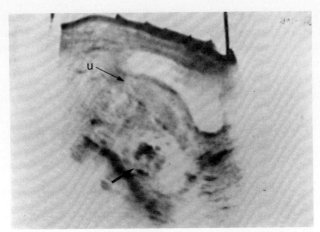

Figure 2-10C. Ruptured ectopic pregnancy (longitudinal, midline). This patient presented with a history of one-month amenorrhea and what was thought to represent a retroflexed uterus. On the sonogram, the uterus (u) is displaced anteriorly by a complex mass in the region of the cul-de-sac (*large arrow*).

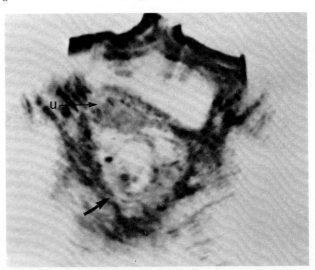

Figure 2-10D. Same patient as in Figure 2-10C (transverse, 4 cm above symphysis pubis). A rounded, complex mass, predominantly cystic, is seen in the cul-de-sac (*arrow*) which is surrounded by an echogenic collection representing clotted blood. The uterus (u) is displaced anteriorly by the mass, and no evidence of an intrauterine gestational sac is seen. This patient was found to have a ruptured ectopic tubal pregnancy that was surrounded by clotted blood.

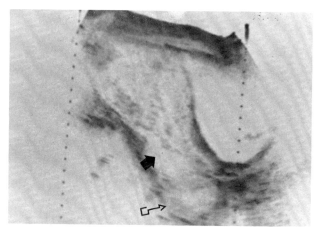

Figure 2-10E. Ruptured ectopic pregnancy with hemoperitoneum (longitudinal, mid-line). This patient presented with a six-hour history of acute lower abdominal pain, vaginal bleeding, and hypotension. A culdocentesis was performed and failed to detect any free blood in the cul-de-sac. The sonograms reveal a sonolucent collection (*solid arrow*) posterior to what appears to be the uterus, as well as an ill-defined, echogenic mass in the cul-de-sac (*open arrow*). The echogenic mass in the cul-de-sac was found to represent clotted blood from a ruptured ectopic pregnancy.

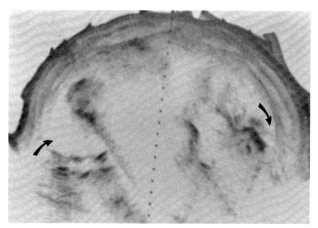

Figure 2-10F. Same patient as in Figure 2-10E (transverse view, 6 cm below xiphoid). This abdominal sonogram reveals sonolucent areas in the paracolic recesses representing free blood in the peritoneal cavity (*curved arrows*). This patient was found to have 2 liters of unclotted blood resulting from a ruptured ectopic pregnancy.

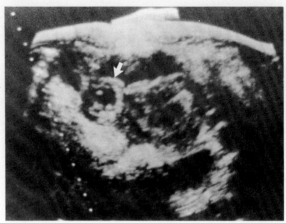

Figure 2-10G. Interstitial ectopic pregnancy (transverse, 4 cm above symphysis pubis). There is a gestational sac within the uterine outline (*white arrow*). However, the markedly eccentric location of the gestational sac within the uterus suggests the presence of an interstitial ectopic pregnancy. When rupture occurs, massive bleeding can ensue because of its proximity to the larger uterine vessels. (Courtesy of Thomas Lawson, M.D., Medical College of Wisconsin, Milwaukee, Wisc.)

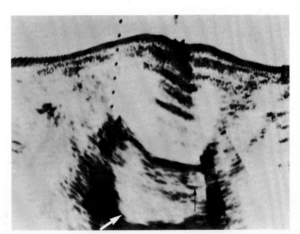

Figure 2-10H. Ovarian ectopic pregnancy (transverse, 6 cm above symphysis pubis). The ill-defined, rounded left adnexal mass was found to represent an ectopic pregnancy within the left ovary (*black arrow*). The sonographic appearance of this rare type of ectopic pregnancy is indistinguishable from that of ectopic tubal pregnancy. Unclotted blood within the cul-de-sac (*white arrow*) was also seen resulting from ovarian rupture by the ectopic pregnancy. (Courtesy of Thomas Lawson, M.D., Medical College of Wisconsin, Milwaukee, Wisc.)

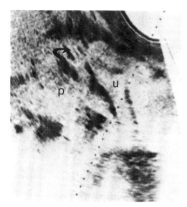

Figure 2-10I. Abdominal ectopic pregnancy (longitudinal, 4 cm to right of midline). A fetus (*curved arrow*) and placenta (p) are delineated separate from the uterus (u). This rare type of ectopic pregnancy probably occurred as the result of abortion of the fetus and products of conception into the abdomen and subsequent reestablishment of blood supply from the mesentery or omentum. The fetus and products of conception must be identified outside the uterus in order to suggest the diagnosis of an abdominal ectopic pregnancy. (Courtesy of Roger Sanders, M.D., Johns Hopkins University, Baltimore, Md.)

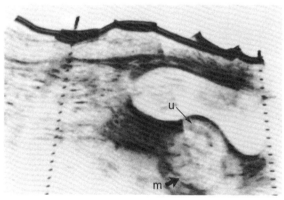

Figure 2-10J. Chronic ectopic pregnancy (longitudinal, midline). This patient was evaluated for sporadic fever, intermittent lower abdominal pain, and a palpable pelvic mass. The sonogram reveals an ill-defined, echogenic mass (m) displacing the uterus (u) anteriorly. This was found to represent hematoma from a ruptured ectopic pregnancy. Hematomas adjacent to the uterus may result in the "indefinite uterus sign". This is a term used to denote apparent enlargement of the uterine outline by masses that are adjacent to the uterus and have a similar echo pattern. Also, no interface between the mass and the uterus can be demonstrated. In this case, the hematoma was the result of a ruptured ectopic pregnancy that occurred approximately six months prior to this examination.

adnexal mass consisting of a chorionic and amniotic cavity and fetal parts within a distended tube is frequently encountered (Figs. 2-10A,B). The circular muscular layers of the oviduct may result in an apparent rim around the gestational sac, giving a "pseudogestational sac" appearance (24). The hypertrophied endometrium may also reveal a "pseudointrauterine" appearance. However, in these cases, a well-defined embryonic pole cannot be delineated.

The sonographic features of a ruptured ectopic pregnancy consist of a complex adnexal mass that is frequently associated with sonographic signs of unclotted intraperitoneal blood or cul-de-sac hematoma. Unclotted intraperitoneal blood can be observed as sonolucent areas within the paracolic recesses (Figs. 2-10C, D). Clotted blood in the cul-de-sac usually appears as a sonolucent structure, depending on the amount of clot organization. Fresh unclotted blood is sonolucent, whereas organized clot appears echogenic. The uterus may be displaced to one side by the adnexal mass. In addition, hypertrophy of the endometrium can be observed secondary to the stimulatory effect of estrogen. Hypertrophied endometrium appears as thickening of the interfaces arising from the center of the uterus. The uterus in patients with ectopic pregnancy is also slightly enlarged.

If the embryo and chorionic tissue survive abortion into the abdomen and trophoblastic cells derive vascular nutrition by attaching to the omentum or mesentery, an abdominal ectopic pregnancy can result. In order to derive adequate blood supply, the chorionic tissue usually implants on the mesentery or omentum. If uncomplicated, an abdominal pregnancy can progress to term without producing symptoms and therefore may be unsuspected. Occasionally, only when difficulty in delivery occurs will the possibility of abdominal pregnancy be considered. In order to establish this diagnosis, the slightly enlarged uterus should be defined on ultrasound study as a separate structure from the fetus and placenta.

An unusual type of ectopic pregnancy that has serious implications is the interstitial ectopic pregnancy (Fig. 2-10G). In this rare type of ectopic pregnancy, the fertilized zygote implants in the interstitial portion of the oviduct. This part of the oviduct has the smallest caliber and is in close proximity to the large uterine vessels. An interstitial ectopic pregnancy can progress for three to four months without producing symptoms. However, when the tube reaches its maximal point of distension, rupture occurs with profuse bleeding from the large uterine vessels that are in the area of the interstitial part of the oviduct. Sonographically, an interstitial ectopic pregnancy can be recognized by the unusually eccentric location of the gestational sac within the cornu of the uterus (24). This is best demonstrated on transverse scans as a gestational sac that lies in an unusually asymmetrical location with respect to the uterus.

Chronic ectopic pregnancy may be difficult to detect both sonographically and clinically (Fig. 2-10J). Clinically, the patients often present with a history of sporadic fever together with a palpable pelvic mass. Since the echogenicity of hematomas in retrouterine areas may be similar to that of the uterus, the outline of the uterus may appear to be enlarged by the mass. This has been referred to as the "indefinite uterus sign" that is associated with diagnostic error in evaluation of pelvic masses (49). If one suspects a chronic ectopic pregnancy, the posterior aspect of the uterus should be completely delineated and one should try to demonstrate an interface between the uterus and any masses that may surround it. Although extremely rare, an intrauterine gestation can occur concomitantly with ectopic pregnancy. The incidence of this condition is estimated to be only 1 in 30,000 pregnancies (29). Patients who take fertility drugs may have an increased incidence of this condition.

EVALUATION OF PLACENTAL LOCATION AND TEXTURE

Ultrasound has an important role in the evaluation of placental location as well as in detecting morphological changes in its texture. Sonography has afforded visualization of the dynamics of placental development to an extent that has not been possible by any other imaging modality. This technique is of clinical importance particularly in patients who present with third trimester bleeding and in whom placenta previa is considered. For instance, sonography can also be used to establish the presence of placental abruption.

Placentation refers to the process of formation of the placenta into an organ that functions as a means for transferring maternal nutrients to the fetus. The placenta is formed by trophoblastic cells that implant within the endometrium. The earliest form of the placenta that can be recognized sonographically is the chorion frondosum. This structure appears as localized echogenic area along the periphery of the gestational sac. This localized thickening can often be delineated in gestational sacs of four to five weeks' menstrual age. In a normal pregnancy, localized thickening representing the chorion frondosum should be well defined and its contour smooth.

At 10 to 11 weeks, the placenta appears as a thickened band of echoes that covers the majority of the endometrial surface (Fig. 2-11A). Placental growth is greatest during the last portion of the first trimester and maximal during the second trimester. In late first and second trimesters, the placenta can cover the entire uterine surface. Conversely, the rate of uterine enlargement reaches a peak around the second and third trimesters. This results in differential growth

Figure 2-11. PLACENTAL POSITION

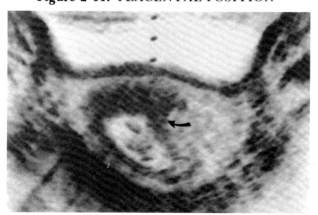

Figure 2-11A. Circumferential placenta at 10 weeks (transverse, 4 cm above symphysis pubis). The early placenta encompasses the entire endometrial surface and appears as a circumferential thickening at the periphery of the gestational sac (*curved arrow*).

rate in a gradual diminution of the proportion of the uterine surface that the placenta occupies (1).

With the advent of sonography, the dynamics of placentation have become apparent. As previously discussed, the term "placental migration" has been used to describe an apparent change in location of the placenta as pregnancy progresses (16). Although this term implies that the placenta changes its site of implantation during pregnancy, the placenta may appear to change its position, probably as a result of stretching of the lower uterine segment as term approaches. Arteriographic studies of the placenta do show small changes in the location of the placenta during pregnancy, and this may account for change in position of the placenta during the third trimester (18). As we have noted, this phenomenon has been referred to as "placental ascension," which is a descriptive term depicting movement of the placenta from the lower uterine segment as it elongates. The phenomenon of "placental migration" or "ascension" is clinically relevant in those patients who are scanned in the second trimester who appear to have low-lying placentae (Figs. 2-11B,C). Serial studies of the same patient usually reveal that the placenta moves away from the internal cervical os as term is approached. Therefore, if a patient appears to have a placenta previa or low-lying placenta on an examination performed in the second trimester, the examination should be repeated near term to exclude placenta previa. If significant bleeding occurs prior to the third trimester, the patient should be rescanned at any time significant bleeding occurs.

Profuse bleeding can occur as a result of separation of the placenta from the maternal myometrium when the uterus contracts in patients with placenta previa. This condition is important to recognize by diagnostic studies before labor ensues (Figs. 2-11D,E). Placenta previa generally refers to a condition in which the placenta is between the presenting part of the fetus and the internal cervical os. A partial placenta previa is said to exist when the placenta covers a portion of the internal cervical os. A complete placenta previa refers to a placenta that entirely covers the lower uterine segment and the internal cervical os.

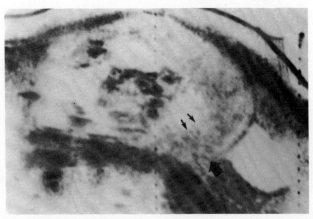

Figure 2-11B. Low-lying placenta during mid-second trimester (longtudinal, midline). This patient had not experienced vaginal bleeding prior to the examination. The placenta (*small arrows*) appears to extend to the region of the internal cervical os (*large arrow*).

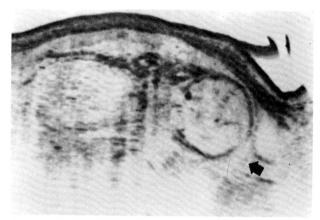

Figure 2-11C. Placental "ascension" (longitudinal, midline) in the same patient as seen in Figure 2-11B. A repeat sonogram obtained four weeks later shows that the placenta has ascended out of the lower uterine segment. The fetal head is now well within the lower uterine segment and in close proximity to the internal cervical os (*large arrow*). This apparent movement of the placenta as term is approached should not be considered abnormal. It most probably is due to differential growth of the lower uterine segment as the pregnancy approaches term.

Initial evaluation for placenta previa should include a series of scans performed with the patient's bladder full and then partially full. This is done in order to evaluate the lower uterine segment in various degrees of compression. Over-distension of the bladder may compress the lower uterine segment and placenta, resulting in a sonographic appearance of placenta previa. For this reason, patients with a possible placenta previa should also be scanned after voiding. The region of the cervical canal can be identified usually within 1 to 2 cm of midline on longitudinal scans as a thickened echogenic line which represents the mucus

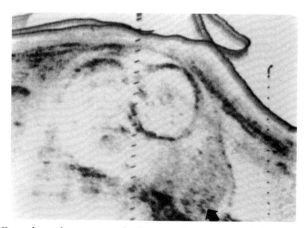

Figure 2-11D. Complete placenta previa (longitudinal, midline). The placenta covers the area of the internal cervical os (*arrow*) and lies between the internal cervical os and the fetal presenting part. The fetal head is elevated out of the lower uterine segment by the placenta previa.

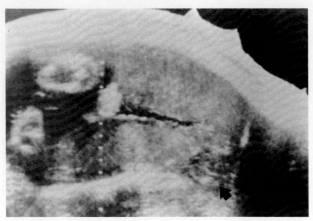

Figure 2-11E. Complete placenta previa (longitudinal, 2 cm to right of midlone; white-on-black image). The placenta covers the entire area of the cervical canal (*arrow*).

plug within the canal (Fig. 2-11B). The collapsed vagina can be delineated; it appears as three parallel lines immediately beneath the posterior aspect of the bladder. The cervical portion of the uterus is demonstrated as a tubular echogenic extension of the uterine outline which is continuous with the posterior fornix of the vagina (Fig. 2-11B).

Placenta previa on sonography appears as diffusely echogenic tissue that covers the internal cervical os. Areas of hemorrhage in the region of placental tears are depicted as areas of irregular sonolucency and disruption in the normally homogeneous texture of the placenta in this region.

Textural changes of the placenta that may reflect normal changes in maturation of the placenta, as well as changes in the texture of the placenta in a variety of disorders, are depicted by sonography (Figs. 2-12A,B,C,D). Certain structural changes in the placenta appear normally as the placenta approaches term. These

Figure 2-12. PLACENTAL TEXTURE

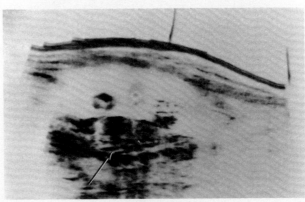

Figure 2-12A. Venous channels of the placenta (longitudinal, 6 cm to left of midline). There are tubular sonolucent structures along the posterior aspect of the placenta representing the venous lakes that drain the placenta (*arrow*).

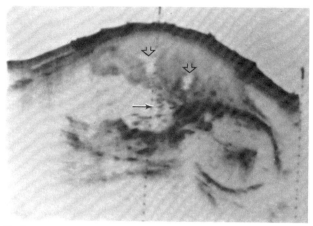

Figure 2-12B. Hydropic areas within the placenta (longitudinal, midline). This anterior placenta contains sonolucent areas within it representing areas of hydropic villi (*open arrows*). The number of villi in these areas is also diminished. This finding can be encountered in normal patients as the pregnancy approaches term. The umbilical cord (*closed arrow*) is depicted at its origin from the placenta.

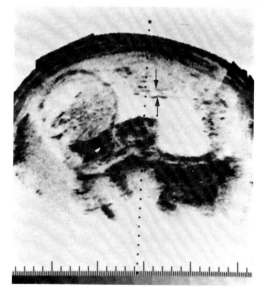

Figure 2-12C. Subchorionic fibrinoid collection (transverse, 10 cm above symphysis pubis). There is a sonolucent collection beneath the chorionic plate of the placenta representing subchorionic fibrinoid degeneration (*arrows*). This is thought to occur as a sequela to placental thrombosis. Since the placenta lacks the ability to form granulation tissue, collections of fibrinoid material can be found. The placenta has a large reserve diffusion capacity; therefore, this process does not appear to endanger the pregnancy.

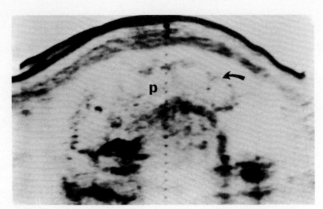

Figure 2-12D. Calcification of basal plate and septa (longitudinal, 2 cm to right of midline). There is increased echogenicity along the basal plate and septa of the placenta (p) (*arrow*) representing deposition of calcium in these areas. The significance of this finding is unknown but may be encountered in normal pregnancies as well as eclampsia.

include calcification along the basal plate and septum of the placenta, as well as areas of diminished numbers of villi corresponding to areas of sonolucency. Fluid-filled spaces in the placenta may also be detected and represent pooling of blood in the intervillous spaces or localized areas of hydropic villi (Fig. 2-12B). Structural changes of the placenta may be seen in normal placentas, but these changes should be correlated with serologic titers of estradiol to assess their physiological significance.

Marked thinning of the placenta is seen in patients with intrauterine growth retardation (IUGR) and hydramnios. Thinning of the placenta may be a manifestation of placental vascular insufficiency. Areas of subchorionic fibrinoid degeneration may also be observed in patients with IUGR. The significance of the sonolucent subchorionic collections is unclear.

Although placental abruption may be difficult to diagnose sonographically, there are several suggestive signs (Fig. 2-12E). The blood that accumulates in the retroplacental location appears as a sonolucent or mildly echogenic band between the placenta and maternal myometrium. In order to establish the diagnosis of placental abruption, one must be able to differentiate this condition from the sonolucent band usually located in the same area that represents the venous pool of the placenta. In general, a separation from the placenta and basal plate of more than 4 cm should be considered suggestive of this condition.

Other conditions that cause textural changes in the placenta include marked thinning of the placenta and placental insufficiency that is associated with intrauterine growth retardation. In this condition, the thickness of the placenta is reduced to less than 3 cm in width. As previously noted, marked thinning of the placenta can be observed in cases of long-standing hydramnios. In these cases, the greatest width of the placenta is only 1.5 to 2 cm. At the opposite end of the spectrum, patients with Rh-isoimmunization disease or erythroblastosis fetalis may have an unusually thick placenta whose dimensions extend from the anterior to the posterior aspect of the uterus (Fig. 2-12F). Hydropic swelling of the placenta is often seen as a relatively early sign of intrauterine fetal demise. In these patients, the placenta appears contracted and more sonolucent than normal due to edema.

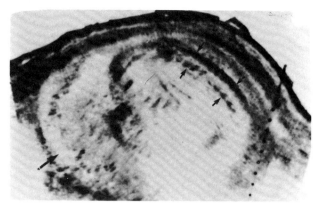

Figure 2-12E. Placental abruption (longitudinal, 4 cm to left of midline). This patient was in a motor vehicle accident and presented with a firm uterus. There is a sonolucent band between the placenta and the maternal myometrium (*large arrow*) representing collection of blood behind the placenta. The vertebrae of the fetal spine are well delineated (*small arrows*). (Courtesy of Gordon Hixon, M.D. Tri-counties Hospital, Fort Olgethorpe, Ga.)

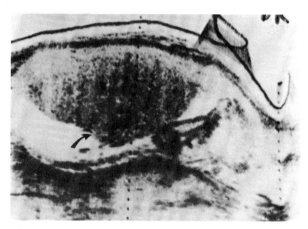

Figure 2-12F. Thickened, edematous placenta in Rh-isoimmunization (longitudinal, 8 cm to right of midline). The placenta (*arrow*) covers an area from the anterior aspect of the uterus to the posterior and measures approximately 10 cm in thickness. A thick placenta is frequently found in patients with Rh-isoimmunization.

MASSES OCCURRING WITH PREGNANCY

Patients who have a mass coexistent with pregnancy become clinically manifest when these masses produce abdominal pain or result in abnormal labor. On physical examination, a pelvic mass may be suspected when the uterus is too-large-for-dates or when a mass in the pelvis is palpated. In general, patients who are found to have a pelvic mass during pregnancy are managed according to the size of the mass and whether or not there is enlargement. Surgical exploration is usually performed in those patients whose masses appear to enlarge during pregnancy or whose masses are over 5 cm in diameter. In addition, surgery may be indicated for those pelvic masses that cause intractable pain and/or obstruct normal or surgical delivery.

Table 2-8. Sonographic Features of Some Common Pelvic Masses Occurring During Pregnancy

Mass	Sonographic Features
Uterine	
Leiomyoma	Variable echogenicity depending on composition, type of degeneration
Extrauterine	
Dermoid cyst	Cystic to complex appearance, depending upon composition
Cystadenoma	Unilocular or septated
Corpus luteum cyst	Sonolucent, echogenic if contain organized clot
Theca lutein cyst	Multilocular, bilateral; associated with hydatidiform mole
Other	
Pelvic kidney	Reniform configuration

Because of its noninvasive quality, sonography has a very important role in establishing the size and consistency of a pelvic mass that occurs in pregnancy, as well as in documenting whether there is serial enlargement or regression. Ultrasound is important in distinguishing between benign cystic structures, such as corpus luteum cysts and malignant masses (Tables 2-7, 2-8). Sonography is also helpful in establishing whether or not a mass is fixed or on a pedicle. Fixed masses have an increased incidence of rupture during labor. Masses that are not fixed in the pelvis may change position if the patient is scanned before and after full distension of the bladder (Figs. 2-13A, B).

Figure 2-13. PELVIC MASSES OCCURRING WITH
INTRAUTERINE PREGNANCY

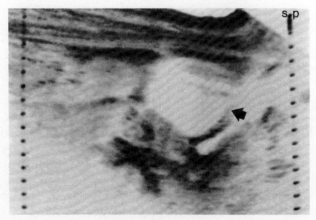

Figure 2-13A. Corpus luteum cyst (longitudinal, midline). There is a 6-cm, predominantly sonolucent mass anterior to the uterus and superior to the bladder (*arrow*). The intrauterine gestational sac is not well demonstrated on this sonogram.

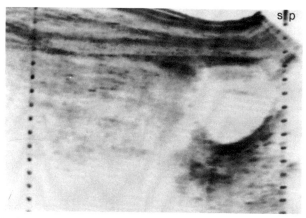

Figure 2-13B. Mobility of corpus luteum cyst seen in Figure 2-13A after patient voided (longitudinal, midline). In order to assess the mobility of the mass, the patient was re-scanned after voiding. The mass moved approximately 5 cm caudally, using the symphysis pubis as a reference (sp). Corpus luteum cysts are frequently encountered during the first trimester of pregnancy. Their internal consistency depends on the presence of clotted blood or liquefied hematoma. When the cyst contains organized hematoma, it appears echogenic. When the clot is liquefied, it appears sonolucent.

In general, if surgical exploration of patients with masses during pregnancy is indicated, it should be performed during the second trimester. There is less likelihood of inducing premature labor at this time. Sonography is also helpful in establishing the age of the pregnancy so that surgery can be performed at the appropriate time.

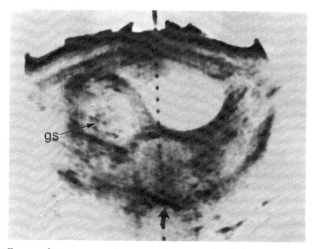

Figure 2-13C. Corpus luteum cyst that contains organized clot (transverse, 3 cm above symphysis pubis). There is an echogenic pelvic mass associated with a first trimester pregnancy and intact gestational sac (gs). Its echogenic appearance (*large arrow*) is related to the presence of organized internal clot.

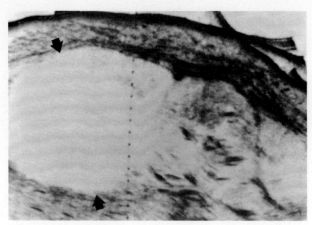

Figure 2-13D. Mucinous cystadenoma coexistent with a 14-week intrauterine pregnancy (longitudinal, midline). There is a large cystic mass anterior to the gravid uterus (*arrows*).

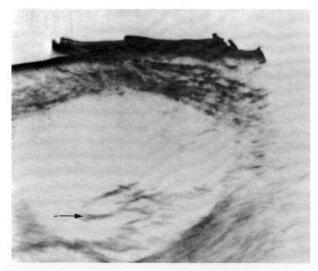

Figure 2-13E. Same patient as in Figure 2-13D (longitudinal, 3 cm to left of midline). On this sonogram, the mass is more completely delineated. There are thin internal septations (*arrow*) within the mass, suggesting the diagnosis of mucinous cystadenoma. This was confirmed at surgery, which was performed during the second trimester of pregnancy. The pregnancy progressed normally after surgical resection of the mass.

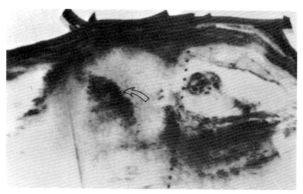

Figure 2-13F. Dermoid cyst coexistent with a 16-week intrauterine pregnancy (longitudinal, 4 cm to right of midline). Anterior to the gravid uterus is an ill-defined mass that contains a central area of high-amplitude echoes with posterior acoustical shadowing (*open arrow*). This mass was a dermoid cyst that contained fatty contents and radiographically demonstrable calcification. The most frequent location for a dermoid cyst is anterior and superior to the uterine fundus. These masses are usually pedunculated and displaced from the pelvis by a gravid uterus. (Courtesy of Bill Wilson, M.D., Calloway County Hospital, Murray, Ky.)

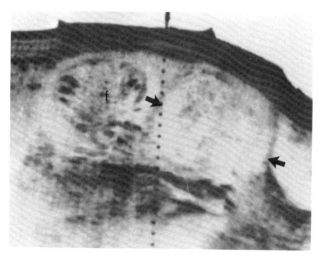

Figure 2-13G. Intramural leiomyoma coexistent with a 20-week pregnancy (longitudinal, 4 cm to left of midline). There is a large, mildly echogenic mass originating in the wall of the lower uterine segment (*arrows*). The fetal body is imaged in transverse section (f). An intramural leiomyoma was present, and its position in the lower uterine segment prohibited vaginal delivery.

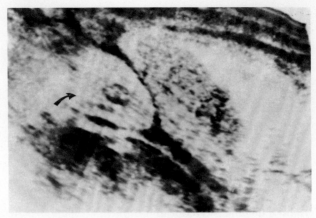

Figure 2-13H. Ectopic kidney with intrauterine pregnancy (longitudinal, 2 cm to right of midline). There is a fusiform mass (*curved arrow*) posterior to the uterine fundus. The mass has a central linear echogenicity corresponding to the renal pelvis. (Courtesy of Dean Birdwell, R.D.M.S., Nashville General Hospital, Nashville, Tenn.)

Solid Masses

The most common solid mass occurring with pregnancy is the uterine leiomyoma. Uterine leiomyomas tend to enlarge during pregnancy because of the stimulatory effect of estrogen and maternal hormones (Fig. 2-13G). The sonographic appearance of leiomyomas ranges from totally sonolucent to moderately echogenic, as described in Chapter 3. Leiomyomas that have undergone internal hyaline or myxoid degeneration appear as sonolucent to complex masses with areas of irregularity within them. Leiomyomas may also have an increased tendency toward necrosis during pregnancy. Ischemia within the tumor can cause tissue necrosis leading to abdominal pain. A myomectomy is sometimes indicated when the patient experiences intractable pain during pregnancy or when the myoma obstructs normal delivery.

Other less common solid masses encountered during pregnancy include solid ovarian tumors, such as adenocarcinoma, and solid masses created by the nongravid horn of bicornuate uterus. Solid ovarian tumors can be distinguished from other uterine masses by their extrauterine location. A nongravid horn of a bicornuate uterus may appear as a focal bulge of the uterine contour with a texture similar to that of the myometrium.

Complex Masses

Complex masses that are frequently encountered during pregnancy include dermoid cysts and cystic tumors that have solid components within them. The most common complex mass associated with pregnancy is a dermoid cyst (Fig. 2-13F). These masses usually exhibit an echogenic texture, which most likely emanates from the sebaceous components within them. They can be diffusely echogenic, which prohibits complete delineation of these masses since sebum may be highly reflective. Dermoid cysts are commonly pedunculated and will cause pain when they undergo torsion about their axis. Pedunculated dermoid cysts are often located anterior to the uterus. Pelvic kidney may also appear as a complex mass in the pelvis associated with pregnancy (Fig. 2-13H).

Cystic Masses

Some common cystic masses associated with pregnancy include corpus luteum cysts and serous cystadenomas (Figs. 2-2C, 2-13A,B,C,D,E). As stated previously, corpus luteum cysts are normal structures that usually undergo regression before the 14th week of pregnancy.

Corpus luteum cysts appear as sonolucent or echogenic pelvic masses, depending on the consistency of their internal components. In the first 8 to 10 weeks of pregnancy, these masses usually contain organized hemorrhage. Therefore, they appear as echogenic masses. However, after liquefaction of the clot occurs, these masses appear sonolucent because they contain serous fluid (Figs. 2-13A,B). Cystic ovarian masses, such as serous cystadenomas, may also be encountered with pregnancy. As in the nongravid patient, cystic ovarian tumors may contain separations and solid components and if malignant, produce material ascites. Cystic masses of the spleen, liver, and kidney may also be encountered in gravid patients. The nature of these cystic masses can become evident when the organ of origin is identified.

CONGENITAL ANOMALIES

With the recent improvement in resolution afforded by gray scale image processing, several major organs of the fetus can be routinely delineated in utero. As a consequence, several anatomical anomalies that affect these organs can be recognized sonographically in utero. Sonographic examination of the fetus is helpful when an anomaly is suspected on the basis of family history or laboratory studies such as alpha-fetoprotein.

Some of the fetal structures that can be routinely visualized in a fetus in the third trimester include the distended, urine-filled bladder, fluid-filled loops of bowel, the falx cerebri, lateral ventricles and thalami, and the vertebral bodies of the fetal spine (Fig. 2-12C). The fetal kidneys, liver, aorta, heart, and external genitalia can also be delineated (Figs. 2-5A,B,C,D).

Because the circulation and distribution of the amniotic fluid depend on its absorption through the gastrointestinal tract and production in the kidney and normal swallowing reflex, an excessive or decreased amount of amniotic fluid may suggest fetal anomalies. In particular, maternal hydramnios is associated with atresias and/or obstruction of the gastrointestinal tract (Fig. 2-14D), such as esophageal atresias, duodenal atresias, and imperforate anus. Hydramnios is associated with diminished or altered fetal swallowing mechanism, which may also be secondary to a central nervous system abnormality. Although the cause in about one-half of patients with hydramnios will not be known, this condition is most commonly associated with systemic disorders, such as diabetes mellitus, rh incompatibility, and viral infection in utero. Hydramnios is also associated with fetal tumors that obstruct venous return, such as the mediastinal teratoma seen in

Figure 2-14. CONGENITAL ANOMALIES

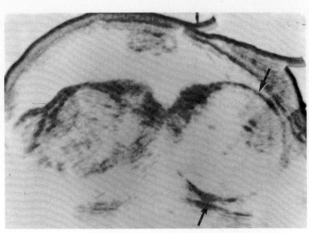

Figure 2-14A. Hydrocephalus (longitudinal, midline). Fetal biparietal diameter measured 11.7 cm. The mother was hydramniotic. Recognition of these features suggested the diagnosis of hydrocephalus. Hydrocephalus should be considered when the BPD is greater than 11 cm. Maternal hydramnios may result from altered fetal swallowing, which implies a central nervous system malfunction or gastrointestinal tract obstruction.

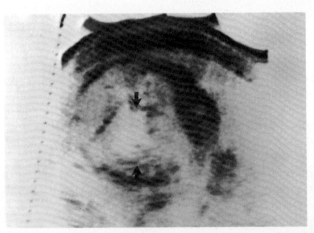

Figure 2-14B. Same patient as in Figure 2-14A (transverse, through fetal head). This image was obtained in the region of the lateral ventricles, which are markedly distended (*arrows*). These findings further document the presence of hydrocephalus.

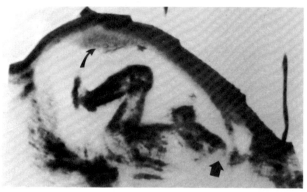

Figure 2-14C. Anencephaly (longitudinal, 4 cm to left of midline). There were no demonstrable cranial structures in this fetus (*straight arrow*). The fetal leg is completely delineated. The mother had hydramnios, and the placenta (*curved arrow*) is markedly thinned. This condition can result from rubella contracted during the first trimester of pregnancy.

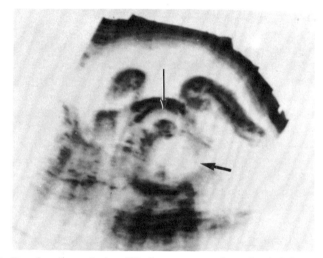

Figure 2-14D. Duodenal atresia (modified transverse, along fetal abdomen). The mother had hydramnios. Two persistent cystic masses were seen in the fetal abdomen. One was rounded (*large arrow*) and the other tubular and C-shaped (*small arrow*). These findings suggested the diagnosis of duodenal atresia. Amniography was unsuccessful because of esophageal atresia associated with duodenal atresia and an imperforate anus.

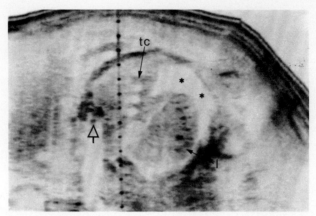

Figure 2-14E. Fetal ascites (modified transverse, across fetal abdomen). There is a sono-lucent area around the fetal liver (1) representing ascitic fluid (*asterisks*). In addition, a fluid-filled portion of the splenic flexure of the transverse colon can be identified (tc). The fetal lumbar vertebrae appear highly echogenic, producing complete acoustical shadow (*open arrow*). This fetus was later found to have a mediastinal teratoma that obstructed venous return, thus leading to ascites.

Figure 2-14E, fetal renal hamartoma, as well as infantile polycystic kidney disease. Other causes of fetal ascites include congestive heart failure and renal and liver disease (Table 2-9).

Diminished amount of amniotic fluid is associated with defects in renal development, such as in Potter's syndrome. In this syndrome, there is agenesis of the kidneys. The normally prominent adrenals in a mature fetus may simulate the configuration of kidneys. Because of the importance of amniotic fluid to lung development, renal agenesis is also associated with hypoplasia of the lung.

Hydramnios may be an indication of atresia and/or obstruction of the gastrointestinal tract. In particular, atresias of the duodenum, esophagus, and other areas of the bowel are usually associated with hydramnios. In duodenal atresia, the stomach and proximal portion of the duodenum can be identified as fluid-filled structures in the upper abdomen of the fetus (Fig. 2-14D). An imperforate anus can produce fluid-filled loops of distal colon in the lower abdomen which have their longest axis corresponding to the fetal trunk. Other fetal gastrointestinal tract abnormalities include gastroschisis, which results from a failure of normal development of the abdominal musculature and resultant herniation of the fetal bowel in an eccentric manner. Omphaloceles are the result of herniation of the fetal bowel outside the fetal abdomen into the umbilical cord. This disorder appears as a midline bulge of the anterior abdominal wall. As stated previously, the fetal bowel is usually fluid-filled and can be recognized as sonolucent tubular structures (Fig. 2-5D). Herniation of bowel into the thorax, such as in hernias through the foramina of Bochdalek and Morgagni, may appear as tubular, sonolucent structures within the thorax.

Several intracranial anomalies of the fetus can be detected by sonography (Figs. 2-14A,B,C). These include hydrocephalus, porencephaly, and anencephaly. In advanced hydrocephalus, the fetal BPD is usually greater than 10.7 cm. The diameter of the head usually increases toward the vertex. In a hydro-

Table 2-9. Some Common Causes of Hydramnios, Oligohydramnios, and
Fetal Ascites

Condition	Sonographic Features
Hydramnios	
Diabetes	Large fetus for dates
Intracranial disorder	Altered fetal swallowing
Anencephaly	Underdeveloped cranium
Porencephaly	Cystic areas within brain
Idiopathic	
Oligohydramnios	
Renal agenesis	Fetal renal structures or bladder not identifiable
Intrauterine fetal demise	Edematous soft tissue of fetus; swollen placenta
Fetal ascites	
Rh-isoimmunization	Thick, edematous placenta
Congestive heart failure	Fetal anasarca
Bowel obstruction	Distended, fluid-filled proximal bowel loops
Posterior urethral valves	Bilateral hydronephrosis
Viral infection	
Idiopathic	

cephalic fetus, the head is usually at least 2 to 3 cm larger in circumference than the fetal body. The width of the body of the lateral ventricles in a third trimester fetus varies from 0.8 to 1.1 cm and the ratio of lateral ventricles to hemisphere is 0.25 to 0.34 (36). When this ratio is increased, this suggests the presence of hydrocephalus. Cystic areas within the fetal brain, such as those due to liquefactive necrosis in hydranencephaly and porencephaly, can occasionally be recognized in utero (42). Anencephaly may be associated with rubella infection during the first trimester. Lack of a well-formed fetal head can be demonstrated by ultrasound. The cranial portions of such a fetus are recognized as only a small area of soft tissue (Fig. 2-14C). Since these central nervous system abnormalities frequently affect the fetal swallowing reflex, there is usually an associated maternal hydramnios.

Disorders of the genitourinary system, such as hydronephrosis and/or bladder outlet obstruction, can also be diagnosed in utero by ultrasound study (37). Distension of the renal pelvis appears as cystic areas within the fetal abdomen. The bladder will often appear as a rounded cystic structure in the lower abdomen that occupies the entire abdomen if bladder outlet obstruction is present.

Sonography is also a sensitive detector of fetal ascites. Although there are several causes of fetal ascites, the most common one is hydrops of the fetus seen in Rh-isoimmunization (Fig. 2-14E). Other causes of fetal ascites include congestive heart failure, bowel obstruction, posterior urethral valves, and viral infection. As in the adult, excessive fluid within the abdomen can be detected as sonolucent areas that surround the liver and bowel and tend to collect in the dependent portions of the body.

Other fetal anomalies that can be identified in utero include meningomyelocele and maldevelopment of the fetal extremities (35). Open neural tube defects may cause localized disruption of the normal "picket fence" appearance of the spine. Real-time sonography can be used to delineate the entire fetal spine. Disproportionately small limbs can be recognized in some types of dwarfism by ultrasound studies.

Real-time sonography can be used for rapid and accurate assessment of several of the major organs in the body, as well as for localization of the fetal parts for interventional procedures such as intrauterine transfusion. By using real-time ultrasound, the exact position of the fetus can be determined in a dynamic manner, and also the location of the needle within the fetus. The air that is trapped at the end of the needle can be observed to rise within the fetal abdomen by using real-time scanning. Fetal heart motion can be observed as dynamically moving structures in the region of the midthorax. Peristaltic motion of the bowel can also be recognized by using this method.

INTRAUTERINE FETAL DEMISE

Although ultrasound can be used to confirm the diagnosis of intrauterine fetal demise, it may be of greater clinical importance to detect signs that precede intrauterine fetal demise or may indicate severe fetal distress in utero. Signs of fetal distress include the double-ring sign associated with edema of the soft tissues particularly about the cranium (3).

Real-time Doppler examinations may be combined to evaluate fetal viability in the first and second trimesters. Even though the fetus may be quite small, some motion of the fetal heart should be identifiable. As the fetus is delineated, fetal motion can be recognized secondary to motion of the fetal extremities and heart (40). The fetal heart rate is almost twice that of the mother, allowing differentiation. Abnormal cardiac contractions or valvular motion of the fetus can be monitored with M-mode echocardiography or with real-time scanning.

In general, the sonographic features of intrauterine fetal demise can be identified earlier in the course of the disorder than the radiographic signs. The signs become apparent approximately five days to two weeks after intrauterine fetal demise (Figs. 2-15A,B). Marked edema of the soft tissue around the fetal head, as well as abdomen, is the earliest sign of intrauterine fetal demise and may be seen in severe fetal distress (Figs. 2-15A,B). Eventually, edema of the fetal scalp can become so pronounced as to develop a double-ring sign (3). Edema surrounding the abdomen may be noted with fetal anasarca. The double-ring sign refers to two concentric rings that are separated by at least 4 mm representing interfaces emanating from the cranial structures and the outer border of edematous soft tissue. This sign may, however, be seen in other causes of intrauterine fetal distress, such as sickle cell disease, diabetes mellitus, and hydrops of the fetus secondary to Rh-isoimmunization disease.

In the late stages of intrauterine fetal demise, overlapping of the fetal sutures can be seen by ultrasound as well as on radiographic studies. Other findings associated with intrauterine fetal demise include loss of the falx cerebri echo complex, as well as hydropic swelling of the placenta.

Figure 2-15. INTRAUTERINE FETAL DEMISE

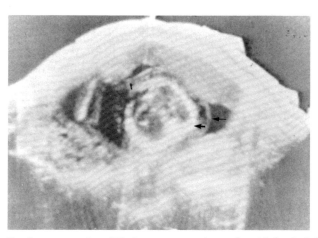

Figure 2-15A. Fetal anasarca (modified transverse through mid-fetal abdomen; white-on-black image). There is edema of the soft tissue surrounding the fetal abdomen demonstrated by abnormal separation between the deep (*large arrow*) and subcutaneous soft tissue layers and skin (*small arrow*). This is seen in fetal anasarca, as well as in fetal demise. Edema may be encountered secondary to conditions that cause severe fetal distress, such as hydrops fetalis, diabetes, and sickle cell anemia.

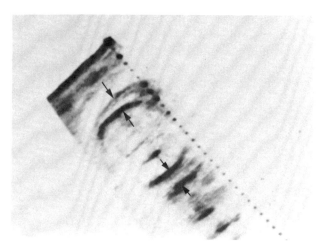

Figure 2-15B. Scalp edema (transverse, through bi-parietal plane). Edema of the fetal scalp is depicted as a double outline of the fetal cranium (*arrows*). This "double ring" sign is seen in severe fetal distress, fetal anasarca, and fetal demise.

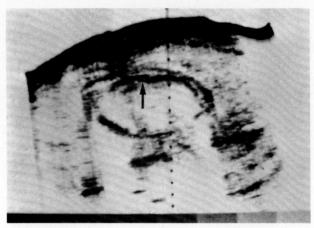

Figure 2-15C. Overlapping sutures (transverse, through fetal head). The outline of the fetal head is flattened, and there is evidence of overlapping of the cranial bones consistent with fetal demise (*arrow*). This condition was also radiographically demonstrable. Overlapping of the fetal cranial bones occurs several days to two weeks after fetal demise has occurred.

MATERNAL COMPLICATIONS

Since exposure to ionizing radiation during pregnancy should be minimized, sonography is a very useful modality for the evaluation of certain maternal conditions. Although distension of the maternal renal pelvis and ureter occurs normally during pregnancy, it may be associated with an increased incidence of pyelonephritis and acute costovertebral angle pain secondary to urine stasis. In these patients, sonography can be useful in establishing hydronephrosis and hydroureter (Figs. 2-16A,B). This is detected by separation of echoes emanating

Figure 2-16. MATERNAL COMPLICATIONS

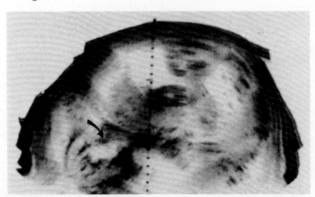

Figure 2-16A. Hydronephrosis of pregnancy (transverse scan through maternal upper abdomen). The right renal pelvis is dilated (*curved arrow*), consistent with hydronephrosis. This condition is normally encountered during the second and third trimesters of pregnancy. Gravid uterus is seen in transverse section.

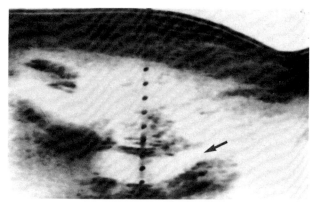

Figure 2-16B. Same patient as in Figure 2-16A (longitudinal, 4 cm to left of midline). The distended ureter appears as a tubular structure posterior to the uterus (*arrow*). It can be differentiated from distended placental venous structures by its large size and characteristic course extending to the posterior medial aspect of the bladder.

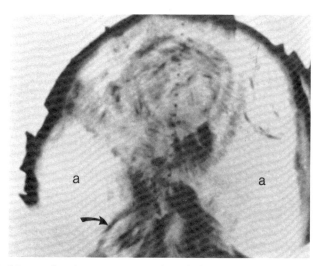

Figure 2-16C. Maternal ascites (transverse, 6 cm below xiphoid). This gravid patient had a markedly distended abdomen. Sonography revealed collections of ascitic fluid on both sides of the gravid uterus (a). This condition was not suspected clinically and was later found to be secondary to an ovarian carcinoma. The right kidney (*curved arrow*) is also seen to be medially displaced by the ascitic fluid.

from the maternal renal pelvis. Hydroureter appears as a tubular structure that has a longitudinal course and inserts into the posterior aspect of the bladder wall.

Upper abdominal pain during pregnancy can also be evaluated by ultrasound. Cholecystitis, especially when it is associated with gallbladder calculi, can be established diagnostically by this technique. Acute pancreatitis can be demonstrated as overall enlargement and diminished echogenicity of the pancreas.

If the patient's condition permits, other conditions, such as rupture of splenic gland and hepatic artery aneurysm, can be initially evaluated by ultrasound before

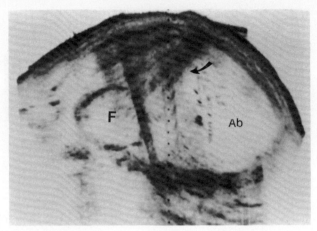

Figure 2-16D. Intraabdominal abscess secondary to Crohn's disease coexistent with second trimester pregnancy (transverse, F = fetus). Patient presented with a history of intermittent fever. She had been placed on steroids because of Crohn's disease discovered during an exploratory laparotomy performed during the first trimester of pregnancy. In the longitudinal scan, there is a large cystic mass (Ab) lateral to the uterus which contained highly reflective components hampering delineation of the uterine fundus (*arrow*). With real-time scanning, the echoes within this mass could be seen to float. This later proved to be a large abscess secondary to perforation of bowel as a sequela to Crohn's disease. The echoes within the mass represented gas contained within the abscess.

more invasive studies are contemplated. Maternal ascites secondary to chronic renal or cardiac failure may be recognized as fluid collections on either side of the enlarged uterus (Fig. 2-16C). This disorder may be difficult for the obstetrician to detect, for the uterus is enlarged and palpation of the abdomen difficult.

POSTPARTUM APPLICATIONS

Ultrasound studies are helpful in evaluating certain conditions in the postpartum period. Most commonly, sonography is used to evaluate the uterus that fails to involute. Failure of the uterus to involute may be secondary to problems created by retained products of conception or intrauterine hematoma (Figs. 2-17A,B). Retained placenta can be distinguished from other intrauterine masses by its increased echogenicity when compared to the myometrium. Hematomas within the uterus appear as localized areas of relative sonolucency.

Sonography can also be useful in the evaluation of suppurative endometritis that may occur in the postpartum period. Postpartum endometritis usually results from infection that ascends from the vaginal area. In this condition, the uterine lumen may be irregularly distended on the sonogram.

Figure 2-17. POSTPARTUM DISORDERS

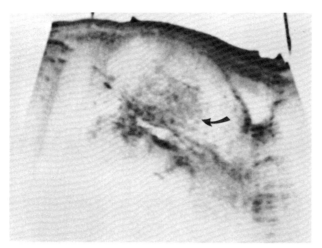

Figure 2-17A. Retained placenta (longitudinal, 2 cm to left of midline). This scan was performed five days after delivery. There is an echogenic area along the posterior uterine wall (*curved arrow*) representing retained placenta.

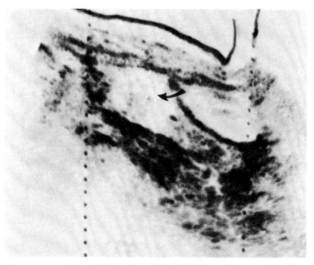

Figure 2-17B. Hematoma (longitudinal, midline). There is a relatively sonolucent area in the region of the uterine fundus (*curved arrow*). This patient was two months post cesarean section. The sonolucent area was found to represent persistent hematoma in the region of the uterine fundus.

SUMMARY

Thus, there are numerous applications of ultrasound in obstetrics. Ultrasound is more widely used in obstetrics than in any other medical field and has achieved great clinical acceptance. Recent improvements in the resolution of real-time scanning have afforded better depiction of fetal structures. Detection of fetal anomalies will assume a more important role when in utero surgical intervention becomes feasible.

REFERENCES

General

1. *Ultrasonography in Obstetrics and Gynecology*. R. Sanders, A. E. James, Jr., eds. Second ed. New York: Appleton-Century-Crofts, 1980.
2. Hobbins, J., Winsberg, F.: *Ultrasonography in Obstetrics and Gynecology*. Baltimore: Williams and Wilkins, 1977.
3. Sanders, R., Conrad, M.: Sonography in obstetrics. *Radiol. Clin. N. Am.* 13(4):435–455, 1975.

Technique

4. Bartrum, R., Crow, H.: Examination in pregnancy. In *Gray Scale Ultrasound: A Manual for Physicians and Technical Personnel*. Philadelphia: Saunders, 1977, pp. 154–174.
5. Zemlyn, S.: The effects of the urinary bladder on obstetrical sonography. *Radiology* 128:169–175, 1978.

Fetal Growth and Maturity

6. Chilcote, W., Asokan, S.: Evaluation of first trimester pregnancy by ultrasound. *Clin. Ob./Gyn.* 20:253–256, 1977.
7. Robinson, H.: Sonar measurement of fetal crown rump length as means of assessing maturity of first trimester of pregnancy. *Br. Med. J.* 4:28–31, 1973.
8. Campbell, S., Newman, G.: Growth of fetal biparietal diameter during normal pregnancy. *Br. J. Ob./Gyn.* 78:513–519, 1971.
9. Sabbagha, R., Hughey, M., Depp, R.: The assignment of gross adjusted sonographic age (GASA): A simplified method. *Am. J. Ob./Gyn.* 126:485, 1976.
10. Wiener, S., Flynn, J., Kennedy, A., Bonk, F.: A composite curve of ultrasonic biparietal diameters for estimating gestational age. *Radiology* 122:781–786, 1977.
11. Campbell, S., Wilkin, D.: Ultrasonic measurement of fetal abdomen circumference in the estimation of fetal weight. *Br. J. Ob./Gyn.* 82(9):165–174, 1975.
12. Campbell, S., Wilkin, D.: Ultrasonic measurement of fetal abdomen circumference and estimation of fetal weight. *Br. J. Ob./Gyn.* 82:689–697, 1976.
13. Campbell, S., Thomas, A.: Ultrasonic measurement of fetal head to abdominal circumference ratio and assessment of growth retardation. *Br. J. Ob./Gyn.* 84:165–174, 1977.
14. Flamme, P.: Ultrasonic fetal cephalometry: Percentiles curve. *Br. Med. J.* 3:384–385, 1972.

Placenta

15. Fisher, C., Garrett, W., Kossoff, G.: Placental aging monitored by gray scale echograpy. *Am. J. Ob./Gyn.* 124 (5):483–488, 1976.
16. King, D.: Placental migration demonstrated by ultrasonography: A hypothesis of dynamic placentation. *Radiology* 109:167–170, 1973.

17. Haney, A., Trough, D.: Changes in placenta. Presented at meeting of American Institute of Ultrasound in Medicine, San Diego, California, 1978.

18. Young, G.: The peripatetic placenta. *Radiology* 128:183–188, 1978.

19. Goldberg, B.: Identification of placenta previa (Opinion). *Radiology* 128:255–256, 1978.

20. Bowie, J., Rochester, D., Kadkin, A., Cooke, W., Kuntzman, A.: Accuracy of placenta localization by ultrasound. *Radiology* 128:177–180, 1978.

Uterus

21. Sample, W.: The unsoftened portion of the uterus. *Radiology* 126:227, 1978.

22. Steel, W.: The gravid uterus: A dynamic organ. Presented at meeting of American Institute of Ultrasound in Medicine, San Diego, California, 1978.

23. Hobbins, J., Winsberg, F.: *Ultrasonography in Obstetrics and Gynecology.* Baltimore: Williams and Wilkins, 1977, p. 160.

Ectopic Pregnancy

24. Lawson, T.: Ectopic pregnancy: Criteria and accuracy of ultrasonic diagnosis. *Am. J. Roentgenol.* 131:153–156, 1978.

25. Schoenbaum, S., Rosendorf, L., Cappleman, N., Rowan, T.: Gray scale ultrasound in tubal pregnancy. *Radiology* 127:757–761, 1978.

26. Maklan, N., Wright, Z.: Gray scale ultrasonography in the diagnosis of ectopic pregnancy. *Radiology* 126:221–225, 1978.

27. Rogers, W., Shaub, M., Wilson, R.: Chronic ectopic pregnancy: Ultrasonic diagnosis. *J. Clin. Ultrasound* 54:257–260, 1977.

28. Fleischer, A., Boehm, F., James, A.: Sonographic evaluation of ectopic pregnancy, in *Ultrasonography in Obstetrics and Gynecology.* Second ed. R. Sanders, A. E. James, Jr., eds. New York: Appleton-Century-Crofts, 1980.

29. Burger, M., Taymor, M.: Simultaneous intrauterine and tubal pregnancies following ovarian induction. *Am. J. Ob./Gyn.* 113 (6):812–813, 1972.

Abortion

30. Donald, I., Morley, P., Barnett, E.: The diagnosis of blighted ovum by sonar. *Ob./Gyn. Br. Comm.* 79:304–310, 1972.

Trophoblastic Disease

31. Fleischer, A., James, A., Krause, D., Millis, J.: Sonographic patterns of trophoblastic disease. *Radiology* 126:215–220, 1978.

Multiple Pregnancy

32. Levi, S.: Ultrasonic assessment of the high rate of human multiple pregnancy in the first trimester. *J. Clin. Ultrasound* 413–519, 1977.

33. Laveno, K., Santos-Rhamos, R., Duenhoelter, J., Whally, P.: Sonar cephalometry in twins: A comparison with single fetus and in evaluation of twin disordancy. Presented at meeting of American Institute of Ultrasound in Medicine, San Diego, California, 1978.

Masses with Pregnancy

34. Bezjian, A., Carretero, M.: Ultrasonic evaluation of pelvic masses in pregnancy. *Clin. Ob./Gyn.* 20 (2):325–338, 1977.

116   Obstetrical Sonography

Congenital Anomalies

35. Shaff, M., Blumenthal, B., Coetze, M.: Meningo-encephalocele: Pre-partum ultrasonic and fetoamniography findings. *Br. J. Radiol.* 50:754–757, 1977.
36. Johnson, M., Mack, L., Gottsfeld, K., Rashbaum, C., Dunne, M.: Fetal M-mode echoencephalography. Presented at meeting of American Institute of Ultrasound in Medicine, San Diego, California, 1978.
37. Garrett, W., Gossoff, G.: Selection of patients by ultrasonic echography for fetal and immediate neonatal surgery. *Australia Pediat. J.* 12:313–318, 1976.
38. Lee, T., Blake, S.: Prenatal fetal abdominal ultrasonography and diagnosis. *Radiology* 124:475–477, 1977.
39. Shaub, M., Wilson, R.: Erythroblastosis fetalis: Ultrasonic diagnosis. *J. Clin. Ultrasound* 41:19–21, 1977.
40. Birnholtz, J., Stevens, J., Faria, M.: Fetal movement patterns: A possible means of defining neurologic development *in utero*. *Am. J. Roentgenol.* 130:537–540, 1978.
41. Lee, T., Warren, L.: Antenatal ultrasonic demonstration of fetal bowel. *Radiology* 124:471–474, 1977.
42. Fleischer, A., Brown, M.: Hydramnios associated with fetal hydrencephaly: A case report. *J. Clin. Ultrasound* 5 (1):41–43, 1976.
43. Bean, W., Calonje, M., Aprill, C., Geshner, J.: Anal atresia: A prenatal ultrasonic diagnosis. *J. Clin. Ultrasound* 6:111–112, 1978.

Miscellaneous

44. Anderson, J., Lee, T., Nagel, N.: Ultrasound diagnosis of nonobstetric disease during pregnancy. *Ob./Gyn.* 48 (3):359–362, 1976.
45. Cooperberg, P., Carpenter, C.: Ultrasound as an aid in intrauterine transfusion. *Am. J. Ob./Gyn.* 128:439–441, 1977.
46. *Williams' Obstetrics*. L. Hellman, J. Pritchard, eds. New York: Appleton-Century-Crofts, 1971, p. 199.
47. Goldberg, B., Ziskin, M., Kotler, M., Waxham, R.: *Diagnostic Uses of Ultrasound*. New York: Grune and Stratton, 1975.
48. Guttman, P.: In search of the elusive benign cystic teratoma: The "tip of the iceberg" sign. *J. Clin. Ultrasound* 5:403–406, 1976.
49. Bowie, J.: Ultrasound of gynecologic pelvic masses: The indefinite uterus and other patterns associated with diagnostic error. *J. Clin. Ultrasound* 5 (5):323–328, 1977.

3
Gynecological Sonography

GENERAL COMMENTS

In the field of gynecology, sonography has its greatest clinical application in the evaluation of pelvic masses. In general, the variety and morphologic complexity of these pelvic masses make gynecologic sonography more challenging and difficult than obstetrical ultrasound. Gray scale image processing affords better delineation of the internal morphological detail of soft tissue masses and interfaces around these masses than could be previously obtained by B-mode bi-stable images. Hence, the introduction of gray scale instrumentation has noticeably broadened the role of diagnostic ultrasound in the evaluation of gynecologic disorders. However, since the sonographic features of many pelvic masses are nonspecific, ultrasound pattern must be combined with the clinical data for an accurate diagnosis.

Although the relative efficacy of sonography for the evaluation of gynecological disorders is yet to be determined, its proved value and noninvasive and atraumatic qualities justify its inclusion as a useful test among those used for complete evaluation of pelvic masses. Rather than depicting indirect signs, such as deviation or partial obstruction of the ureter as demonstrated by excretory urography, or displacement of the bowel as seen on contrast gastrointestinal series, sonography provides direct evaluation of the size, location, sometimes origin, and internal consistency of a mass within the pelvis. This does not mean that the barium enema and excretory urogram are not important studies that document involvement of the ureter and bowel by a pelvic mass. Also, by detecting small amounts of free intraperitoneal fluid and hepatic or peritoneal and omental metastases, sonography contributes to the total evaluation of a pelvic mass. Serial ultrasound examinations can be performed since they apparently do not produce any significant biological effects (1).

The relative nonspecificity of the sonographic patterns of pelvic masses (Table 3-1) emphasizes the importance of considering the clinical assessment in formulating a differential diagnosis. Instead of attempting to provide a specific histological diagnosis on the basis of ultrasonography, one should evaluate the features that are clinically important in a patient with a pelvic mass. Sonography is valuable for the following:

1. Confirming the existence of a mass that is suspected from pelvic examination
2. Delineating the size, consistency, and contour
3. Establishing the origin and anatomic relationship to other structures
4. Documenting involvement of other organs
5. Establishing the presence or absence of ascites or metastatic lesions

Table 3-1. Pattern Specificity of Pelvic Masses[a] (9)

Mass	No. of Cases[b]	Common Sonographic Features	Total No. of Masses with Pattern	No. of Specific Masses with Pattern	Percent Pattern Specificity for Specific Masses[a]
Ovarian mucinous cystadenoma	19	Predominantly cystic Pelvoabdominal Septated	20	18	90
Uterine leiomyoma	27	Mildly to moderately echogenic Nodular uterine enlargement	28	25	89
Endometrioma(s)	12	Multiple cysts of various sizes	14	10	71
Tubo-ovarian abscess	18	Complex, predominantly cystic Adnexal	21	13	61
Dermoid cyst	17	Complex with echogenic focus	18	9	50
Ectopic pregnancy	19	Complex Extrauterine	35	14	40
Physiological ovarian cyst	18	Cystic Adnexal	52	17	33
Serous cystadenoma	16	Cystic Adnexal	52	12	23
Hydrosalpinx	12	Cystic Adnexal	52	10	20

[a]Defined as ratio of number of times a particular mass displayed a certain sonographic appearance divided by the total number of times that pattern was encountered.

[b]Masses for which there were fewer than 10 cases not included in this table.

INDICATIONS

In addition to evaluation of these features of a pelvic mass, ultrasound studies have been helpful in:

1. Establishing the presence or absence of lymphadenopathy associated with a pelvic mass
2. Establishing intrauterine location of contraceptive device
3. Performing serial examinations of a pelvic mass during or after therapy
4. Confirming cystic breast masses (described in Chapter 8)
5. Establishing treatment fields and doses when an intracavitary device is used (discussed in Chapter 8)

SONOGRAPHIC FEATURES OF NORMAL PELVIC STRUCTURES AND SCANNING TECHNIQUE

Prior to the ultrasound study, the patient's urinary bladder should be distended so that an "ultrasonic window" is created for adequate delineation of the pelvic structures. A full bladder is obtained by having the patient drink two to four glasses of water or tea approximately one hour before the examination. If the patient's oral intake is restricted, catheterization of the bladder, using aseptic technique, may be necessary. Since large pelvic masses usually elevate the bladder trigone, complete distension of the bladder may not always be possible in patients with large pelvoabdominal masses. A fully distended bladder also serves as a standard for comparison of the echogenicity of a pelvic mass. If one is interested only in evaluating the location and consistency of a large pelvic mass, the patient can be examined without completely filling the bladder.

In most nonobese adults and pediatric patients, a 3.5-MHz transducer with a medium or long (9- to 11-cm) focus is optimal for pelvic scanning. In obese patients, scanning may be performed with a 2.25-MHz transducer with long internal focus. After the routine series of longitudinal and transverse scans is completed, additional views oblique to the longitudinal and transverse planes or with a transducer of higher frequency can be obtained if clinically necessary. Penetration of sound through soft tissue (solid) masses is an indicator of the overall attenuation of the incident beam to the mass. Less penetration through the solid mass will be obtained when a transducer of higher frequency is used.

When interpreting a gynecologic ultrasound study, one should be aware of the normal size, shape, and location of the uterus, ovary, and adnexal structures (7). Knowledge of the region of interest is mandatory before the patient is scanned, so that evaluation of this area can be as complete as possible. Normal pelvic structures, especially the uterus, must be identified before pelvic masses are evaluated. As discussed in detail elsewhere, establishing the uterine or extrauterine location of a mass is of primary importance in formulating the correct differential diagnosis.

Meticulous scanning technique is crucial in evaluating pelvic masses (4). In order to retrieve echoes emanating from within the mass or discontinuities of parenchymal texture, an attempt should be made to orient the transducer perpendicular to the surface or structure that is to be evaluated. Many diagnostic errors can be attributed to an improper transducer angle relative to the area of interest. In general, patients do not need to be in suspended respiration for ultrasound imaging of the pelvic organs. The pelvic side walls and uterus are best evaluated by a simple sector scan with a transducer held lateral to the midline. Evaluation of the structures on one side of the pelvis is best obtained by using a simple sector scan with the transducer placed on the opposite side of the midline.

The gain settings that are used for evaluation of pelvic structures should be adjusted to emphasize the recording of low-level echoes so that parenchymal detail can be demonstrated and the "noise" level can be distinguished from echoes emanating from acoustical interfaces. The time gain compensation (TGC) curves should be set so that unimportant echo interfaces such as the anterior abdominal wall are de-emphasized. Compound scanning may be used for the delineation of soft tissue interfaces around pelvic masses, whereas simple sector scanning usually affords the most information concerning the attenuation of the incident beam through a mass.

One usually begins the sonographic examination of the pelvic organs by obtaining a longitudinal scan starting at the midline with the patient in the supine position. Real-time scanning can be used initially to define the location of organs and the greatest longitudinal axis of the uterus for orientation. Transverse scans should be obtained starting at the symphysis pubis, with a 5- to 10-degree cephalic angulation of the transducer. The cephalic angulation of the transducer optimizes delineation of the "genital axis," since it usually lies oblique to the anterior abdominal wall. The "genital axis" refers to a sling of peritoneal structures that contains the oviducts, ovaries, and uterus oriented in a "hammock-like" arrangement (31). Full distension of the bladder produces convex curvature of these structures and separation of the ovaries to either side of the uterus.

On longitudinal scans, the uterus lies immediately posterior to the bladder. The uterine fundus is often slightly anterior to the cervix, but retroflexion of the uterus can be seen normally in patients who are multigravidas. The size of the uterus (length, anterior-posterior and transverse widths) varies from approximately 3 × 2 × 2 cm in prepubertal girls to 6 × 3 × 3 cm in postpubertal women, 8 × 6 × 5 cm in multigravidas, and 4 × 2 × 2 cm in postmenopausal women (Figs. 3-1A,B,C,D,E) (7,18). The uterus changes from a tubular structure with the cervix wider than the fundus during infancy to a more pear-shaped organ with the fundus wider than the cervix in postpubertal women. The change in shape of the uterus as the young girl approaches puberty can be quantitated by the ratio of the cervix to the fundus, measured in the anterior-posterior and transverse dimensions (7). The normal uterus has a smooth contour. Any nodularity or convexity of the uterine outline should be delineated in at least two scanning planes. By using these ultrasound criteria, the focal bulge or convexity

Figure 3-1. NORMAL UTERUS AND ADNEXA

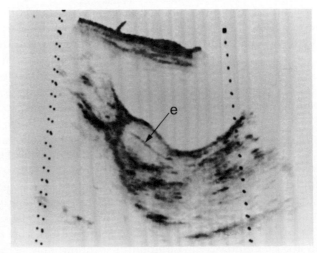

Figure 3-1A. Normal, nulliparous uterus (longitudinal, midline). The uterus is a tubular structure and the endometrium (e) is seen as a linear interface within the center of the uterus prior to menstruation.

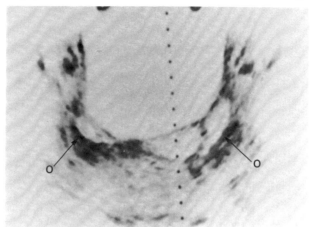

Figure 3-1B. Normal, nulliparous uterus and ovaries (transverse, 4 cm above symphysis pubis). The ovaries (o) lie to either side of the uterus. They are elliptical in shape and may measure up to 4 cm in length.

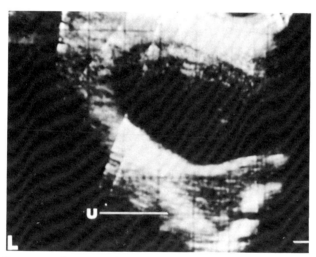

Figure 3-1C. Retroverted uterus (longitudinal, midline). This demonstrates nodular shape and retroflexion of the uterus. A retroverted uterus is commonly seen in multiparous patients.

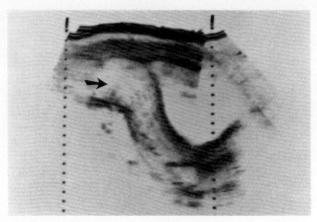

Figure 3-1D. Multiparous uterus (longitudinal, midline). The uterus (*arrow*) is larger in multiparous women than in nulliparous women. Its outline is often more nodular, probably due to variations in muscle growth during pregnancy.

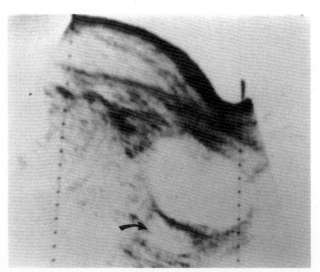

Figure 3-1E. Postmenopausal uterus (longitudinal, midline). The uterus (*arrow*) in postmenopausal women is smaller than in premenopausal individuals. The size approximates that of a prepubertal uterus.

of the uterus such as seen in partial duplication or bicornuate uteri can be differentiated from an adnexal mass or uterine leiomyoma.

In normal women, the myometrium has a finely echogenic texture. The endometrium can be recognized as a 3- to 4-mm sonolucent band around the central echogenic interface arising from the endometrial surface. When menstruation occurs, the endometrial cavity becomes echogenic, probably the result of the numerous interfaces created by sloughed endometrium and blood. The echogenic endometrium that is seen during menstruation can serve to identify the location of the uterus in relation to a pelvic mass. For example, if the intra- or extrauterine location of a pelvic mass can not be readily determined, the patient can be requested to return during menstruation so that the uterus can be outlined relative to the mass.

Changes in the endometrium and uterine texture as well as the transient presence of free intraperitoneal fluid in the cul-de-sac have been documented as changes that occur during the normal menstrual cycle (8). As previously stated, the endometrial area is particularly echogenic during menstruation probably due to the multiple interfaces that emanate from the sloughed endometrium and blood clots. The endometrium becomes accentuated as an echogenic line approximately one week before menstruation when the endometrium is hypertrophied and edematous. The edematous endometrium can be identified as a sonolucent band immediately beneath the lumen, but as menstruation occurs, the endometrium becomes echogenically prominent. In addition to the changes in the endometrium during the menstrual cycle, small amounts of free intraperitoneal fluid can be seen in the cul-de-sac at the time of ovulation. This fluid appears to regress later in the menstrual cycle (8).

Because of the echogenicity of the endometrium during menstruation, it may be difficult to localize an intrauterine contraceptive device (IUCD) at this time. However, the echogenic nature of the metal or plastic in the IUCD can usually be identified by its acoustical shadowing. The sonographic appearance of the various IUCDs that are commonly used, as well as a technique for localization, will be discussed in a later section in this chapter.

Because of the ovaries' loose attachment to the peritoneum, their position is variable and may change according to the patient's position during the study. The ovaries are elliptical structures that usually lie to either side of the uterine corpus and are best visualized on transverse scans (Figs. 3-1B, 2A); only rarely are both ovaries identified on the same transverse scan. They also can be seen posterior to the uterus or anterior to the fundus on longitudinal scans. The greatest length of the ovary should be no more than one-third to one-half the transverse diameter of the uterine corpus (31). Occasionally, follicles within the ovaries can be identified as small cystic structures of approximately 5 to 15 mm located within the ovary. Like the uterus, the ovaries can be observed to vary in size and consistency according to the patient's menstrual cycle and endocrinologic status (8) (Figs. 3-2B,C).

Ovaries of prepubertal girls may be difficult to delineate sonographically because of their small size. In postpubertal and ovulatory women, the ovaries measure from 2.5 to 4 cm along their greatest axis. Since the ovaries in postmenopausal women should be atrophic and not readily detected by palpation, adnexal masses that measure more than 3×5 cm or are easily palpable suggest a pathologic mass. Polycystic ovaries are seen as bilateral masses greater than 3 cm in diameter and have a complex sonographic appearance emanating from the multiple follicles that are contained within the ovary.

The fallopian tubes, or oviducts, are approximately 5 mm wide and have a serpiginous course. For these reasons, they are only infrequently visualized when they are not dilated. However, if these structures are distended with fluid, their fusiform shape and orientation through the "genital axis" can be recognized (Fig. 3-2D). They usually lie in a slightly oblique orientation lateral to the uterus and usually can be distinguished from fluid-filled small bowel loops by their lack of peristaltic motion and mucosal folds (Fig 4-16A) (24).

Figure 3-2. CYSTIC ADNEXAL MASSES

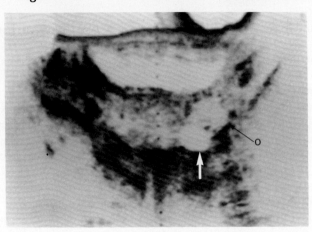

Figure 3-2A. Ovarian follicle before ovulation (transverse 3 cm above symphysis pubis). This transverse sonogram demonstrates a 1.5-cm cystic mass (*arrow*) in the periphery of the ovary (o), which represents a mature ovarian follicle. Serial examinations by ultrasound can be used to evaluate follicular maturation.

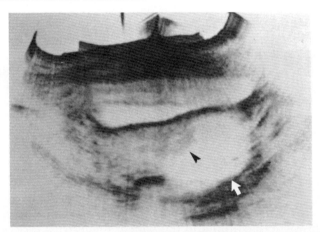

Figure 3-2B. Physiologic ovarian cyst (transverse, 4 cm above symphysis pubis). This cyst was 6 × 8 cm in size and regressed after estrogen therapy. The unaffected portion of the ovary is also seen (*arrowhead*). Serial sonograms can be used to document enlargement or regression of pelvic masses during and after appropriate therapy.

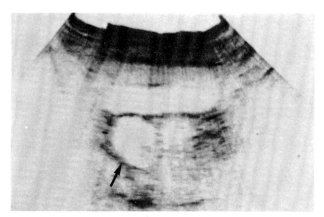

Figure 3-2C. Serous cystadenoma (transverse view, 4 cm above symphysis pubis). This cystic adnexal mass (*arrow*) failed to regress after estrogen therapy but has a sonographic appearance similar to that of an ovarian cyst. The combination of estrogen therapy and serial imaging aids in the differential diagnosis.

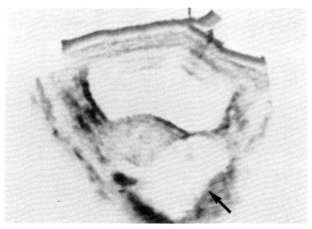

Figure 3-2D. Unilateral hydrosalpinx (transverse, 6 cm above symphysis pubis). This transverse pelvic sonogram demonstrates a tubular, sonolucent, distended oviduct filled with serous inflammatory fluid (*arrow*) to the left of the uterus.

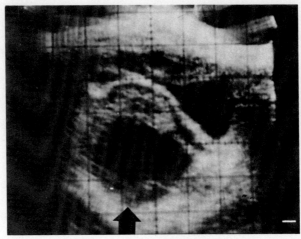

Figure 3-2E. Clear cell carcinoma in an endometrioma (transverse, 4 cm above symphysis pubis, white-on-black image). The thick posterior wall of this mass (*arrow*) suggested a neoplastic process. The thick wall could be distinguished from cellular debris within the mass since it did not change configuration when the patient was scanned in the decubitus position. The echogenic structure between the bladder and the cyst is the normal uterus.

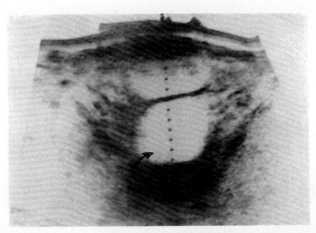

Figure 3-2F. Lymphoma metastatic to ovary (transverse, 4 cm above symphysis pubis). Even though this was a solid mass, its lack of interstitial components explains its sonolucent texture (*arrow*). Masses that are highly cellular and lack interstitial tissue, such as lymphomas and sarcomas, may exhibit a sonolucent texture.

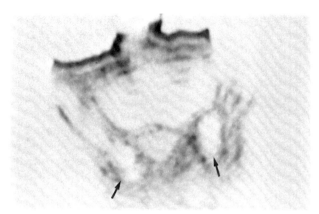

Figure 3-2G. Bilateral hydrosalpinx (transverse, 4 cm above symphysis pubis). Bilateral cystic fusiform masses are present on each side of the uterus (*arrows*). These can be differentiated from fluid-filled bowel loops because there are no mucosal markings.

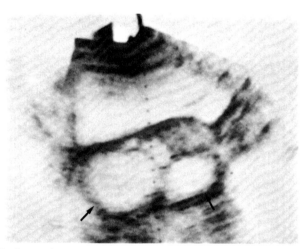

Figure 3-2H. Endometriomas (transverse, 6 cm above symphysis pubis). The multiple cystic adnexal masses (*arrows*) represent several endometriomas. They may contain echoes from hemorrhage and can rarely occur in patients without an abnormal menstrual history.

There are several other structures within the pelvis that may be identified on routine pelvic sonograms. Most important is the fluid-filled small bowel, which frequently mimics the sonographic appearance of a cystic pelvic mass. However, distended, fluid-filled loops of small bowel are usually fusiform and may demonstrate linear echoes emanating from their mucosal folds (24). Real-time scanning can be used to distinguish distended fluid-filled bowel from cystic pelvic masses since bowel will show evidence of peristaltic contractions. Peristaltic contraction of the bowel appears as a rapidly changing, echogenic pattern arising from trapped gas and succus entericus being passed through the bowel. If the sonogram is suggestive of the presence of distended, fluid-filled loops in the pelvis, one may obtain a supine and upright abdominal radiograph in order to determine if the radiographic signs of distended, fluid-filled bowel are present.

Recognition of the sonographic appearance of fluid-filled bowel is particularly useful, when a water enema technique is administered, for better evaluation of pelvic anatomy (6).

Vascular structures such as the internal iliac vein and distended lower ureter can also appear as tubular structures in the pelvic side walls. The veins will be seen to bifurcate on the longitudinal scan and appear as sonolucent dots related to the lateral pelvic wall on the transverse scan (Figs. 3-1C,D).

One should occasionally alter the scanning technique to increase the diagnostic information regarding a pelvic mass. If the patient is suspected of having a malignant pelvic mass, the liver and abdomen should be scanned to exclude the presence of metastatic deposits and/or ascites. Similarly, one may scan the patient in the Trendelenburg and decubitus position or with or without a distended bladder in order to ascertain the mobility of a mass within the pelvis. Masses that are attached to the anterior abdominal wall or the pelvic wall will not change their location after the bladder is empty. If the two masses can be delineated, the mass is probably extrauterine (5). Thus, maneuvers designed to gain specific information utilizing the capabilities of ultrasound can provide significant information about pelvic masses.

EVALUATION OF PELVIC MASSES

The following specific features seen on a sonographic image of a pelvic mass should be evaluated in order to formulate a proper differential diagnosis (Table 3-2). The major criteria that have been established for the sonographic evaluation of pelvic masses include:

1. Size, location, and organ of origin
2. Internal consistency
3. Definition of margins
4. Presence or absence of ascites or other metastatic lesions

Each of these will be discussed in detail, since they all pertain to the differential diagnosis of pelvic masses.

Size and Location

Visualizing the size of a pelvic mass assists in the differential diagnosis, in that only a few masses such as mucinous cystadenomas characteristically attain pelvoabdominal dimensions. Although it may be difficult to identify the origin of a large mass that distorts the pelvic landmarks, its location can be determined sonographically. As stated previously, whether a mass is uterine or extrauterine is of primary importance in establishing a proper differential diagnosis. In some patients, the organ of origin is difficult to identify, and the mass should be considered "indeterminate" in origin (Figs. 3-10A–F). Masses in this category include those created by bowel, fat, or lymphoma, and should be considered in the indeterminate category (22).

Recognition of the location of displaced bowel may suggest the major direction of growth of a pelvic mass and thus assist in the determination of its pelvic or

Table 3-2. Criteria for Sonographic Categorization of Pelvic Masses

Location, organ of origin, and size — unilateral or bilateral — adnexal / uterine / pelvoabdominal[a] / indeterminate

Internal consistency:
- cystic — homogeneous / fluid-fluid level / septated / solid foci
- complex — predominantly cystic / predominantly solid
- solid — mildly echogenic / moderately echogenic / markedly echogenic

Margins — well-defined / moderately well-defined / poorly defined

Ascites or other metastatic lesions — present / absent

[a]Can be uterine or extrauterine.

abdominal origin. For example, pelvic masses that enlarge in a cephalic direction displace bowel superiorly, whereas masses that enlarge from the abdomen in a caudal direction and displace bowel manifest inferior shadowing. As stated previously, the echogenic lumen of the uterus observed in menstruating patients can be used as a landmark for localizing a pelvic mass in relation to the uterus. The pelvic component of a large pelvoabdominal mass must be delineated so as not to confuse it with a large abdominal mass. Bilaterality can similarly favor a particular group of pelvic masses, such as Krukenberg tumors or polycystic ovary disease, which tend to involve both ovaries.

Internal Consistency

Gray scale sonography affords gross evaluation of the internal consistency of a mass (9). Cystic masses can be subdivided into those that are homogeneously cystic or septated, or those that exhibit internal solid foci (Figs. 3-2A–H, 3-3A–D, 3-4A–E). Complex masses can be subdivided according to the predominant internal component, that is complex, predominantly solid mass or complex predominantly cystic mass. Solid masses can be subdivided into those that are mildly, moderately, or markedly echogenic.

The echogenicity of a solid mass seems to be related to the amount, arrangement, elasticity of stromal components (collagen framework), degree of degeneration, and vascular supply (2). For example, lymphomas tend to be sonolucent,

Figure 3-3. COMPLETELY CYSTIC PELVOABDOMINAL MASSES

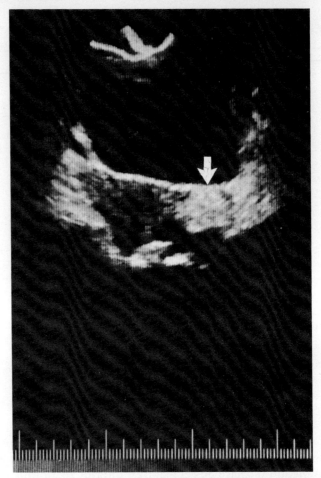

Figure 3-3A. Dermoid cyst (longitudinal, midline, white-on-black image). This dermoid cyst contained a hair ball and fat which appear as an echogenic focus (*arrow*).

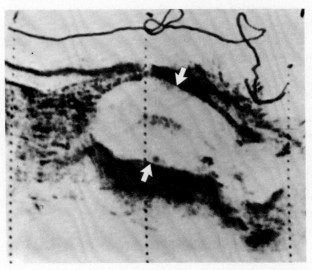

Figure 3-3B. Corpus hemorrhagicum (longitudinal, 2 cm to right of midline). This large cystic pelvoabdominal mass (*arrows*) originated from the ovary and represented chronic bleeding into an enlarging ovarian follicle. These masses can attain huge dimensions.

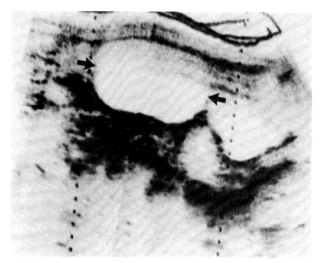

Figure 3-3C. Paraovarian cyst (longitudinal, 2 cm to right of midline). This cystic pelvic mass (*arrow*) was not related to the ovary but to a remnant of the Wolffian system or Gartner's duct.

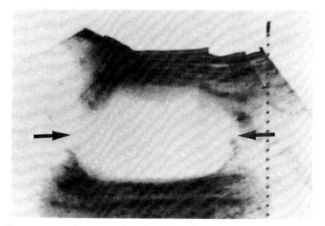

Figure 3-3D. Serous cystadenoma (longitudinal, 7 cm to left of midline). These masses present as large cystic pelvoabdominal masses (*arrows*) with a sonographic appearance similar to that of other benign conditions, such as dermoid cysts and corpus hemorrhagicum. The patient's age and clinical presentation are more important differential features than the sonographic pattern.

which probably reflects their high degree of cellularity and paucity of interstitial components. On the other hand, the majority of uterine leiomyomas have an echogenic texture. This feature probably reflects their dense arrangement of connective tissue and smooth muscle fibers. Sebum within a dermoid cyst, organized clot, pus, or soft tissue debris can also produce echoes within masses. Occasionally, pus and fluid within the cellular debris of inflammatory masses such as a tubo-ovarian abscess will exhibit an echogenic interface emanating from the fluid-pus layer (3). Cellular debris within a mass will be observed to change in position with patient movement, thus aiding in its differentiation from an unusually thick wall.

Figure 3-4. PREDOMINANTLY CYSTIC PELVIC MASSES WITH INTERNAL ECHOES

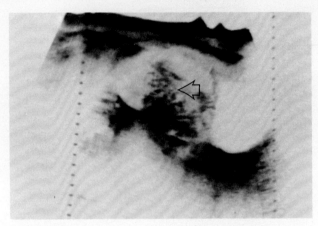

Figure 3-4A. Endometrioma containing clotted blood (longitudinal, 4 cm to left of midline). This transverse scan demonstrates the appearance of an endometrioma which contains clotted blood. Within the mass (*open arrow*) there are echoes arising from the clotted blood.

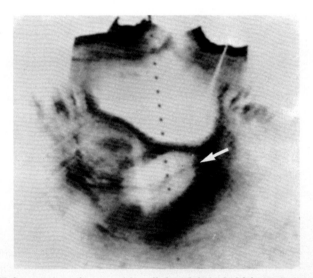

Figure 3-4B. Tubo-ovarian abscess with cellular debris-fluid layer (transverse, 4 cm to right of midline). This transverse scan demonstrates an interface arising from the cellular debris-fluid layer within the tubo-ovarian abscess (*arrow*). Echoes within a cyst are most commonly due to cellular debris, organized hemorrhage, sebum, or neoplasm.

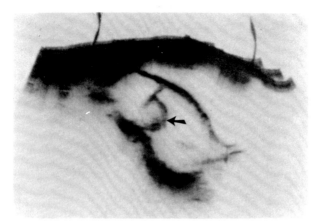

Figure 3-4C. Pelvic inflammatory disease entrapping bowel (longitudinal, 2 cm to right of midline). This pelvic inflammatory mass has surrounded the bowel, producing a cystic appearance with a focal area of echogenicity. The bowel loop is seen "end on" (*arrow*).

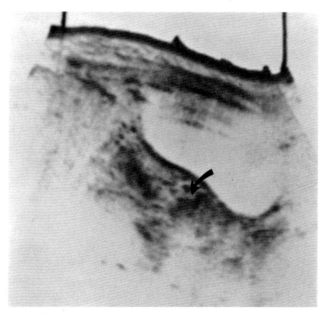

Figure 3-4D. Dermoid cyst (longitudinal, 2 cm to right of midline). This dermoid cyst contains sebum-producing echoes (*arrow*) as well as serous fluid, which appears sonolucent. The echogenic properties of the sebum prohibit adequate delineation of the mass. Only the most proximal portion of the dermoid cyst is demonstrated, resulting in the "tip of the iceberg" effect.

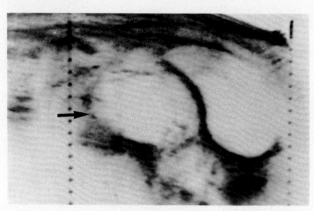

Figure 3-4E. Ectopic pregnancy (longitudinal, midline). Superior to the uterus is a sono-lucent mass, with focal soft tissue echoes arising from the embryonic pole of the gestational sac. An ectopic pregnancy should be considered when an adnexal mass associated with abdominal pain is encountered in a woman of reproductive age.

In general, the sonographic appearance of a pelvic mass is not a reliable indicator of its benign or malignant potential. As a rule, the more soft tissue components that can be identified within a cystic mass, the greater the likelihood that it is malignant. Another sonographic feature that suggests malignancy is the presence of ascites. Rarely ascites can be associated with benign ovarian masses such as ovarian fibroma that results in Meig's syndrome. Peritoneal or omental implants that appear as moderately echogenic, ill-defined areas along the peritoneum and omentum also suggest the presence of a malignant process.

Definition of Margins

The continuity of the soft tissue interfaces surrounding a mass is an important feature to evaluate by ultrasound. Marked irregularity of the border of the pelvic mass may suggest localized inflammatory or infiltrative process (Fig. 3-2E). Conversely, benign masses usually reveal a smooth border due to concentric compression of surrounding soft tissue. An example is an ovarian adenocarcinoma that had invaded the rectosigmoid colon and exhibited a markedly irregular border and indistinct mass-soft tissue interface. The thick irregular posterior wall of an endometrioma depicted in Figure 3-2E was correctly interpreted as a neoplasm. On pathological examination, this area was found to contain a focus of clear cell carcinoma.

Assessement of the margination of a mass by sonography may also suggest the presence of malignancy. For example, solid masses that cannot be separated from the bladder or colon suggest a malignant process. However, the margination of a mass as depicted by sonography cannot be relied upon for the absolute assessment of the malignant potential of a mass. When compared to sonography, computed body tomography (CBT) may better delineate invasion into surrounding organs. This can be seen by disruption or obscuring of fat planes that surround a mass. However, computerized body tomography (CBT) cannot always determine whether or not there is invasion of other organs because of the artifacts produced by partial volume averaging effect (15).

Presence or Absence of Ascites or Other Metastatic Lesions

Ultrasound studies can detect small amounts of intraperitoneal fluid. Fluid within the peritoneum appears as a sonolucent region, which if nonloculated tends to settle in the most dependent portions of the body. When the patient is supine, fluid tends to localize in the paracolic recesses, cul-de-sac, or the hepatorenal recess (Morrison's pouch). Loculated pockets of ascites can collect within the cul-de-sac or in Morrison's pouch and may simulate the sonographic features of a cystic mass.

Metastatic involvement of the omentum can occasionally be recognized as a relatively sonolucent band beneath the anterior abdominal wall (28). The omental band results from thickening of the omentum secondary to metastatic infiltration by neoplastic cells. Metastatic disease involving the omentum is most commonly encountered in ovarian carcinoma.

DIFFERENTIAL DIAGNOSIS OF PELVIC MASSES

The following discussion of the sonographic evaluation of pelvic masses is organized into three main categories according to the predominant appearance of the mass by ultrasound (See Tables 3-3A,B,C). Only the most common pelvic masses in each category will be discussed, with the uncommon and rare masses considered as they relate to the differential diagnosis of certain categories of common pelvic masses. Masses that are difficult to localize to a particular organ or category are considered "indeterminate."

The schemes for differential diagnosis of pelvic masses are organized in a similar manner to the "Gamut" approach of Reeder and Felson for radiologic differential diagnoses (26). Although exceptions to these schemes will undoubtedly occur, it is again emphasized that one should attempt to assess all clinically relevant features of a pelvic mass rather than endeavor to provide a specific diagnosis. Instead of listing diagnostic possibilities, one should confine the differential diagnosis to the most probable based on sonographic and clinical findings. Since pelvic masses exhibit a variety of sonographic appearances, certain ones are listed in more than one category. Clinical features that may be helpful in distinguishing the different types of pelvic masses are mentioned in the discussion.

Cystic Masses

Although physiologic (functional) ovarian cysts are the most frequently encountered type of cystic pelvic mass, several different types of masses reveal a similar sonographic appearance (9). For example, a follicular cyst (Figs. 3-2A,B), serous cystadenoma (Fig. 3-2C), and markedly distended oviduct from pelvic inflammatory disease or so-called hydrosalpinx (Fig. 3-2D) are sonographically indistinguishable from one another. Inflammatory or neoplastic cystic masses can be occasionally differentiated from benign cystic lesions by their unusually thick walls or low-level internal echoes that correspond to internal areas of hemorrhage, soft tissue debris, or proteinaceous material (3). A markedly thickened cyst wall secondary to torsion is demonstrated in some cases.

Table 3-3A. Sonographic Differential Diagnosis of Gynecological Pelvic Masses

		CYSTIC	
Location	Adnexal	Pelvoabdominal	Adnexal or pelvoabdominal
Internal consistency	Homogeneous	Septated	Solid foci
Definition of borders	Well-defined	Well- to moderately well-defined	Well- to moderately well-defined
COMMON	Physiological ovarian cyst	Mucinous cystadenoma (carcinoma)[a]	Dermoid cyst
	Serous cystadenoma[a]		Ectopic pregnancy
	Hydrosalpinx		
	Endometrioma(s)[b]		
UNCOMMON	Dermoid cyst	Serous cystadenoma (carcinoma)[a]	Tubo-ovarian abscess[a]
	Paraovarian cyst	Loculated lymphocele	
		Loculated pelvic abscess	
RARE	Lymphocele		
	Appendiceal abscess[b]		
	Mesenteric cyst[a]		
	Peritoneal inclusion cyst		
	Ureterocele[b]		

[a]May present as pelvoabdominal mass.
[b]Can be multiple

Solitary cysts in the pelvis can be differentiated from multiple cystic pelvic masses. Solitary cystic pelvic lesions are frequently ovarian cysts. Multiple cystic masses can be differentiated from those that contain numerous cysts. For example, polycystic ovaries reveal several follicles within the outline of the ovary, as opposed to the numerous cystic masses of various sizes seen in some patients with endometriosis. Multiple follicular cysts of the ovary simulate the findings of multiple cystic endometriomas, and are encountered most frequently in patients taking fertility drugs. Multiloculated cysts can be differentiated from masses that have numerous cysts within them, since multiloculated cystic areas will be contained within the outline of the mass, as opposed to multicystic masses that will contain several rounded masses within a single organ.

Homogeneous, Adnexal

Physiological Ovarian Cysts. Physiological or functional ovarian cysts usually appear as well-circumscribed, spherical, sonolucent masses that average 3 to 4 cm

Table 3-3B. Sonographic Differential Diagnosis of Gynecological Pelvic Masses

		COMPLEX		
Location	Uterine	Uterine	Extrauterine	Extrauterine
Internal consistency	Predominantly cystic	Predominantly solid	Predominantly cystic	Predominantly solid
Definition of borders	Variable	Well- to moderately well-defined	Moderately well-defined	Well- to moderately well-defined
COMMON	Intrauterine pregnancy	Uterine leiomyoma[a]	Tubo-ovarian abscess[a]	Degenerated or partially cystic solid ovarian tumor[a]
			Ectopic pregnancy Ovarian cystadenoma (carcinoma)[a]	
UNCOMMON	Pyometrium	Uterine leiomyosarcoma	Fluid-filled loops of bowel	
	Adenomyosis	Endometrial carcinoma[a]		
RARE	Invasive trophoblastic tumor		Polycystic ovaries[b]	

[a]May present as pelvoabdominal mass.
[b]Usually bilateral.

Table 3-3C. Sonographic Differential Diagnosis of Gynecological Pelvic Masses

		SOLID	
Location	Uterine	Extrauterine	Indeterminate
Internal consistency	Moderately echogenic	Mildly to moderately echogenic	Variable
Definition of borders	Well-defined	Moderately well-defined	Variable
COMMON	Uterine leiomyoma[a]	Solid ovarian tumor (fibroma, teratoma, adenocarcinoma)[a]	Bowel
UNCOMMON	Endometrial carcinoma or sarcoma	Pedunculated leiomyoma	Lymphadenopathy[b]
	Uterine leiomyosarcoma	Lymphoma[a]	Intraperitoneal fat
RARE			Retroperitoneal tumor
			Ectopic pelvic kidney

[a]May present as pelvoabdominal mass.
[b]Usually multiple.

in diameter (Figs. 3-2A,B). Cystic non-neoplastic masses of the ovary can reach pelvoabdominal dimensions, such as masses created by large corpus hemorrhagicum. In some patients, hemorrhage or clot within the cyst is identified by echogenic areas within the mass (Fig. 3-4A). The regression of functional ovarian cysts after a clinical trial of estrogen suppression or during the menstrual cycle can be documented by serial sonographic examination. Because the signs of torsion are often subtle, this condition is difficult to detect sonographically. However, if torsion has been present for a few days, thickening of the cyst wall, as well as a fluid-clot level within the cyst, will sometimes be demonstrated.

Serous Cystadenomas. In general, serous cystadenomas and other epithelial ovarian tumors occur most frequently in postmenopausal women. Clinically, a serous cystadenoma may be suspected clinically in a patient with a palpable cystic adnexal mass that fails to regress after a trial of estrogen suppression. The type of cystadenoma (mucinous or serous) depends on the consistency of the material that is elaborated by the epithelium of the cyst. Another variant of an epithelial ovarian cystic tumor is the papillary serous cystadenoma. Papillary projections can be recognized within the mass. These neoplasms tend to have a significant solid component.

As stated previously, serous cystadenomas of less than 5 cm usually exhibit a sonographic appearance that is indistinguishable from that of other cystic adnexal masses (Fig. 3-2C). Serous cystadenomas tend to appear as sonolucent masses without septations. Large serous cystadenomas can occasionally be differentiated from mucinous cystadenomas since internal septations are somewhat less common in the serous variety. Serous types are more frequently bilateral (15% of cases) than the mucinous (30). A corpus hemorrhagicum that is large may also simulate the sonographic appearance of a large serous cystadenoma (Figs. 3-3B,C,D).

Hydrosalpinx. The fallopian tubes or oviducts, because of their small caliber (approximately 5 mm) and serpiginous course, cannot be routinely delineated in the nondistended state. However, when they become distended with inflammatory material or serous secretions as a result of tubal inflammation, these structures are seen as fusiform sonolucent adnexal masses (Fig. 3-2D). Unilateral hydrosalpinx is found with increasing frequency as a sequela to pelvic inflammation associated with intrauterine contraceptive devices (IUCD) or previous tubal surgery. When the oviducts become massively distended with serous fluid, they will have the appearance of cystic adnexal masses or fluid-filled loops of small bowel. Peristalsis can be demonstrated in a bowel loop by real-time scanning. In addition, the echoes emanating from the mucosal folds and small bowel will not be delineated in distended oviducts.

Multiple, Extrauterine

Endometriomas. Endometriosis is usually encountered in women in their second and third decades. They may be infertile, and often present with a complaint of dysmenorrhea. Sonographically, endometriomas exhibit a similar appearance to that of other cystic adnexal masses except that they are usually multiple and of various sizes (from 0.5 up to 15 cm) (Fig. 3-2H). Low-level echoes can be observed within endometriomas when they contain organized clot. Low-level internal echoes may also be encountered in tubo-ovarian abscesses secondary to pus and dermoid cysts where the echoes arise from the sebum within the mass. In some patients with endometriosis, no definite sonographic abnormality will be demonstrated, although there is strong clinical evidence. In these patients, extensive fibrosis in the pelvis is seen at laparoscopy. Another pattern that is frequently encountered on ultrasound studies of endometrioma is a septated pattern. Because its appearance is similar to that of a cystadenoma, these two entities may be sonographically indistinguishable (13).

Septated, Extrauterine

Mucinous Cystadenomas. Patients with mucinous cystadenoma are usually post-menopausal and experience asymptomatic abdominal enlargement. Sonographically, the numerous thin septations seen within these cystic pelvic and pelvoabdominal masses are highly specific for this entity (greater than 90% pattern specificity) (9). The multiplicity of the internal septations does not appear to correlate with the degree of malignancy since masses with a complex internal arrangement can be benign (Fig. 3-5C, D). Mucinous cystadenomas often contain low-level echoes; a reflection of the mucinous material within the mass that has a high protein content.

Predominantly cystic pelvoabdominal masses that contain irregular internal septations or are associated with ascites are more frequently malignant than benign (Figs. 3-5A–G). Collections of ascitic fluid are most commonly found in the perihepatic, paracolic recess or in the cul-de-sac. The number of septations within a cystadenoma does not reflect its malignant potential but seems to correlate with the rate of growth of the mass.

Solid Foci, Extrauterine

Dermoid Cyst. Dermoid cysts of the ovary are commonly encountered in 15- to 30-year-old women. The masses do not usually cause symptoms unless they undergo

Figure 3-5. SEPTATED CYSTIC MASSES

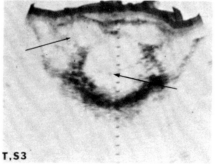

T,S3

Figure 3-5A. Endometrioma (transverse, 3 cm above symphysis pubis). Endometriomas commonly contain internal septation (*arrows*). They may also be sonolucent or contain focal echoes arising from clotted blood.

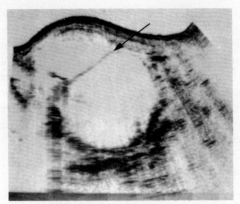

Figure 3-5B. Dermoid cyst (transverse, 4 cm above symphysis pubis). Dermoid cysts may also contain internal septations (*arrow*).

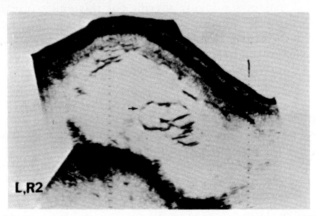

Figure 3-5C. Mucinous cystadenoma (longitudinal, 2 cm to right of midline). This is the typical appearance of a mucinous cystadenoma with multiple septations, (*small arrow*) in a predominantly cystic pelvoabdominal mass.

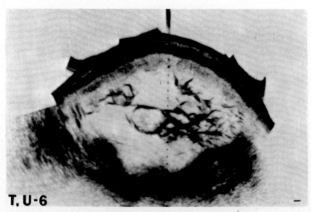

Figure 3-5D. Mucinous cystadenoma (transverse, 4 cm above symphysis pubis, same patient as in Figure 3-5C). This scan demonstrates the numerous septations within the mass (*small arrow*). The number of septations does not correlate with malignancy.

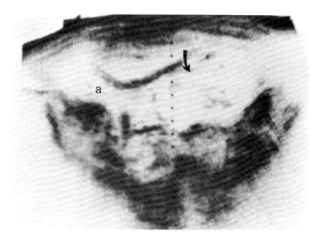

Figure 3-5E. Mucinous cystadenocarcinoma (transverse, 4 cm above symphysis pubis). This cystic pelvoabdominal mass (*curved arrow*) was associated with ascites (a).

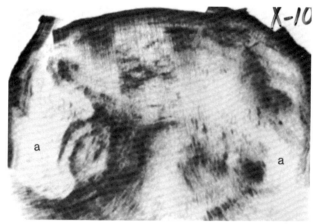

Figure 3-5F. Mucinous cystadenocarcinoma (transverse, 10 cm below xiphoid). Upper abdominal transverse sonogram demonstrates ascites as fluid collections in both paracolic recesses (a). The presence of ascitic fluid and a pelvic mass suggests malignancy.

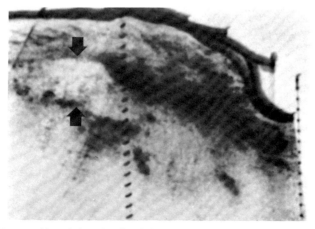

Figure 3-5G. Omental band (longitudinal, 2 cm to right of midline). The mildly echogenic mass immediately beneath the anterior abdominal wall represents infiltration of the omentum by tumor cells (*arrow*). This is frequently associated with ovarian carcinomas.

torsion. Since the majority of dermoid cysts are pedunculated, they are commonly located anterior to the uterine fundus. This is felt to be movement into available space. Dermoid cysts may also be discovered for the first time during pregnancy, when they become readily palpable due to elevation out of the pelvis by a large uterus.

The appearance of dermoid cysts on ultrasound images varies from completely sonolucent to homogeneously echogenic masses, depending on internal consistency (Figs. 3-3A, 3-4D, 3-5D). Dermoid cysts that are lined by neuroectoderm secrete a cerebrospinal fluid-like fluid that is completely sonolucent. Some dermoid cysts contain a soft tissue pole within a predominantly cystic mass. Because of the favorable imaging circumstance, this can be outlined sonographically. The most common pattern for dermoid cysts is a complex pelvic mass that has areas of high echogenicity with posterior acoustical shadowing within it. The areas of high echogenicity and posterior acoustical shadowing correspond to calcification within the dermoid cyst, whereas the sebaceous material is moderately to highly echogenic. This component can be so highly reflective as to result in the inability to delineate the posterior aspect of the mass to produce the "tip of the iceberg" effect (12). Dermoid cysts will occasionally be encountered when a pelvic mass is palpable but no mass lesion is defined on sonography. In these cases, the sebum within the dermoid cysts may simulate the sonographic appearance of a gas-filled loop of bowel and, thus, fail to be detected. A pelvic radiograph may be helpful in detecting signs of radiolucency or calcifications associated with a dermoid cyst in those patients for whom a sonogram fails to define an abnormality (32).

Complex Masses

In general, complex masses contain both fluid, which appears as a sonolucent collection, and solid components, which are echogenic. Consequently, this group of pelvic lesions consists primarily of soft tissue masses that have undergone cystic internal degeneration or cystic masses that contain soft tissue, organized clot, and/or cellular debris (Figs. 3-6A–E). Granulosa cell tumors and dysgerminomas are examples of tumors that characteristically undergo cystic degeneration as they enlarge and thus appear sonographically as complex structures having both components of soft tissue and fluid appearances (30).

Predominantly Cystic, Extrauterine

Ectopic Pregnancy. Clinically, patients with an ectopic pregnancy usually present with a palpable adnexal mass and if rupture or intraperitoneal bleeding has occurred, acute blood loss and/or physical signs of peritoneal irritation. Because approximately three out of four patients with an ectopic pregnancy will have uterine bleeding, the presentation of patients with this condition is frequently perplexing. A positive pregnancy test can be found in most patients with an ectopic pregnancy. Therefore, it is important in evaluating a complex mass in the pelvis to know whether or not the patient has a positive pregnancy test and what type of pregnancy test was performed.

Whenever a complex adnexal mass is encountered in a woman of reproductive age or in a woman who has a history of pelvic inflammatory disease and is amenorrehic, an ectopic pregnancy should be considered (Fig. 3-4E). Because gestational sacs formed outside the uterus do not usually exhibit the rounded, well-defined appearance of an intrauterine gestational sac, this condition can be easily confused with other complex-appearing adnexal masses (9). In some patients, only secondary signs of an ectopic gestation, such as a cul-de-sac hematoma, free intraperitoneal fluid, unclotted blood, or a slightly enlarged uterus with an echogenic lumen, can be documented. For this reason, one should not be dissuaded from further evaluation in patients with a clinically suspected ectopic pregnancy in whom ultrasound studies are not diagnostic since rupture may lead to profuse intraperitoneal bleeding.

As stated in the section devoted to sonographic evaluation of patients with first trimester bleeding in Chapter 2, the sonographic appearance of an ectopic pregnancy depends on whether or not rupture of the oviduct and bleeding have occurred. Patients with chronic ectopic pregnancies frequently present for the first time with intermittent fever and a pelvic mass. These patients may not have a history of abdominal pain. Sonographically, chronic ectopic pregnancies usually appear as a mildly echogenic, ill-defined retrouterine mass that causes an apparent enlargement of the uterine outline. This is due to failure to delineate the interface between the hematoma posterior to the uterus and the uterus itself.

Tubo-ovarian Abscess. When inflammatory fluid or cellular debris is contained within a distended oviduct, a complex mass containing an echogenic material within a tubular adnexal structure is seen (Fig. 3-4B). The inflammatory fluid will sometimes layer out, causing a fluid-cellular debris interface within a predominantly cystic mass. At present, tubo-ovarian abscesses cannot be reliably differentiated from a hydrosalpinx that is contained entirely within the oviduct. Distended, fluid-filled loops of small or large bowel may also simulate the sonographic findings observed in tubo-ovarian abscesses, although the mucosal folds

Figure 3-6. COMPLEX PELVIC MASSES

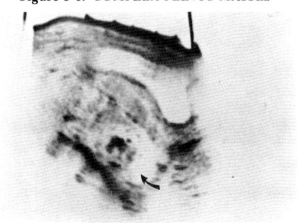

Figure 3-6A. Ruptured ectopic pregnancy (longitudinal, midline). Scan demonstrates a complex mass posterior to the uterus (*curved arrow*). The gestational sac and fetal parts are demonstrated with a uterus imposed between the bladder and the mass.

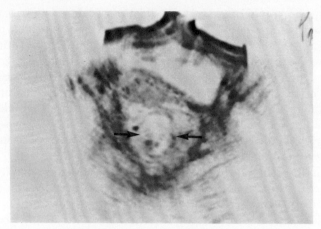

Figure 3-6B. Ruptured ectopic pregnancy (transverse, 4 cm above symphysis pubis, same patient as in Figure 3-6A). This scan again demonstrates the complex mass outside the uterus which corresponds to a gestational sac (*arrows*) and hematoma around the ruptured ectopic pregnancy.

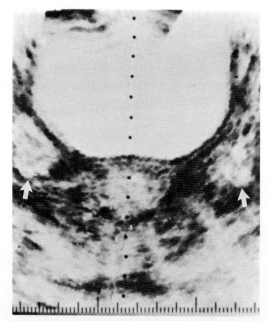

Figure 3-6C. Polycystic ovaries (transverse, 4 cm above symphysis pubis). This scan demonstrates bilateral enlargement of the ovaries, which contain well-defined cystic follicles (*arrow*). The patient had Stein-Leventhal syndrome.

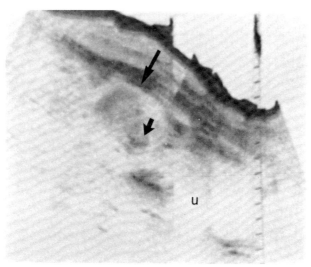

Figure 3-6D. Dermoid cyst (longitudinal, midline). Dermoid cyst (*large arrow*) contains large forms of echogenic sebum (*small arrow*) and is located anterior to the uterus (U).

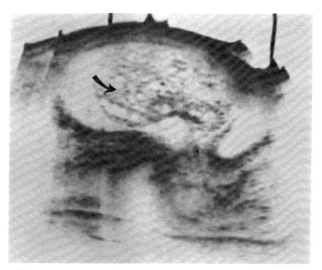

Figure 3-6E. Papillary ovarian cystadenocarcinoma (longitudinal, midline). This complex mass contains numerous septations and solid areas (*arrow*). In general, the more solid the components of a complex mass, the more likely it is malignant.

will not be evident (29). Bowel loops are sometimes trapped within tubo-ovarian abscesses, which results in a complex echo pattern consisting of a cystic mass with an echogenic area within it.

Predominantly Solid, Extrauterine

Ovarian Tumors. As stated previously, dermoid cysts demonstrate a wide variety of sonographic patterns. About one-third of dermoid cysts exhibit a complex, predominantly solid sonographic appearance containing at least one focus of high-level echoes (Fig. 3-6D). The sebaceous material within a dermoid cyst causes the diffuse echo pattern and occasional difficulty in delineating its posterior wall (12).

Other ovarian tumors that exhibit an echogenic or complex appearance include granulosa cell tumors, dysgerminomas, and teratocarcinomas. The latter usually contain cystic areas within the mass. Papillary serous cystadenomas appear as predominantly solid masses but also exhibit a complex sonographic pattern. Markedly irregular internal architecture of a mass suggests a malignant process.

Solid Masses

The majority of soft tissue masses exhibit an echogenic texture that can be enhanced by increasing the sensitivity or gain setting. Scans using a transducer of higher frequency (3.5- and 5-MHz) may also show diminished penetration of a solid mass when compared with scans obtained with standard transducers (2.25-MHz). As stated previously, the echogenicity of solid masses seems to be related to the amount and arrangement of their interstitial components (2) (Figs. 3-7A–D).

Uterine

Uterine Leiomyoma. In general, the sonographic appearance of uterine leiomyomas depends on the amount and type of internal degeneration within the mass. The echogenicity of the leiomyomas depends on the relative amount of collagen and smooth muscle, as well as the presence and type of degeneration (Figs. 3-8A,E). When leiomyomas contain a large connective tissue component, they usually

Figure 3-7. SOLID, EXTRAUTERINE PELVIC MASSES

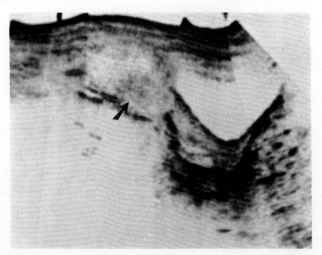

Figure 3-7A. Ovarian teratoma (longitudinal, 2 cm to right of midline). Solid ovarian mass (*arrow*) is located adjacent to the uterine fundus and results in apparent enlargement of the uterine outline ("indefinite uterus sign").

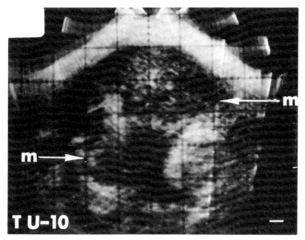

Figure 3-7B. Krukenberg tumors (transverse, 10 cm above symphysis pubis, white-on-black image). This patient had a primary tumor of the colon, and bilateral solid pelvic masses (m) were demonstrated on sonography. These masses were found to represent bilateral ovarian metastases from the colonic tumor.

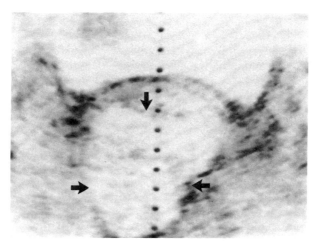

Figure 3-7C. Ovarian adenocarcinoma (transverse magnified view, 4 cm above symphysis pubis). There is a solid mass in the adnexae (*arrows*) representing adenocarcinoma of the ovary.

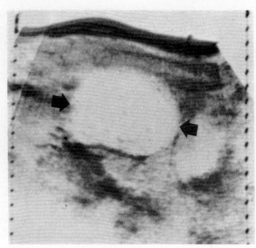

Figure 3-7D. Lymphoma metastatic to the ovary (longitudinal, 2 cm to right of midline). This patient had a known B-cell lymphoma and presented with a pelvic mass (*arrows*). The mass demonstrates no internal echoes and poor through transmission of ultrasound. This feature is frequently encountered in lymphomatous masses and is probably due to their highly cellular composition.

appear as echogenic. Leiomyomas that consist of primarily smooth muscle and are very vascular frequently appear only mildly to moderately echogenic. Areas of hyaline and cystic degeneration within leiomyomas are demonstrated as areas of relative sonolucency with increased through transmission by comparison with the myometrium. Calcification within leiomyomas is depicted as areas of high-level echogenicity with posterior acoustical shadowing.

Ultrasound is of clinical importance in the evaluation of a leiomyoma because it makes it possible to establish the location and size of these lesions. For example, a pedunculated subserosal leiomyoma can be differentiated from an intramural one. Intramural leiomyomas are contained within the wall of the uterus and tend to cause nodular enlargement of the uterine outline, whereas pedunculated leiomyomas do not change the shape of the uterus but are attached by a pedicle. The pedunculated nature of the mass can sometimes be documented by scans taken with a small amount of pressure placed over the mass in an attempt to separate the mass from the uterus (5). In addition, an intramural leiomyoma can be detected as an area of diminished echogenicity by comparison with the moderately echogenic myometrium.

Because the sonographic appearance of leiomyomas is indistinguishable from that of other uterine tumors such as uterine sarcoma and endometrial carcinoma, differentiation between these entities may not always be reliable. Similarly, predictions concerning the benign or malignant properties of uterine leiomyomas based on the sonographic appearance are not always accurate. The spectrum of ultrasound patterns of leiomyomas is discussed in detail in the section devoted to uterine masses. Sonography can also be helpful in localizing an intrauterine tandem when radiotherapy is applied to the uterus (33).

Figure 3-8. UTERINE LEIOMYOMATA

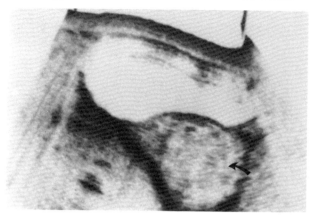

Figure 3-8A. Intramural leiomyoma (longitudinal, 1 cm to left of midline). There is an echogenic mass (*curved arrow*) within the uterine outline representing an intramural leiomyoma. Tumors of this kind frequently appear as echogenic masses that cause nodular enlargement of the uterine outline.

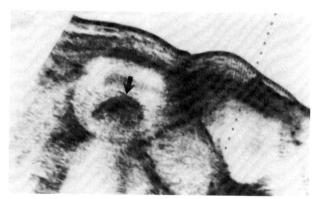

Figure 3-8B. Calcified uterine leiomyoma (longitudinal, 6 cm to right of midline). Calcification within the leiomyoma appears as an echogenic area (*arrow*) associated with distal acoustical shadowing. (Courtesy of Roger Sanders, M.D.)

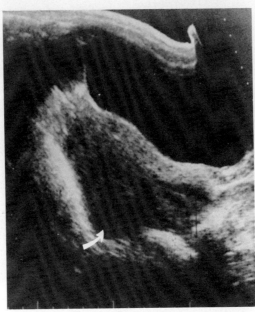

Figure 3-8C. Leiomyoma containing hyaline degeneration (longitudinal, midline, white-on-black image). This intramural leiomyoma exhibits a sonolucent area (*curved arrow*) that represents hyaline degeneration. (Courtesy of Thomas Lawson, M.D.)

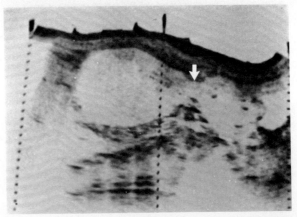

Figure 3-8D. Pedunculated subserosal leiomyoma (longitudinal, midline). There is a solid mass that appears to be attached to the uterine fundus (*arrow*).

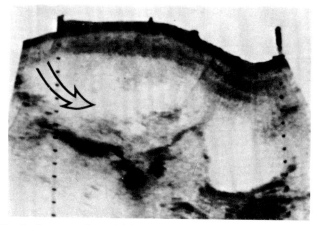

Figure 3-8E. Cystic degeneration within a "parasitic" leiomyoma (longitudinal, 4 cm to right of midline). There is a complex mass, separate from the uterus, which contains a cystic component (*open arrow*). This mass was found to represent a leiomyoma that had become "parasitic", deriving its blood supply from the omentum. There was cystic material within the mass from internal degeneration.

Solid, Extrauterine

Solid Ovarian Tumor. In general, soft tissue ovarian tumors are less common than cystic ones. Small solid ovarian tumors can sometimes be difficult to delineate because they have the same acoustical properties as surrounding soft tissue (Fig. 3-7C). Benign solid ovarian tumors include ovarian fibromas (Brenner tumor) and thecomas, whereas adenocarcinomas, metastatic ovarian tumors (including Krukenberg tumor), and solid teratomas represent malignant varieties. The Krukenberg tumor, which is defined as metastatic involvement of the ovary from a gastrointestinal tract neoplasm, produces many internal echoes and moderately good through-transmission (Fig. 3-7B). This is thought to be related to its mucinous matrix (16). Even though metastatic involvement of the ovary by lymphoma produces a solid mass, a lymphomatous ovarian mass is usually seen as an area of low echogenicity. This appearance reflects a paucity of stromal elements and a high degree of cellularity.

Solid, Indeterminate

Lymphomatous Masses. Lymphadenopathy is a general term used to signify pathologic enlargement of the lymph nodes. This may be due to benign hyperplasia but may also be due to neoplastic involvement. The sonographic appearance of lymphadenopathy is discussed in detail in Chapter 4. Whether or not lymphadenopathy is present is important in evaluating gynecologic tumors because it may alter therapy. However, sonography is not a reliable method for establishing the presence of small- to medium-size lymph nodes within the pelvis; large nodes measuring at least 1.5 cm can be detected by ultrasound. Enlarged nodes in the para-aortic chain are readily delineated. Mesenteric lymphadenopathy can be differentiated from para-aortic nodes based on the oval shape and proximity to the root of the mesentery (27). This is discussed in detail in Chapter 4.

Lymphomatous masses usually produce low-level internal echoes which, as we have stated, reflects their high degree of cellularity and paucity of interstitial components. As in the patient with metastatic B-cell lymphoma to the ovary, lymphomatous masses may even appear completely sonolucent (Fig. 3-10G).

Bowel. Occasionally, collapsed, mucous-containing or fecal-filled small and large bowel or gastrointestinal tract neoplasms are misdiagnosed as a complex or solid pelvic mass (24). Frequently, bowel tumors appear as a complex mass with a central area of echogenicity and a sonolucent halo. Fluid-filled bowel appears as a sonolucent tubular structure and may occasionally be identified by the presence of its mucosal folds. Peristalsis can be recognized using real-time sonography. The nature of a mass arising in the colon can be documented by using a water enema technique (6). Another advantage of this technique is that it enables the sonologist to evaluate the uterine cervix; fluid within the bowel and the uterus can surround the lower uterine segment and cervix, making it sonographically accessible.

DIAGNOSTIC ACCURACY

When combined with clinical and laboratory data, gray scale sonography can determine the presence, size, location, and consistency of a pelvic mass with approximately 90% accuracy (14). However, the specificity of this method in determining the histologic type of a pelvic mass is only 60 to 70% accurate. Ultrasound studies portray the morphology of a mass and do not directly reflect histologic consistency at present. Specific diagnosis can be formulated on the basis of the sonographic pattern and clinical presentation.

Certain sonographic patterns have proved to be quite specific. The most notable of these is the septated pattern seen almost exclusively in mucinous cystadenomas and mucinous cystadenocarcinomas. The majority of pelvic masses, however, exhibit nonspecific sonographic features. This makes it very important to combine clinical data from the patient with information desired from the sonographic pattern to formulate the most likely diagnosis.

In general, false-positive and false-negative sonographic examinations of pelvic masses are less than 5% (9,14). The majority of errors that occur can be attributed either to poor scanning technique (such as improper angulation of the transducer) or gain setting or to lesion size below the scanning resolution (less than 2 cm) (9,14). Small, solid pelvic masses whose acoustical properties are similar to those of surrounding soft tissue can also be the source of the false-negative diagnosis. Misinterpretation of a collapsed or fluid-filled bowel can be a frequent cause of diagnostic errors.

EVALUATION OF UTERINE MASSES

The uterus can be evaluated by a number of direct and indirect techniques, including pelvic examination, histology, hysteroscopy, and hysterosalpinography. Ultrasound studies are not as clinically important in analysis of the uterus as in

Table 3-4. Sonographic Features of Various Uterine Disorders

Tumors	
Leiomyoma	Nonhomogeneous mass that causes nodular enlargement of the uterine outline
	Cystic degeneration emanates focal areas of sonolucency
	Calcification depicted as echogenic areas with shadowing
	Becomes more sonolucent with pregnancy
	Enlarges during pregnancy
Leiomyosarcoma	Indistinguishable from benign leiomyoma
Adenocarcinoma of the endometrium or uterine sarcoma	Irregular enlargement of uterine outline
	Various degrees of internal degeneration
	Distorted parenchymal texture
	Contiguous involvement of bladder, colon may occur
Inflammatory conditions	
Pyometritis	Sonolucent and irregularly widened uterine lumen
Congenital	
Hemato (hydro) metrocolpos	Distended uterus and vagina with sonolucent mass
	May contain echogenic areas due to organized clot
Bicornate uterus	Binodular uterine outline, especially seen on transverse scan
Acquired	
Adenomyosis	"Swiss cheese" appearance of myometrium

evaluation of adnexal lesions. The role of ultrasound is sometimes limited because of the lack of specificity of the sonographic findings in many of the uterine neoplasms. Ultrasound is frequently helpful in establishing that a mass is uterine rather than adnexal in origin. Also, with ultrasound we are able to visualize the parenchymal texture of the uterus. This may be important in detecting certain pathological entities at an earlier stage than was previously possible in that neither distortion of the organ outline nor the formation of a recognizable mass need to have taken place (Table 3-4).

By far the most common uterine mass that will be encountered is the leiomyoma or so-called fibroid. This tumor consists of connective tissue and smooth muscle in variable distribution and is present in approximately one out of four women of reproductive age (30). Since leiomyomas frequently enlarge during pregnancy, sonography is particularly useful in evaluating leiomyomas, that are found in gravid patients. These masses can be serially examined by ultrasound for enlargement and/or extent of internal degeneration and necrosis.

The ultrasound patterns associated with leiomyomas range from sonolucent to moderately echogenic, depending on their composition, type, and extent of internal degeneration (13). The most common ultrasound pattern observed in leiomyomas reveals a moderately echogenic mass that distorts the uterine outline. Leiomyomas that consist primarily of smooth muscle are seen as almost totally sonolucent masses and sometimes appear almost identical to cystic masses (Fig. 3-8C). However, this type of leiomyoma does not exhibit the posterior wall enhancement that commonly is seen in cystic uterine masses. Therefore, scanning using different techniques may be helpful. Leiomyomas that consist of equal composition of smooth muscle and connective tissue appear as moderately echogenic masses that can be distinguished from the normally mildly echogenic myometrium by a fairly subtle difference in texture pattern. The echoes will be coarser and not so closely spaced. These masses may also have a moderately well-defined margin due to their fibrous reaction around the tumor. Intramural leiomyomas are frequently recognized by their nodular enlargement on the uterine outline (Figs. 3-8A,B). Subserosal leiomyomas may be pedunculated and have a tendency to undergo necrosis. They are occasionally seen on ultrasound outside the uterus and may be confused with other adnexal or solid lesions. Leiomyomas that are subserosal become "parasitic" when they derive their blood supply from surrounding bowel and mesentery. In general, leiomyomas that are observed to extend into the uterine lumen may be better evaluated by hysterosalpingography.

Cystic degeneration within leiomyomas is depicted as an irregular area of sonolucency in a mass that shows posterior wall enhancement. Hyaline degeneration will also appear as a sonolucent area within the leiomyoma but usually does not exhibit posterior acoustical enhancement as areas of cystic necrosis. Calcific degeneration within leiomyomas is seen as focal areas of high-amplitude echoes with posterior acoustical shadowing. If the calcification is located along the anterior aspect of the mass, it may be difficult to outline the remainder of the mass because of shadowing. Therefore, one should be very cautious in estimating size and extent of this type of leiomyoma.

Pedunculated leiomyomas usually appear as masses separate from the uterus. If a pedunculated leiomyoma is thought to be present, one can use the technique of placing gentle pressure between the mass and uterus. This pressure should only be sufficient to delineate the pedicle of the mass (6).

A bicornuate or partially septated uterus will simulate an intramural or subserosal leiomyoma on ultrasound. However, during menstruation, both lumina will be echogenic, giving an appearance distinctly unlike that of a leiomyoma. One horn of the bicornuate uterus may be obstructed, giving an enlarged outline. In general, the bicornuate uterus has a binodular outline, especially noted on the transverse sonogram (Fig. 3-9A).

Benign and malignant uterine masses are so similar in presentation that it is impossible to distinguish leiomyosarcomas and other malignant uterine tumors from benign leiomyomas in ultrasound studies (Figs. 3-9B,C). Endometrial carcinomas, uterine sarcomas, and leiomyosarcomas demonstrate enlargement of the uterus and an inhomogeneous internal texture (Fig. 3-9D). Areas of localized hemorrhagic necrosis in the myometrium, such as seen in cases of chorioadenoma destruens or choriocarcinoma, are visualized as irregularly outlined areas

Figure 3-9. UTERINE DISORDERS

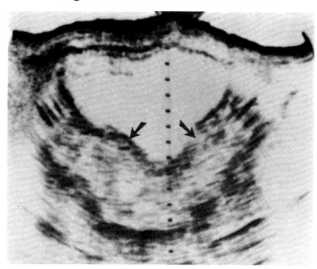

Figure 3-9A. Bicornuate uterus (transverse, 4 cm above symphysis pubis). On this scan, the binodular appearance of the uterus is demonstrated (*arrows*). This pattern may simulate the findings of subserosal leiomyomas. Serial scans during the menstrual cycle may demonstrate the endometrium as an echogenic intraluminal interface.

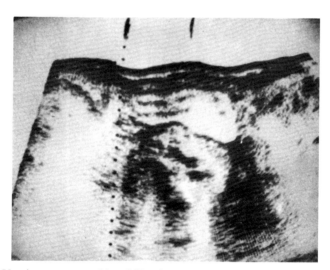

Figure 3-9B. Uterine sarcoma with calcification (transverse, 4 cm above symphysis pubis). The appearance of this tumor is similar to that of a leiomyoma with calcification. (Courtesy of Thomas Lawson, M.D.)

155

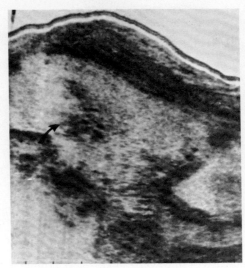

Figure 3-9C. Adenocarcinoma of the uterus (longitudinal, midline). The uterus is markedly enlarged and shows disordered parenchymal texture (*curved arrow*). (Courtesy of Roger Sanders, M.D.)

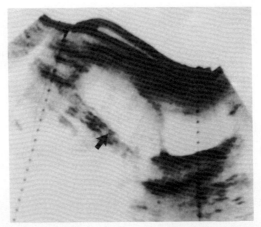

Figure 3-9D. Hematometra resulting from adenocarcinoma of the uterus (longitudinal, midline). This represents another pattern associated with uterine adenocarcinoma. Hematometra results from collection of blood and secretions within the uterus secondary to stenosis of the cervical canal by tumor.

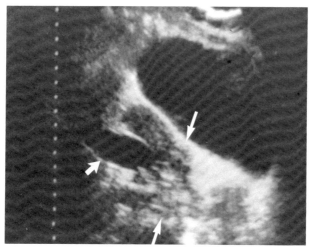

Figure 3-9E. Carcinoma of the cervix with obstruction of the distal ureter (longitudinal, 2 cm to left of midline). This mass (*large arrows*) appears to invade the bladder as well as to cause obstruction of the distal ureter, which is shown as a tubular sonolucent structure on the posterior aspect of the bladder (*small arrow*). (Courtesy of M. Louis Weinstein, M.D.)

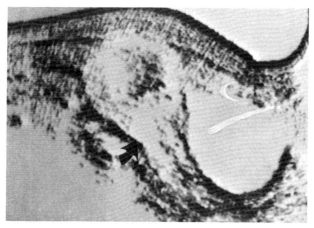

Figure 3-9F. Adenomyosis (longitudinal, midline). This condition, which is due to in-growth of endometrial tissue into the myometrium, produces an inhomogeneous uterine texture (*arrow*) and enlargement of the uterus.

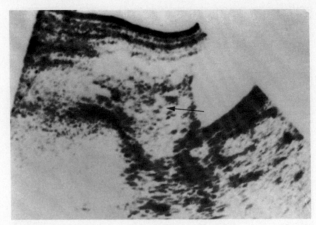

Figure 3-9G. Endometritis (longitudinal, 2 cm to right of midline). The uterine lumen is irregular and distended (*arrow*). This patient had a septic abortion and subsequently developed endometritis. (Courtesy of Thomas Lawson, M.D.)

of sonolucency surrounded by high-amplitude echoes (Fig. 2-9G). A similar pattern may also be encountered in adenomyosis secondary to myometrial implantation of endometrium (Fig. 3-9F). Although disseminated choriocarcinoma may be present, it is often difficult to detect, because the change in the uterine texture in this disorder may be subtle.

Inflammatory conditions of the endometrium usually present in the postpartum period or secondary to septic abortion and result from bacterial invasion of the endometrium. In pelvic inflammatory disease, the endometrium is sometimes unusually well demonstrated. Similarly, in pyometritis, the uterine lumen may be enlarged and irregular as a result of inflammatory components in the uterine lumen.

Although there has been interest in the sonographic evaluation of patients with cervical carcinoma, the role of ultrasound in this condition appears limited because of the inability to definitively document parametrial disease (Fig. 3-9E). Many types of devices have been advocated for evaluation of cervical carcinoma, including transducers that are introduced transvaginally or transrectally. None of these methods has achieved widespread use, probably secondary to the poor image quality and lack of patient acceptance. The uterine cervix may be evaluated using a technique in which water is introduced into the rectum and fills the rectosigmoid colon. The water in the bladder and in the rectum lies on both sides of the lower uterine segment, thereby increasing sonographic accessibility. CT often provides superior information concerning parametrial extension because of greater delineation of the fat planes surrounding the cervix. Parametrial invasion can be seen as an ill-defined area of increased echogenicity on either side of the uterus. Further clinical experience is needed in order to assess the value of sonography in revealing this condition.

Carcinoma of the oviduct is rare and is seen on sonography as a complex pelvic mass. Bowel may be involved by the neoplasm, giving rise to a large, complex abdominal mass.

Figure 3-10. INDETERMINATE MASSES

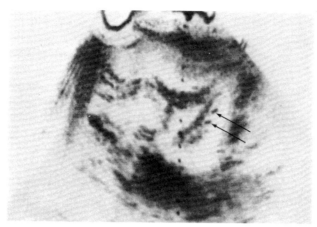

Figure 3-10A. Fluid-filled jejunum (transverse, 4 cm above symphysis pubis). This patient presented with a left pelvic mass. Because of the characteristic mucosal fold pattern (*arrows*), the diagnosis of mechanical small bowel obstruction was suggested by ultrasound.

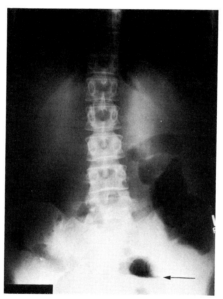

Figure 3-10B. Upright radiograph of same patient showing air-fluid level in distended jejunum (*arrow*).

159

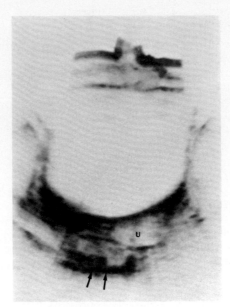

Figure 3-10C. Fecal-filled rectosigmoid colon simulating a solid pelvic mass (transverse, 4 cm above symphysis pubis). A transverse scan of this patient demonstrates an ill-defined echogenic mass (*arrows*) in the right adnexa (u = uterus). (Courtesy of Anthony Dowling, M.D.)

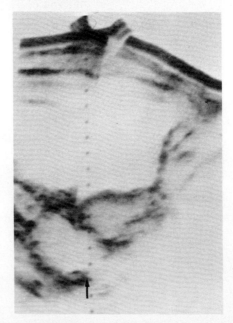

Figure 3-10D. Same patient as in Figure 3-10C after water enema (transverse, 4 cm above symphysis pubis). After water enema was performed, this "mass" became cystic, indicating that it was part of the rectosigmoid colon.

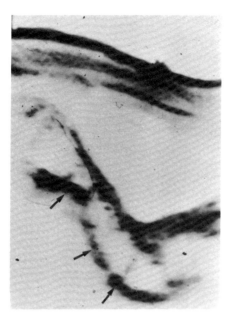

Figure 3-10E. Fluid-filled rectosigmoid colon (longitudinal, 2 cm to left of midline, same patient as in Figure 3-10C and 3-10D). The rectosigmoid colon is recognized during a water enema as a tubular, sonolucent structure with periodic mucosal folds (*arrows*).

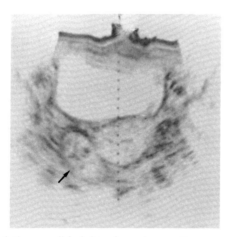

Figure 3-10F. Fat simulating a solid right adnexal mass (transverse, 4 cm). This patient was found to have a mass of fat (*arrow*) that herniated through the posterior peritoneum. This condition is sometimes described as Allen-Masters syndrome. (Courtesy of M. Louis Weinstein, M.D.)

LOCALIZATION OF INTRAUTERINE CONTRACEPTIVE DEVICE (IUCD)

Sonography can be used to locate an intrauterine contraceptive device that is thought to be in an abnormal location. Concern often arises because the strings cannot be located protruding from the cervical os. In these cases, an IUCD can be localized as an echogenic linear interface within the uterus. Ultrasound studies may be also employed in evaluating the size and configuration of the uterus prior to IUCD insertion. Sonography is least helpful in locating an IUCD when

Figure 3-11. INTRAUTERINE CONTRACEPTIVE DEVICES (IUCD)

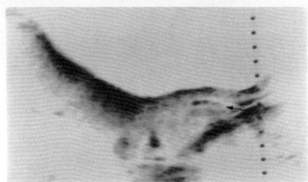

Figure 3-11A. Copper-7 IUCD in lower uterine segment (longitudinal, midline). This longitudinal scan demonstrates a linear echogenic interface with a focal echogenicity representing the IUCD (*arrow*). The shaft of the IUCD is located too low in the lower uterine segment to be effective.

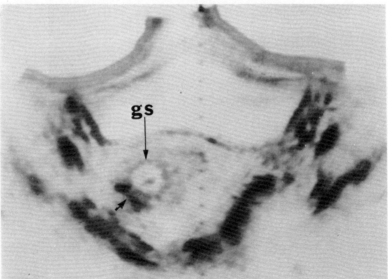

Figure 3-11B. Intrauterine contraceptive device with intrauterine pregnancy (transverse, 4 cm above symphysis pubis). A Copper-7 IUCD is seen (*arrow*) lateral to a small gestational sac (gs).

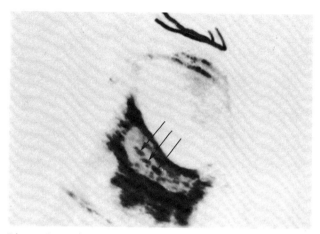

Figure 3-11C. Lippes loop IUCD (longitudinal, midline). Multiple echogenic interfaces are seen emanating from the periodic curves of a Lippes loop device (*arrows*).

it lies outside of the uterus; bowel gas and structures prevent specific delineation of the IUCD. In these cases, a pelvic radiograph may be necessary for localization, the difficulty here is that one does not always directly visualize the uterus.

Intrauterine contraceptive devices have a variety of sonographic appearances, depending on their configuration and metallic or plastic composition. The copper-7 device is seen as an echogenic line and dot when imaged along its longitudinal axis (Fig. 3-11A,B). On the transverse scans, this intrauterine contraceptive device is difficult to demonstrate, since only a small area will be in the proper relation to produce a characteristic pattern. Another commonly used device is the Lippes loop, which is demonstrated as a series of regularly spaced echoes within the uterine lumen and associated localized posterior acoustical shadowing (Fig. 3-11C).

Sonography can be helpful in revealing an intrauterine contraceptive device that may coexist with an intrauterine pregnancy. In these rare cases, the IUCD can usually be identified beneath the chorionic and embryonic membranes (Fig 3-11B).

SUMMARY

Ultrasound studies have many applications in gynecology. In particular, sonography is helpful in the evaluation of pelvic masses. The similarity of the morphologic features of these masses, however, limits the specificity of the sonographic findings.

REFERENCES

Biological Effects

1. Baker, M., Dalrymple, G.: Biological effects of diagnostic ultrasound: A review. *Radiology* 126:479–484, 1978.

Diagnostic Principles

2. Fields, S., Dunn, F.: Correlation of the echographic visualization of tissue with biological composition and physiological state. *J. Acous. Soc. Am.* 54(3):809–812, 1973.
3. Cunningham, J., Worten, W., Cunningham, N.: Gray scale echogenicity of soluble proteins and protein aggregates (an *in vitro* study). *J. Clin. Ultrasound* 4(6):417–419, 1976.

Technique and Normal Anatomy

4. Bartrum, R., Crow, H.: Examination of the pelvis, in *Gray Scale Ultrasound: A Manual for Physicians and Technical Personnel.* Philadelphia: Saunders, 1977, pp. 145–153.
5. Bezjian, A., Carretero, M.: Ultrasonic evaluation of pelvic masses in pregnancy. *Clin. Ob./Gyn.* 20(2):325–338, 1977.
6. Rubin, C., Hertz, A., Goldberg, B.: Water enema: A new technique for defining pelvic anatomy. *J. Clin. Ultrasound* 6(1):78–83, 1977.
7. Sample, W.: Gray scale ultrasonography findings of normal female pelvis. *Radiology* 125:477–478, 1977.
8. Hall, D., Hann, L., Ferrucci, J., et al.: Sonographic morphology of the normal menstrual cycle. *Radiology* 133:185–188, 1979.

Pelvic Masses

9. Fleischer, A., James, A. Jr., Millis, J., Julian, C.: Differential diagnosis of pelvic masses by gray scale sonography. *Am. J. Roentgenol.* 131:469–474, 1978.
10. Cochrane, W.: Ultrasound in gynecology. *Radiol. Clin. N. Am.* 13(3):457–466, 1975.
11. Fleischer, A., Boehm, F., James, A. Jr.: Sonographic evaluation of ectopic pregnancies, in *Ultrasonography in Obstetrics and Gynecology.* Second ed. R. Sanders, A. E. James, Jr., eds. New York: Appleton-Century-Crofts, 1980.
12. Guttman, P.: In search of the elusive benign cystic teratoma: "Tip of iceberg" sign. *J. Clin. Ultrasound* 5:83–87, 1977.
13. Sandler, M., Karo, J.: The spectrum of sonographic findings in endometriosis. *Radiology* 127:229–231, 1978.
14. Lawson, T.: Diagnosis of gynecologic pelvic masses by gray scale ultrasonography: An analysis of specificity and accuracy. *Am. J. Roentgenol.* 128:1003–1006, 1977.
15. Coulam, C., Julian, C., Fleischer, A.,: Clinical efficacy of CT and sonography in the evaluation of gynecologic tumors. (In press.)
16. Rochester, D., Levin, B., Bowie, J., Kuntzman, N.: Ultrasonic appearance of Krukenberg tumor. *Am. J. Roentgenol.* 129:919–920, 1977.

Uterine Masses

17. Fleischer, A., Julian, C., James, A. Jr.: Sonographic evaluation of uterine disorders, in *Ultrasonography in Obstetrics and Gynecology.* Second ed. R. Sanders, A. E. James, Jr., eds. New York: Appleton-Century-Crofts, 1980.
18. Miller, E., Thomas, R., Lines, B.: The atrophic postmenopausal uterus. *J. Clin. Ultrasound* 5(4):261–263, 1977.
19. Bowie, J.: Ultrasound of gynecologic pelvic masses: The indefinite uterus sign and other patterns associated with diagnostic error. *J. Clin. Ultrasound* 5(5):323–328, 1977.

Misellaneous

20. Whittmann, B., Chow, T.: Diagnostic ultrasound in the management of patients using IUCD. *Br. J. Ob/Gyn.* 83:802–807, 1976.
21. Towne, B., Maholar, H., Wooley, M., Isaacs, H.: Ovarian cysts and tumors in infancy and childhood. *J. Pediat. Surg.* 10(3):311–320, 1975.

22. Schnur, P., Symmonds, R., Williams, T.: Intestinal disorders masquerading as gynecologic problems. *Surg. Obstet. Gynecol.* 128(2):1016–1020, 1969.

23. Fleischer, A., Muhletaler, C., James, A.: Sonographic patterns arising from normal and abnormal bowel. *Rad. Clin. N.A.* 18(2), 1980. (In press.)

24. Fleischer, A., Dowling, A., Weinstein, M., James, A.: Sonographic patterns of distended fluid-filled small and large bowel: Anatomic and radiographic correlation. *Radiology* 133, 1979. (In press.)

25. Yeh, H., Wolf, B.: Ultrasound in ascites. *Radiology* 124:783–790, 1977.

26. Reeder, M., Felson, B.: *Gamuts in Radiology.* Cincinnatti: Audiovisual Aids, 1975.

27. Rochester, D., Bowie, J., Huzman, C., Lester, E.: Ultrasound in staging lymphoma. *Radiology* 124:483–487, 1977.

28. Stein, M.: Omental band: A new sonographic sign of metastases. *J. Clin. Ultrasound* 5(6):410–412, 1977.

29. Meyer, M.: Pathways of ascitic flow, in *Dynamic Radiology of the Abdomen: Normal and Pathologic Anatomy.* New York: Springer-Verlag, 1976, p. 56.

30. Novak, E., Woodruff, R.: *Gynecologic and Obstetric Pathology.* Philadelphia: Saunders, 1977, pp. 243–647.

31. Zatz, L.: Comparison of pelvic ultrasound with pneumography for ovarian size. *J. Clin. Ultrasound* 2(4):337–339, 1974.

32. Zakin, B.: Radiologic diagnosis of dermoid cysts. *Survey Ob./Gyn.* 3:108–114, 1976.

33. Brascho, D., Kim, R., Wilson, E.: Use of ultrasound in placing intracavitarial radiotherapy in endometrial carcinoma. *Radiology* 129:163–167, 1978.

4
Abdominal Sonography

GENERAL CONSIDERATIONS

Ultrasound has proved to be of significant value in the evaluation of the abdomen. It may be used alone or combined with other imaging modalities. In general, sonography is of its greatest use for abdominal problems as a screening procedure in the evaluation of known or suspected abdominal abnormalities. The data obtained by sonographic examination may not only answer the question of normal or abnormal but also localize and morphologically characterize an area of abnormality. If sufficient information pertinent to the clinical problem is obtained by ultrasound, invasive diagnostic tests that are potentially harmful and also add to the length of hospitalization may be avoided. If the ultrasound study fails to delineate or adequately characterize a lesion, further diagnostic procedures are indicated.

Since sonography is but one of many diagnostic modalities for the evaluation of a pathological process in the abdomen, its role relative to other imaging procedures will be emphasized throughout this chapter and examined again in the subsection on efficacy considerations. In most clinical situations, ultrasound examination adequately reveals the size, location, organ or origin, and internal consistency of an abdominal mass; nevertheless, sonographic evaluation of the abdomen is often limited when the incident beam is scattered by gas-filled bowel. When the examination is significantly hindered by gas, other imaging modalities (such as computed body tomography—CBT) may be preferred over continued attempts with ultrasound studies.

INDICATIONS

The most common indications for abdominal sonography include:

1. Screening for an abdominal aortic aneurysm
2. Localization and characterization of suspected or palpable abdominal masses
3. Differentiation of obstructive and hepatocellular jaundice
4. Evaluation of the nonvisualized or "poorly" visualized gallbladder
5. Evaluation of suspected lymphadenopathy and ascites
6. Evaluation of patients with fever of unknown origin or unexplained abdominal pain
7. Evaluation of retroperitoneal masses

With the myriad of diagnostic alternatives for evaluating abdominal disease, the number and order of examinations that are performed on a particular patient should be tailored to the clinical setting. Although CBT is less operator-dependent than sonography and often more accurate in evaluating the extent of a neoplastic or inflammatory process in the abdomen, ultrasound has in some ways a greater potential than CBT in analyzing parenchymal detail of an organ or mass. This chapter provides information that we hope will allow the physician to make priority choices in an appropriate manner in the diagnostic evaluation of abdominal disease.

ABDOMINAL AORTA

General Considerations

Sonographic examination of the abdominal aorta can delineate its contour, course, and size from its entry into the abdomen near the diaphragm to its bifurcation into the common iliac arteries at the level of the umbilicus (Fig. 4-1A). Especially when real-time scanning is employed, sonography is a rapid, noninvasive, and accurate technique that can be used for evaluation of pulsatile abdominal mass(es) that, on a clinical basis, are thought to represent abdominal aortic aneurysms (3).

Patients with an asthenic body habitus frequently will have their abdominal aorta located immediately beneath the anterior abdominal wall, and pulsations from this vessel may be readily palpable. Ultrasound can readily distinguish between pulsations from a normal aorta (or transmitted through structures overlying a normal aorta) and pulsations from an abdominal aortic aneurysm. Sonography not only can identify masses that may lie above the aorta, such as enlarged lymph nodes or tumors of bowel, but also can adequately characterize them.

Figure 4-1. NORMAL ABDOMINAL VASCULATURE

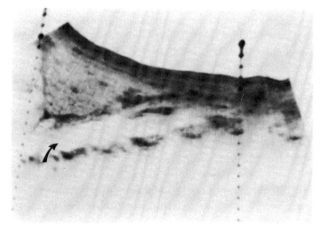

Figure 4-1A. Normal abdominal aorta (longitudinal, 2 cm to left of midline). The abdominal aorta (*curved arrow*) can usually be demonstrated on one longitudinal scan. Its diameter tapers from approximately 3 cm near the diaphragm to 1.5 cm at its bifurcation.

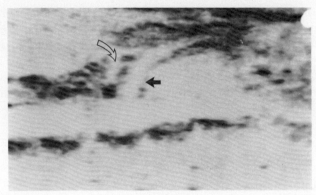

Figure 4-1B. Celiac axis and superior mesenteric artery (longitudinal magnified view, 2 cm to left of midline). The celiac axis appears as a branch from the anterior aspect of the aorta (*open arrow*). The superior mesenteric artery (*solid arrow*) originates a few centimeters caudal to the celiac axis.

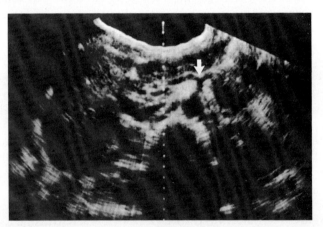

Figure 4-1C. Celiac axis (transverse, 2 cm below xiphoid, white-on-black image). Two arterial branches are seen originating from the anterior aspect of the aorta in a "seagull" configuration (*white arrow*). The branch that courses to the left represents the splenic artery, and the branch that is seen coursing to the right represents the hepatic artery. (Courtesy of Richard Martin, R.D.M.S., Veterans Administration Hospital, Nashville, Tenn.)

The normal aorta lies slightly to the left of the midline in the longitudinal plane and gradually slopes anteriorly to its bifurcation near the umbilicus (Fig. 4-1A). Its outer wall diameter near the diaphragm should be no greater than 3 cm and near the bifurcation no more than 1.5 cm. Its contour should be smooth except for small serrations caused by pulsations. The superior mesenteric artery (SMA) can be routinely visualized at its origin approximately 3 cm below the diaphragm to approximately the level of the umbilicus. Real-time scanning is especially useful in identifying the origin of the SMA. After a short vertical segment at its origin, the SMA courses horizontally. The celiac axis can often be identified on longitudinal scans as a tubular branching structure originating from the anterior aortic surface, then coursing in a vertical direction for a short

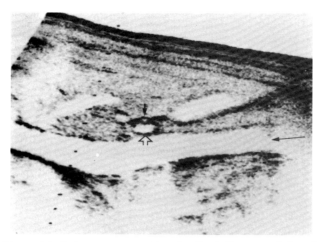

Figure 4-1D. Normal inferior vena cava (longitudinal, 3 cm to right of midline). The inferior vena cava (*straight arrow*) has a more horizontal course than the abdominal aorta. It is best delineated when distended by a Valsalva maneuver. Note that the inferior aspect of the portal vein touches the superior border of the inferior vena cava (*open arrow*). Also shown is the hepatic artery (*small arrow*) anterior to the portal vein. (Courtesy of Thomas Kirkham, R.D.M.S., Xonics Corp., Des Plaines, Ill.)

distance. On abdominal sonograms the larger arterial branches from the aorta, such as the celiac and superior mesenteric arteries, can be delineated and evaluated for aneurysmal dilatation (Fig. 4-1B,C). The common iliac arteries are only occasionally identified on scans made obliquely along their course. The inferior mesenteric artery is infrequently visualized due to overlying intraluminal bowel gas.

On scans made transversely, the abdominal aorta is seen to lie anterior and slightly to the left of the vertebral bodies (Figs. 4-1B,D). The superior mesenteric artery originates approximately 1 to 2 cm inferior to the celiac axis and appears on transverse scans as a circular sonolucent structure posterior to the body of the pancreas. The fat surrounding or adjacent to the SMA is echo-producing, and this is useful in distinguishing it from the slightly larger superior mesenteric vein (SMV) that has a similar course and lies to the right of the SMA. As on longitudinal scans, the inferior mesenteric artery is rarely seen on transverse views due to overlying bowel gas.

Sonographic examination of the abdominal aorta should begin in a longitudinal plane at the midline, centered over the mid-portion of that vessel, which is at a point 4 to 6 cm above the umbilicus. If the aorta is not tortuous, the entire vessel may be delineated on a single longitudinal scan. Bi-stable B-mode scanning can be effectively employed to outline the aortic outer wall. Transverse sonograms should be performed at 1- or 2-cm intervals with particular attention to the size and shape of the aorta in the region of the renal arteries. Overlying bowel may prohibit adequate visualizaton of the entire abdominal aorta. In such cases, patients can be scanned in a decubitus or oblique position with the transducer aimed toward the center of the body; or a scan can be performed in the prone position. Oral ingestion of decanted water and simethicone and use of water enemas to decrease air collection size have been only moderately helpful. Repeat studies on subsequent days are often attempted if clinically reasonable.

Abdominal Aortic Aneurysm

Aneurysms of the abdominal aorta appear as fusiform or saccular dilatations of that vessel. They most frequently begin caudal to the origin of the renal arteries (Figs. 4-2A,B). The aorta should be considered aneurysmal if its anterior-posterior diameter is greater than 3.5 cm in the upper abdomen or 2.5 cm in its distal portion. A patent vessel lumen contains blood and is echo-free, differentiating it from an echogenic, thrombus-filled lumen. An ectatic aorta, because

Figure 4-2. ABDOMINAL AORTA ANEURYSM

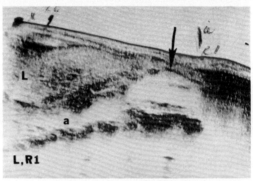

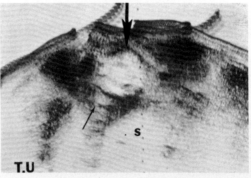

Figure 4-2A. Abdominal aorta aneurysm (longitudinal, 1 cm to right of midline). *Top*: There is aneurysmal dilatation of the distal abdominal aorta (*large arrow*) (a = aorta, L = liver, u = umbilicus, x = xiphoid). The patent lumen appears as a tubular sonolucent area surrounded by echogenic thrombus. *Bottom*: This transverse sonogram (transverse, 12 cm below xiphoid) was obtained across the greatest diameter of the distal abdominal aorta aneurysm (*large arrow*) (s = spine). The patent lumen appears as a sonolucent circle surrounded by a concentric echogenic thrombus. The inferior vena cava is demonstrated along the inferior aspect of the aneurysm (*small arrow*) and simulates the features of a ruptured aortic aneurysm.

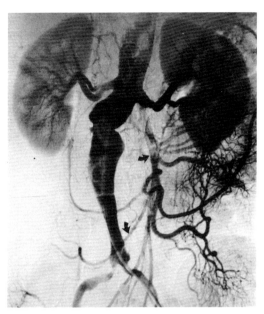

Figure 4-2B. Abdominal aorta aneurysm (angiogram). This aortogram demonstrates draping of the branches of the superior mesenteric arteries over the abdominal aortic aneurysm (*arrows*). There is a short area of narrowing of the abdominal aorta below the renal arteries. The patent lumen only indirectly suggests the presence of aneurysmal dilatation.

of its tortuous course, may be difficult to depict on a single longitudinal scan, making assessment of aneurysmal dilatation difficult. Aneurysms that extend into the branches of the aorta, such as the common iliac arteries, appear as fusiform dilatations.

Acute dissection of an abdominal aortic aneurysm cannot be reliably detected by sonography and is best demonstrated by angiography or CBT. Similarly, the extent of thrombus within major vessels is difficult to ascertain by sonography, again necessitating angiography. Clot within a vessel may be evaluated by using a static imaging device in combination with a gated Doppler attachment. The presence or absence of flow in a vessel is established by detecting a shift in frequency of the incident beam. This shift of frequency can be amplified to create a sound, the absence of which indicates lack of flow in the vessel (52). With the anatomical representation on the static study and the flow determined by Doppler, one can make a diagnosis reliably.

Efficacy Considerations

One advantage of sonography is that it can portray the entire course of the normal abdominal aorta in its longitudinal axis. This makes aneurysmal dilatation more readily apparent than if seen in multiple transverse sections on CBT. In many patients who are found to have an abdominal aortic aneurysm by sonography, angiographic evaluation is indicated in order to define the full extent of aneurysmal dilatation and determine involvement of major arterial branches.

This is particularly important when a patient is evaluated for insertion of a prosthetic aortic Y-graft; one must determine the adequacy of peripheral blood flow. Angiography may also be necessary to evaluate clot within the abdominal aorta. However, using a device capable of static imaging with the Doppler attachment may permit detection of clots within the abdominal aorta and determine flow as well. Sonography is an adjunctive modality for evaluation of patients who are status post-Y-graft to determine the status of the graft as well as the anastomotic site (4). Extravasations and hematomas about the anastomotic site are better delineated by ultrasound and CBT than by angiography, but angiography may be able to detect the movement of blood from the vessel and determine if bleeding is active. Hematomas appear as localized collections of mildly echogenic material around the abdominal aorta.

THE PANCREAS

General Considerations

The relative roles of sonography and CBT in the evaluation of pancreatic disorders are still being assessed (5). Detection of pancreatic masses by both CBT and sonography still depends, in large part, upon recognition of distortion of the pancreatic outline. Sonography is best used as a screening procedure in the initial evaluation of a patient with abdominal pain, jaundice, or a possible pancreatic mass. If the sonographic study does not outline the entire organ or answer the clinical questions posed, CBT is recommended. CBT is less operator-dependent and is not degraded by bowel gas. These factors frequently interfere with the sonographic evaluation of the pancreas. CBT can also detect early invasion of a pancreatic mass into the retroperitoneum by alterations in the appearance of the fat surrounding the pancreas.

Sonography is very accurate in the detection of pseudocyst formation, a rather frequent complication of pancreatitis. Ultrasound has a less important role in establishing the diagnosis of acute pancreatitis. The ileus associated with this disorder can compromise sonographic delineation of the pancreas. Ultrasound images can show the pancreatic texture and delineate the head and portions of the body of the pancreas in most patients. In addition, sonography will frequently detect distension of the pancreatic duct, which may be an early indication of inflammatory or neoplastic obstruction in the pancreatic head region. Dilatation of the pancreatic duct is sometimes encountered as a normal aging phenomenon and in patients with pancreatitis, but its frequent association with pancreatic tumor warrants detailed examination of the organ (12). Dilatation of the pancreatic duct is particularly well demonstrated on transverse scans performed along the length of the pancreas, but may also be demonstrated on longitudinal scans as a small, rounded sonolucent structure in the center of the pancreas (6).

Normal Anatomy and Scanning Technique

Since the pancreas most often lies in the upper abdomen posterior to the left lobe of the liver, it is usually accessible to sonographic evaluation. In most patients, a 3.5-MHz transducer with medium internal focus affords adequate delineation

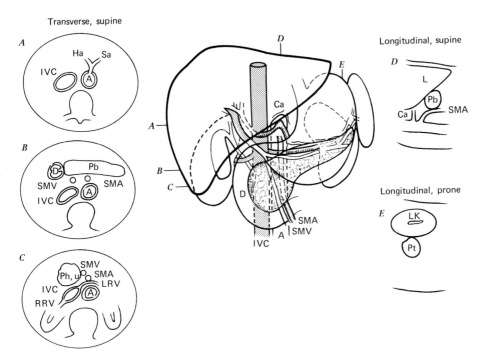

Figure 4-3. Schematic representation of vascular landmarks in the area of the pancreas. (CBD = common bile duct; D = duodenum; IVC = inferior vena cava; A = aorta; SMV = superior mesenteric vein; SMA = superior mesenteric artery; Ha = hepatic artery; Sa = splenic artery; P$_b$ = pancreatic body; P$_{h,u}$ = pancreatic head and uncinate process; RRV = right renal vein; LRV = left renal vein; L = liver; Ca = celiac axis; LK = left kidney; Pt = pancreatic tail). At level *A*, the hepatic and splenic arteries are seen originating from the anterior aspect of the aorta. At level *B*, which is approximately 2 to 3 cm inferior to level *A*, the superior mesenteric artery and superior mesenteric vein appear along the posterior aspect of the pancreatic body. The duodenum has a variable appearance, but is lateral to the pancreatic head. At level *C*, the pancreatic head can be delineated. At this level, the left renal artery usually branches from the inferior vena cava and courses between the superior mesenteric artery and the aorta. In the longitudinal plane designated at *D*, the pancreatic body is seen immediately anterior to the superior mesenteric artery and below the left lobe of the liver. At level *E*, the pancreatic tail is delineated in the region of the left renal hilus as illustrated on a prone scan in the longitudinal plane.

of that organ. The pancreas is usually crescent-shaped with its head being the largest portion. The pancreas usually lies in an oblique plane that extends from the duodenal C-loop to the splenic hilus (Fig. 4-3). On modified transverse scans, the splenic vein can usually be identified along the posterior aspect of the pancreatic body and tail. The superior mesenteric vein outlines the medial aspect of the pancreatic head, whereas the duodenum and gallbladder outline its lateral aspect. Superiorly, the pancreatic head can be delineated by the gastroduodenal artery and, inferiorly, by the common bile duct (Fig. 4-4A).

In most patients, the duodenal bulb (first portion) is recognized as an echogenic area with moderate to marked posterior acoustic shadowing due to the trapped

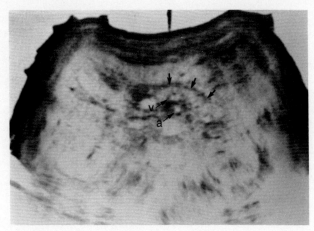

Figure 4-4A. Normal pancreas (transverse, 4 cm below xiphoid). The pancreas appears as a mildly echogenic crescent-shaped structure (*blunt arrows*) which lies anterior to the superior mesenteric vein (v) and superior mesenteric artery (a). The width of the pancreatic body and tail is less than the transverse diameter of the vertebral body (s = spine). The texture of the pancreas usually contains more small, closely spaced echoes than the liver, but this is variable.

gas in the superior portion (2). In other patients, the duodenum may be periodically filled with fluid and recognized as a tubular cystic structure with intraluminal projections corresponding to the valvulae conniventes. When the duodenum is filled with mucus, an echogenic pattern from within the bowel can be recognized. Peristalsis in the duodenal C-loop may also be demonstrated by real-time scanning of the upper abdomen and demonstrates a "to and fro" movement of echoes arising from air bubbles within the bowel segment.

The pancreas can be localized by delineation of certain vascular landmarks (Fig. 4-3); specifically, the body of the pancreas can be identified by the superior mesenteric artery (SMA) that lies immediately posterior to it. The SMA can be recognized by echogenic fat that surrounds the vessel. The superior mesenteric vein (SMV) outlines the medial aspect of the pancreatic head. The SMV has a larger caliber than the SMA and lies above or slightly to the right of the SMA. The pancreatic head and its uncinate process can be identified by localizing the entrance of the left renal vein into the inferior vena cava. When this anatomic configuration is recognized, the pancreatic head should lie within 1 to 2 cm of this area. The uncinate process is the mildly echogenic tissue found lying posterior and medial to the superior mesenteric vein.

Sonography is most reliable for evaluation of the pancreatic head and body, but because the tail is posterior to the gas- or fluid-filled stomach, its delineation may be difficult. The pancreatic tail is sometimes visualized by placing the patient in the prone position and scanning in a longitudinal manner through the left kidney. The stomach may be filled with fluid, such as water or a dilute solution of methylcellulose to provide an acoustic window. The pancreatic tail then appears as a 2- to 3-cm rounded mass anterior and slightly cephalic or caudal to the hilus of the left kidney (8).

As mentioned, distension of the stomach with water may permit delineation of the pancreatic body and tail. This technique involves having the patient drink one to two glasses of water quickly while sitting. After the water is ingested, the patient is placed on his or her left side. Transverse sector scans are obtained of the pancreatic area with the patient placed supine or in the right posterior oblique position. These two positions promote movement of the fluid within the stomach into the duodenum, and this may be helpful in attempts to visualize the pancreatic head and body (Fig. 4-4B). If the pancreas is not adequately demonstrated by these maneuvers, the patient should be requested to drink two to three more glasses of water while upright, and transverse scans can then be obtained in the region of the pancreas. This maneuver allows the gas within the stomach to be collected in the gastric fundus and water to collect in the antrum that overlies the pancreas.

The normal size of the pancreas can be approximated by comparing it to the transverse diameter of the second lumbar vertebral body; however, the contour of the pancreas is less important than its size. A mild degree of nodularity may be seen in the pancreatic outline of normal persons. Localized nodularity may also be found in patients with documented focal pancreatitis. The width of the normal pancreas should taper toward the tail, as a generalization. The body and tail of the pancreas should be no greater than two-thirds of the transverse diameter of the second lumbar vertebra.

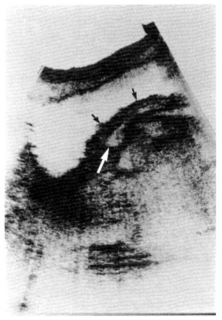

Figure 4-4B. Normal pancreas with patient in right posterior oblique position following water ingestion (transverse along course of pancreas). The fluid-filled stomach appears as a sonolucent structure anterior to the pancreas (*black arrows*). A tubular structure that joins the common bile duct (*white arrow*) is present in the middle of the pancreas representing the pancreatic duct.

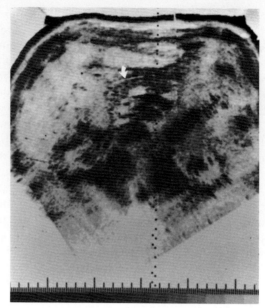

Figure 4-4C. Normal pancreas demonstrating pancreatic duct (transverse, 2 cm below xiphoid). The pancreatic duct (*white arrow*) appears as a tubular structure within the pancreas. This configuration can also be created by the interface of the posterior wall of the gastric antrum and pancreas.

In summary, the following procedures are recommended for sonographic evaluation of the pancreas:

1. Routine series
    a. Longitudinal scans at 1-cm intervals from approximately 8 cm to right to approximately 4 cm to left of midline
    b. Transverse scans at 1-cm intervals from 2 cm to 12 cm below xiphoid
    c. Modified transverse scans from duodenal C-loop (pancreatic head) to splenic hilus (pancreatic tail)
    d. Prone, longitudinal scans through left kidney at 1-cm intervals for delineation of pancreatic tail
2. With water-filled stomach
    a. Have patient drink two to three large glasses of water while sitting
    b. Place patient supine, left posterior oblique position, to collect water in stomach
    c. Determine transverse level of pancreas
    d. Real-time or static scan at level of pancreas with patient in supine and then right posterior oblique positions
    e. If necessary, request patient to drink two to three more large glasses of water or methycellulose while upright
    f. Real-time or static scan at level of pancreas while patient is upright

Pancreatic Disorders

The diagnosis of acute pancreatitis can usually be made clinically. Sonography is most helpful in patients who have continued pain and/or an abdominal mass after an episode of acute pancreatitis should have subsided, because ultrasound is very accurate in demonstrating complications of pancreatitis (Table 4-1). Acute pancreatitis appears as diffuse enlargement of the pancreas with a sonographic texture that is less echogenic than normal. This diminished echogenicity is probably a result of diffuse pancreatic edema (Fig. 4-5A,B) (9). The echogenicity of the normal pancreas is usually greater than or equal to that of the liver parenchyma. When edema involves the pancreas, this is reflected as overall diminished parenchymal echoes associated with enlargement of the pancreatic contour. Dilatation of the pancreatic duct has also been encountered in patients with acute and chronic pancreatitis; nevertheless, its frequent association with pancreatic neoplasms warrants detailed examination of the pancreas for any abnormalities of texture or contour. Acute pancreatitis may be difficult to demonstrate sonographically because of associated ileus, and we have previously suggested certain methods which may help minimize this problem or diagnostic alternative studies.

Pseudocysts of the pancreas, with their predominantly cystic appearance, are readily detected by sonography (Fig. 4-5C). Pseudocysts appear as unilocular or multilocular cystic masses that frequently contain central echoes emanating from pus and cellular debris contained within. Pseudocysts are most commonly located in or immediately adjacent to the pancreas, but can occur anywhere in the abdomen and pelvis and may occasionally extend into the mediastinum. The thickness of the wall of the pseudocyst cannot be reliably assessed by sonography. However, serial examinations are often helpful in monitoring enlargement and/or regression. Spontaneous decompression of a pseudocyst has been observed

Table 4-1. Sonographic Features of Various Pancreatic Disorders

Entity	Sonographic Features
Acute pancreatitis	Diffusely enlarged gland with sonolucent texture
	May be difficult to delineate because of accompanying ileus
	Dilated pancreatic duct may be seen
Chronic pancreatitis	Atrophic pancreas with clusters of calcification
	Dilated pancreatic duct may be seen
Hemorrhagic pancreatitis	Enlarged pancreas with inhomogeneous texture
Suppurative pancreatitis	Enlarged pancreas with fluid collections within pancreas
Pancreatic pseudocysts	Cystic mass(es), either uni- or multiloculated, can decompress spontaneously
Pancreatic carcinoma	Enlarged nodular pancreas with inhomogeneous texture
	Dilated pancreatic and biliary ducts may be seen

Figure 4-5. PANCREATIC DISORDERS

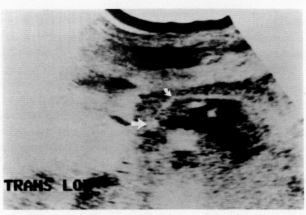

Figure 4-5A. Acute pancreatitis (modified transverse scan along the line of the pancreas). The pancreatic body and tail are enlarged. The pancreatic duct can be demonstrated (*small white arrow*) as it joins the common bile duct (*large white arrow*). Dilatation of the pancreatic duct is encountered in a number of conditions, including pancreatitis and neoplasms. Because of the association of duct dilatation with pancreatic neoplasms, the pancreatic texture should be evaluated when dilatation of the pancreatic duct is present. (Courtesy of B.J. Weinstein, M.D., Presbyterian-University Hospital, Pittsburgh. Penn.)

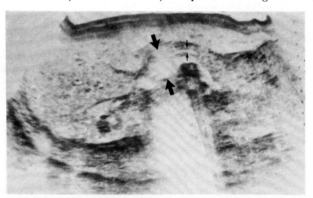

Figure 4-5B. Acute pancreatitis with pseudocyst formation. A pseudocyst is present in the region of the pancreatic head (*large arrows*).This can be differentiated from the fluid-filled duodenum by real-time scanning. The pseudocyst is associated with dilatation of the pancreatic duct (*small arrows*). (Courtesy of Michael Sandler, M.D., Henry Ford Hospital, Detroit, Mich.)

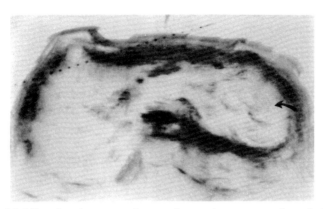

Figure 4-5C. Multiloculated pancreatic pseudocyst (transverse, 4 cm below xiphoid). There is a predominantly cystic, multiloculated mass (*curved arrow*) in the left upper quadrant in a patient with chronic pancreatitis. Pseudocysts may appear as cystic, non-loculated masses, or may have echogenic material within them representing cellular debris, pus, hemorrhage, and/or septations.

by serial ultrasound (11). In rare instances, bowel can overlie a pseudocyst thus hampering its sonographic delineation.

Other complications of acute and chronic pancreatitis, such as formation of pancreatic abscesses and/or the hemorrhage associated with hemorrhagic pancreatitis, can be evaluated by sonography (12) (Figs. 4-5E,F). Sonographically, hemorrhagic pancreatitis appears as a mass with an inhomogeneous texture (Fig. 4-5D). Acute hemorrhage into the pancreas may initially appear sonolucent, but as organization occurs it becomes moderately echogenic. Pancreatic abscesses may have a similar sonographic appearance. Areas of pus within the pancreas will produce a complex sonographic pattern. Areas of gas within the pancreas secondary to abscess can best be detected by CBT (12). The presence of an abscess or hemorrhage can be documented with greater sensitivity by CBT than by sonography because CBT can better demonstrate changes in the retroperitoneal fat planes.

Patients with chronic pancreatitis most often exhibit a small atrophic organ that contains scattered calcifications (Fig. 4-5B). Occasionally, the pancreas may be so small and atrophic that it is difficult to delineate. Calcifications within the pancreas appear as highly to moderately reflective foci with distal acoustical shadowing.

Tumors of the pancreas can be identified by enlargement of the organ, and occasionally a subtle change in the echogenicity of the organ in the region of the tumor can be visualized (Fig. 4-5G). Secondary signs of pancreatic carcinoma include metastases to the liver and/or distension of the extra- and intrahepatic biliary tree. In addition, a dilated pancreatic duct can frequently be found when the tumor causes obstruction in the region of the pancreatic head. Cystic pancreatic tumors are rare but appear as ill-defined, sonolucent masses that may simulate the sonographic patterns of a pseudocyst. Occasionally, pseudocysts may be associated with pancreatic carcinoma secondary to obstruction of the pancreatic duct by tumor.

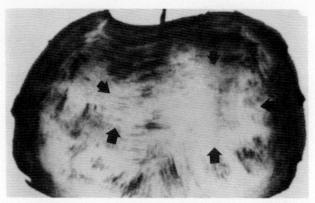

Figure 4-5D. Hemorrhagic pancreatitis (transverse, 4 cm below xiphoid). There is a large, complex, ill-defined mass (*arrows*) in the epigastrium in this patient, who clinically had hemorrhagic pancreatitis. One should be particularly aware of the clinical presentation in these patients since misdiagnosis could lead to unnecessary surgery.

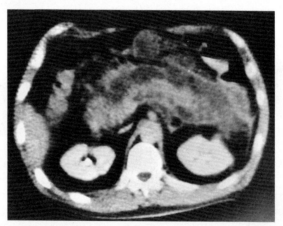

Figure 4-5E. Hemorrhagic pancreatitis (CT scan at level of sonogram in Figure 4-5D). The pancreas is enlarged, and its texture is abnormally inhomogeneous. There are multiple loops of gas-filled bowel anterior to the pancreas which prohibited adequate sonographic delineation of the pancreas. CBT is very useful in evaluating pancreatic hemorrhage and abscess when sonographic studies are hampered by a surrounding ileus.

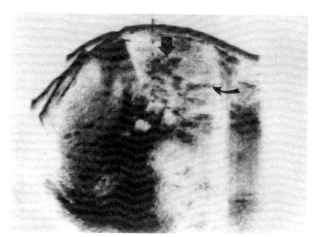

Figure 4-5F. Pancreatic abscess (transverse, 4 cm below xiphoid). This complex epigastric mass (*curved arrow*) contains a focus of high-amplitude echoes which represent a collection of gas within this pancreatic abscess (*large arrow*).

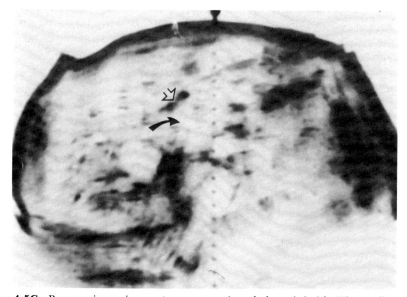

Figure 4-5G. Pancreatic carcinoma (transverse, 4 cm below xiphoid). The outline of the pancreatic head is enlarged (*curved arrow*) representing a tumor in the pancreatic head. The mucus-filled duodenum (*open arrow*) is also displaced anteriorly and laterally by the mass.

Efficacy Considerations

Unfortunately, neither sonography nor CBT can consistently detect carcinoma of the pancreas in its early stages. Evaluation of the pancreas at present is best performed through a multimodality approach with sonography as the primary screening study. Carcinoma of the pancreas may someday be detected by biochemical assay, but imaging techniques will still be required to assess the anatomy and resectability of a lesion.

THE LIVER

Normal Anatomy and Scanning Technique

Sonographic evaluation of the liver should be performed in both longitudinal and transverse planes. To evaluate parenchymal detail, a simple sector scan should be obtained in the longitudinal plane with the patient in suspended inspiration to allow the liver to extend from under the right costal margin (Fig. 4-6A). Transversely, limited sector scans can be obtained between the costal margins. A complete scan can then be obtained by filling in the sides of the scan using simple sector scan technique between the costal margins. In general, however, transverse scans are limited because of the areas of diminished penetration due to the ribs.

Abnormal areas on radionuclide studies can be localized and evaluated sonographically using direct measurements from a ^{99m} Tc sulfur colloid liver/spleen scan or a gallium (^{67} Ga) scan. The xiphoid as well as the right costal margin are noted by lead markers on the radionuclide study, and measurements may be taken directly from the radionuclide image. By using the xiphoid and right coastal margin as landmarks, tailored ultrasound studies can then be made.

Figure 4-6. NORMAL LIVER

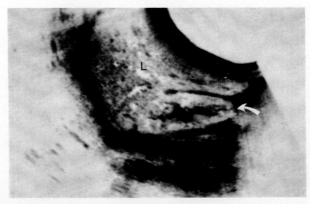

Figure 4-6A. Normal right hepatic lobe (longitudinal, 6 cm to right of midline). The liver (L) appears as a homogeneous, mildly echogenic structure. Its echogenicity is greater than that of the kidney (*arrow*).

When interpreting hepatic sonograms, the vascular structures within the liver must be clearly identified (15). The course and the caliber of an intrahepatic vessel can be particularly well portrayed using real-time scanning. The largest vessels within the liver are the portal vein and the inferior vena cava. One can best delineate the portal vein on transverse sonograms as a tubular, fluid-filled structure that courses in a horizontal fashion to the porta hepatis region. Because the left portal vein has a vertical course, it is frequently difficult to demonstrate. The right portal vein is an extension of the main portal vein and can be used as an anatomical landmark to localize other structures in the liver. The right portal vein is seen as a tubular structure extending into the liver and branching as it passes the porta hepatis region. On longitudinal scans, the right portal vein appears in the mid-portion of the liver as a dumbbell or circular structure with an echogenic collar (Table 4-2). The inferior vena cava is visualized to the right of the abdominal aorta on transverse and longitudinal scans. On longitudinal scans, the inferior vena cava can be seen to enlarge in caliber after it receives blood from both renal veins, and can then be followed in its intrahepatic course.

On transverse scans, the hepatic veins are seen as tubular structures that enlarge as they drain toward the inferior vena cava (Fig. 4-6B). The hepatic veins appear to enlarge on longitudinal scans as they course towards the inferior vena cava in a cephalic direction. The apices of the angles of the hepatic vein branches are oriented toward the inferior vena cava, whereas the branches of the portal veins point to the porta hepatis. The walls of hepatic veins are not as echogenic as those of portal veins because they do not have as much vessel wall collagen and are not enveloped in the portal triad. Branches of the portal vein are echogenic because of their intrinsic connective tissue and the adjacent bile ducts and hepatic arteries that are contained within the portal triad (Fig. 4-6C). Criteria for differentiation of these vascular structures within the liver are summarized in Table 4-2. Punctate foci of echoes within the liver are frequently seen; most likely they arise from collapsed portal veins that contain an echogenic collar of connective tissue.

Table 4-2. Differential Sonographic Features of Tubular Structures Within the Liver

Portal Veins	Hepatic Veins	Dilated Bile Ducts
Enlarge as they course toward porta hepatis	Enlarge as they course toward inferior vena cava	Echogenic "collar" present
		Lobulated shape
Echogenic "collar" of connective tissue, representing fat, hepatic artery, and bile duct which comprise the portal triad	No echogenic "collar"	Ramify over short distance
	Apex of branch points toward inferior vena cava	
Apex of branch points toward porta hepatis		Converge toward porta hepatis in "stellate" pattern

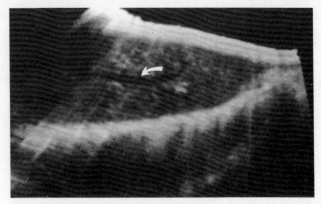

Figure 4-6B. Hepatic vein (longitudinal, 6 cm to right of midline, white-on-black image). The hepatic vein (*arrow*) appears as a tubular branching structure that enlarges as it courses toward the inferior vena cava. These vessels can be differentiated from portal vessels by the lack of echogenic walls.

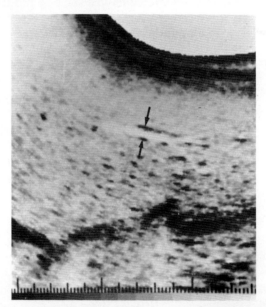

Figure 4-6C. Portal veins (longitudinal, 3 cm to right of midline). A portal vein branch demonstrates an echogenic "collar" (*arrows*).

Hepatic Masses

Ultrasound is useful in detecting hepatic masses as well as in determining their size and internal composition (Table 4-3). In most cases, a suspected liver mass is first evaluated by radionuclide liver/spleen scanning (13). Focal areas of diminished activity that are seen on the more sensitive radioisotope liver/spleen scans can be characterized into cystic, complex, or solid hepatic masses based on their sonographic features. In addition, photon-deficient areas seen in the region of the porta hepatis which may be due to normal structures (such as gallbladder,

Table 4-3. Sonographic Features of Various Hepatic Disorders

Entity	Sonographic Features
Masses	
Simple cysts	Solitary or multiple, sonolucent, well-circumscribed intrahepatic masses with posterior acoustical enhancement
Metastatic foci	Variety of patterns
	"Bull's eye" or "target" pattern frequently associated with adenocarcinoma from gastrointestinal tract
	Sonolucent pattern usually associated with lymphoma and sarcoma
	Mixed pattern may represent central necrosis
	Diffuse disorganization in widespread parenchymal involvement
Abscesses	Intrahepatic mass with predominantly complex pattern depending upon presence of pus or gas
	Irregular borders
Hematoma	Sonolucent if unclotted; echogenic if clot organized
Hepatoma	Complex or echogenic intrahepatic mass with moderately well-defined borders
Parenchymal disorders	
Cirrhosis	Echogenic hepatic texture; peripheral intrahepatic vessels not as easily outlined as in normal patient
	May be associated with splenomegaly
Fatty replacement	Echogenic hepatic texture; peripheral intrahepatic vessels more readily seen than in cirrhotic liver

bile ducts, and vascular structures) can be confirmed on ultrasound studies (15). Since sonography can adequately demonstrate intrahepatic vessels and bile ducts and CBT does not do this as well, the latter is not as helpful as sonography in the evaluation of liver lesions. However, CBT can be used as an adjunct to sonography, especially when sonographic examination is considered nondiagnostic.

Ultrasound is highly accurate in the demonstration of hepatic cysts (16). Several kinds of cysts may exist within the liver, ranging from simple congenital cysts to those seen in polycystic disease that may be coexistent with cysts of the kidneys, spleen, and pancreas. Solitary cysts within the liver appear as round sonolucent masses that exhibit distal acoustical enhancement (Fig. 4-7A,B). Although not as frequent as renal cysts, intrahepatic simple cysts may also be encountered fortuitously. Congenital cysts sometimes contain small amounts of cellular debris that usually layers in the dependent portion of the lesion. The wall of a hepatic

Figure 4-7. LIVER MASSES

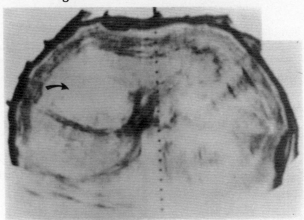

Figure 4-7A. Simple hepatic cyst (transverse, 4 cm below xiphoid). There is a well-defined cystic mass in the right lobe of the liver (*curved arrow*), with a focal collection of echoes in its posterior aspect. The echoes were felt to represent cellular debris layering in a dependent fashion along the posterior aspect of the cyst. Hemorrhage might produce a similar pattern.

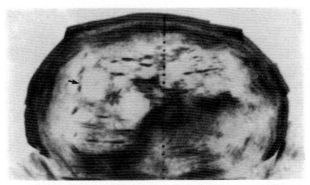

Figure 4-7B. Polycystic liver disease (transverse, 4 cm below xiphoid). There are multiple cysts of various sizes within the liver (*arrow*). This patient also had polycystic kidney disease, which is illustrated in Figure 5-7B.

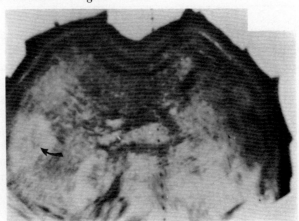

Figure 4-7C. Hemangioma (transverse, 5 cm below xiphoid). There is a moderately well-defined, complex mass in the lateral aspect of the right lobe of the liver (*curved arrow*). This corresponded to a hemangioma. Its echogenic appearance probably arises from the numerous vessels within. A hematoma that has organized clot within may have a similar sonographic appearance.

cyst should be distinct and its shape spherical (Fig. 4-7A). Because of concentric compression of surrounding liver parenchyma, the echoes surrounding the cyst are smooth and well defined. Occasionally, a choledochal cyst may be mistaken for an intrahepatic cyst, but the extrahepatic location can be demonstrated if the patient is scanned upright.

Complex masses in the liver include masses that contain central necrosis and cystic masses in which there is cellular or inflammatory debris. When compared to hepatic cysts, hepatic abscesses tend to have irregular walls and may contain cellular debris and pus within them (Fig. 4-7D). A similar sonographic appearance is seen in necrotic metastases from neoplasms with rapid doubling times. Occasionally an irregularly outlined, predominantly cystic mass is seen as a sequela to rupture of the bile ducts within the liver. Abscesses prior to accumulation of cellular debris may still have an echogenic appearance, particularly if they are secondary to a gas-forming organism (23).

Unusual complex masses within the liver are seen in patients with echinococcal disease and necrotic liver neoplasms (Fig. 4-7C). Traumatic and iatrogenic hematomas can appear as ill-defined, moderately sonolucent to complex masses within the liver. If these patients are studied during the acute stages, an early hematoma appears sonolucent; however, after organization of the clot occurs, it usually appears as a mildly echogenic area.

Solid mass lesions within the liver often represent metastases or primary hepatocellular carcinomas. Hepatomas usually present sonographically as moderately well-defined echogenic masses that are recorded as medium shades of gray within the liver (Fig. 4-7E). Central necrosis can be present; it is seen in the hepatoblastoma of pediatric patients, but less frequently in adult hepatomas and hepatocarcinomas. A tumor thrombus may be detected within the hepatic veins as a result of tumor extension, and can be recognized as an echogenic mass within a major hepatic vein.

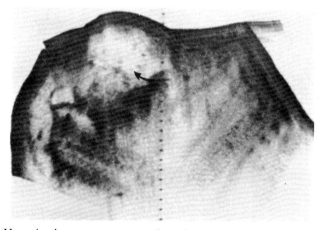

Figure 4-7D. Hepatic abscess (transverse, 6 cm below xiphoid). There is a complex, ill-defined area (*curved arrow*) within the right lobe, with disorganization of the liver texture. This represented a hepatic abscess. Gallium radionuclide study was also positive in this area. (Courtesy of R. Barry Grove, M.D., Veterans Administration Hospital, Nashville, Tenn.)

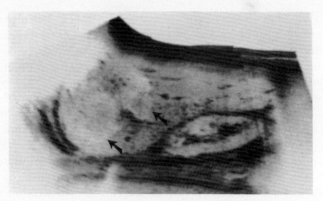

Figure 4-7E. Hepatoma (longitudinal, 6 cm to right of midline). There are two moderately well-defined masses of diminished echogenicity within the right lobe of the liver (*arrows*). This represented a bilobulated hepatoma.

There are several sonographic patterns encountered in metastatic disease of the liver. These do not appear to be accurate indicators of the primary neoplasm (17, 18). At least five patterns of metastases have been described in the current literature:

1. "Bull's eye" or "target" pattern commonly seen from adenocarcinomas of the gastrointestinal tract
2. Echogenic metastases from adenocarcinomas of any origin
3. Predominantly sonolucent metastases from lymphomas, sarcomas
4. Mixed patterns of solid and complex echo consistency
5. Diffuse disorganization pattern with indistinct margins

In some patients, metastatic disease to the liver will cause a diffuse disorganization of the normally homogeneous texture pattern of the hepatic parenchyma (Fig. 4-8D). Echogenic or "bull's eye" and "target" lesions have been associated with adenocarcinoma of the gastrointestinal tract such as colon and carcinoid tumors. This pattern is thought to arise from the echoes of central necrosis surrounded by a sonolucent "halo," representing edema around the central necrosis. Sonolucent metastases from sarcomas tend to undergo degeneration rapidly and produce mixed echo patterns consisting of both fluid-filled and solid components. Thus, it seems that one can reasonably expect to recognize metastases and evaluate their pathophysiology in ultrasound studies; prediction of histology will have to await further advances in tissue characterization.

Parenchymal Disorders

Certain parenchymal disorders of the liver can be readily demonstrated, although their sonographic appearances are not specific. By comparison with normal livers, which have a moderately echogenic pattern, those with cirrhosis tend to have an overall increase in echogenicity, believed due to the greater collagen content and fibrotic reaction. In cirrhosis, the peripheral intrahepatic vessels are not as easily outlined as in normal livers (Table 4-3). This can be a very helpful dif-

Figure 4-8. METASTATIC TUMORS

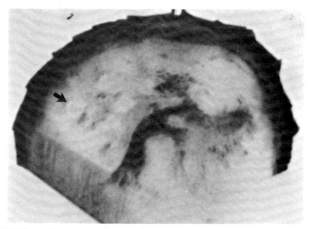

Figure 4-8A. "Bull's eye" pattern from colon carcinoma (transverse, 6 cm below xiphoid). There are numerous rounded masses within the right lobe of the liver which contain central echoes (*arrow*). This pattern is most commonly seen secondary to adenocarcinomas of the gastrointestinal tract, but a number of other causes have been reported.

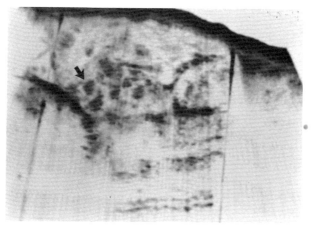

Figure 4-8B. Echogenic metastases from adenocarcinoma of the colon (longitudinal, 6 cm to right of midline). There are numerous echogenic masses within the liver (*arrow*). Some of these metastases have a small sonolucent halo similar to a "bull's eye." This metastatic pattern is most commonly encountered secondary to adenocarcinomas from the gastrointestinal tract. The patient had adenocarcinoma of the colon.

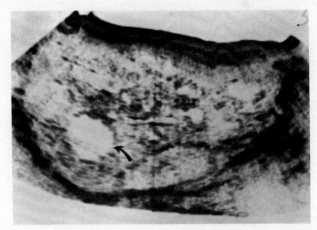

Figure 4-8C. Sonolucent metastases from leiomyosarcoma (longitudinal, 8 cm to right of midline). There are numerous sonolucent masses within the enlarged liver. Focal layering of material within the largest sonolucent mass (*arrow*), representing cellular debris, is seen. Sonolucent metastases most commonly occur from lymphoma and sarcomas.

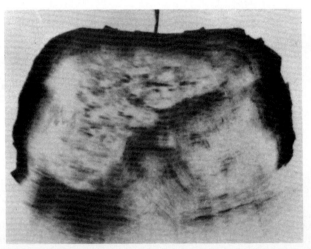

Figure 4-8D. Diffuse disorganization of liver parenchymal echo pattern secondary to metastatic disease from the pancreas (transverse, 1 cm below xiphoid). There is diffuse disorganization of the normally homogeneous hepatic parenchyma. This resulted from diffuse involvement from metastatic pancreatic carcinoma.

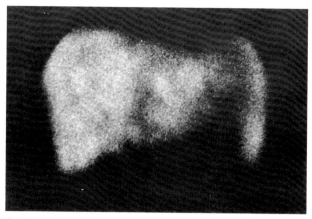

Figure 4-8E. Liver/spleen radionuclide scan of patient in Figure 4-8D (^{99m}Tc sulfur colloid). This liver/spleen scan confirms the impression of diffuse disease of the liver. Detection of the abnormality by radionuclide studies and characterization by ultrasound are very helpful in differential diagnosis.

ferential feature to decide if an increase in echogenicity is due to cirrhosis. Quantification of the reflected echoes will probably be possible in the future for this assessment. Livers that have undergone fatty metamorphosis may also demonstrate increased echogenicity, but the intrahepatic vessels will still be delineated. Secondary signs of cirrhosis should be sought sonographically, such as enlargement of the spleen and/or dilatation of the portal vein. Ascites is also easily delineated and will aid in this differentiation.

Efficacy Considerations

Sonography, CBT, and radioisotopic liver/spleen scanning are complementary procedures for the evaluation of hepatic disorders (19, 20, 21). The radionuclide liver/spleen scan remains the best means of screening for metastatic disease and focal defects in the liver. It is also very helpful in certain diffuse parenchymal disorders. Ultrasound or CBT can then be used as an adjunctive procedure for further characterization of hepatic abnormalities found on the radiocolloid liver/spleen scan. Due to its ability to image a structure in several planes, sonography is superior to CBT in defining intrahepatic structures, such as vessels and biliary ducts that may cause unusual and sometimes questionably abnormal patterns on the liver/spleen scan (Figs. 4-9A,B). Ultrasound can show that a defect is due to an unusual appearance of a normal anatomical structure—this represents a clinically important use of this noninvasive technique.

ABSCESS

Sonography has a complementary role with gallium-67 and CBT studies for the detection of intra-abdominal and pelvic abscesses (25,26), but can effectively be used as the screening procedure to establish the presence or absence of an

Figure 4-9. MISCELLANEOUS HEPATIC DISORDERS

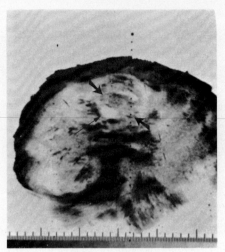

Figure 4-9A. Hepatic artery aneurysm (transverse, 6 cm below xiphoid). There is an ill-defined mass in the left lobe of the liver that contains a central area of sonolucency concentrically surrounded by echogenic material (*large arrows*). At surgery, a large hepatic artery aneurysm was found. The sonolucent area represented the patent lumen (*small arrow*), and the concentric echogenic area around this was caused by thrombus. This pattern simulates that of hepatic abscess.

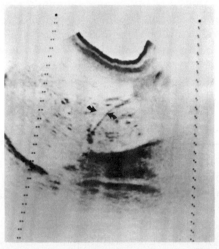

Figure 4-9B. Subhepatic hematoma (longitudinal, 6 cm to right of midline). There is a sonolucent collection in the hepatorenal (Morrison's) pouch (*arrows*). This resulted from liver trauma and a subhepatic hematoma that had not organized.

abscess. If the ultrasound study is equivocal, a gallium scan, which is more sensitive but less specific, may be performed. However, the converse also occurs. An area of abnormal gallium accumulation may be characterized from the anatomical information provided by ultrasound. Since CBT is not compromised by bowel gas, it may be preferred over sonography in patients who have an ileus resulting from an inflammatory intra-abdominal process. Occasionally, gas within an abscess can be delineated by CBT, which may allow the establishment of a specific diagnosis of abscess.

192

The ultrasound pattern of abscesses ranges from a moderately well-defined sonolucency to poorly defined complex mass (Figs. 4-10A,B,C), depending on the internal contents (21). Abscess due to gas-forming organisms can present a sonographic pattern of focal areas of increased echoes without evidence of suppuration (22). The cul-de-sac area and the hepatorenal (Morrison's) pouch should be specifically examined for abscess because of their frequent involvement as drainage sites for inflammatory processes of the abdomen and pelvis (23). Retroperitoneal abscess can be detected by unilateral enlargement of the retroperitoneal and paraspinal muscles (Fig. 4-17C). In general, retroperitoneal abscesses are difficult to detect in an early stage, both clinically and radiographically.

Figure 4-10. ABSCESSES AND ASCITES

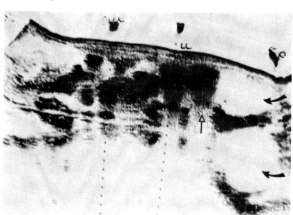

Figure 4-10A. Multiple abscesses (longitudinal, midline). Within the pelvis, there are two sonolucent masses (*curved arrows*) representing abscesses. Barium from gastrointestinal studies was present within the bowel, resulting in echogenic areas and marked acoustical shadowing (*open arrow*) in the region of the bowel. (Courtesy of Anthony Dowling, M.D.)

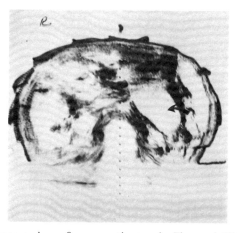

Figure 4-10B. Transverse view of same patient as in Figure 4-10A (transverse, at 8 cm below xiphoid). There is another sonolucent mass in the left upper quadrant (*arrow*) that also represented an abscess.

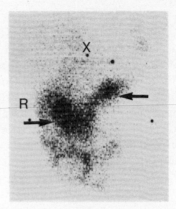

Figure 4-10C. Gallium scan of patient in Figures 4-10A and 4-10B (anterior, xiphoid (X) marked and right (R) marked). There are numerous areas of focal accumulation of gallium (*arrows*) in the areas corresponding to the sonolucent masses seen on abdominal sonography. These masses corresponded to abscesses that contained only serous fluid. (Courtesy of F. David Rollo, M.D., Ph.D., Vanderbilt University Hospital, Nashville, Tenn.)

Efficacy Considerations

Sonography is best used as a screening procedure for the detection of an abscess. If the sonographic pattern establishes the presence of an abscess, additional studies may be avoided. If sonography is inconclusive, additional imaging modalities should be used. Gallium scanning, although sensitive, is not specific and can require up to 72 hours for completion. If an abnormal area is detected, ultrasound and CT can provide important anatomical information. When sonography is inconclusive, CT is very useful because of its excellent anatomical resolution and detection of abnormal collections of gas.

ASCITES

Ascitic fluid is readily detected by abdominal sonography. It appears as sonolucent collections around organs and localizes in the most dependent areas, such as the paracolic recesses, the cul-de-sac, and the hepatorenal or Morrison's pouch (24). Sonograms obtained in the right or left oblique position can be useful in detecting small amounts of ascitic fluid (27). In addition, the patient can be scanned in a supine, partially upright position for collection of ascitic fluid in the cul-de-sac area.

When ascitic fluid is within the paracolic recesses, it results in displacement of the small and large bowel anteriorly and produces what is commonly referred to as the "floating bowel" pattern (Fig. 4-10D). In cachectic persons, matted loops of bowel will often not extend to the anterior abdominal wall. This could be due to a decreased amount of fat around the bowel or due to adhesions. Ultrasound studies can also suggest the diagnosis of malignant ascites when the ascitic fluid appears to be loculated. One should be aware that "floating" bowel that is associated with ascites usually prohibits adequate visualization of any

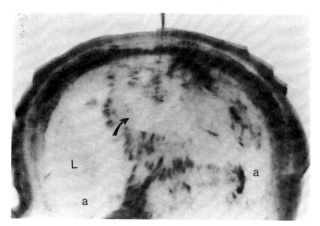

Figure 4-10D. Ascites (transverse, 8 cm below xiphoid). There are sonolucent areas surrounding the liver (L) and in the paracolic recesses. These sonolucent collections represented ascitic fluid (a). The bowel is floating anteriorly (*curved arrow*) and produced a mottled acoustical shadow. (See also Fig. 5-7C).

retroperitoneal structures, including lymph nodes. Therefore, lymphadenopathy can be difficult to establish when bowel is floating anteriorly.

Ascites is associated with a number of systemic disorders, including cirrhosis of the liver, malignant ovarian tumors, and conditions that cause obstruction to the return of lymphatic or venous flow from the mesentery. The sonographic appearance of ascites is indistinguishable from that of the free intraperitoneal blood encountered in rupture of an ectopic pregnancy or abdominal aneurysm. Small collections of intraperitoneal fluid can be identified during the normal menstrual cycle immediately after ovulation in the region of the cul-de-sac (29).

LYMPH NODES

General Considerations

Lymphadenopathy, one should recall, is a term that refers to pathologic enlargement of the lymph nodes which can be due either to benign hyperplasia or to involvement of nodes by a malignant process. A multimodality approach is usually necessary for evaluation of a patient with suspected lymphadenopathy. Sonographic studies can significantly contribute as a screening procedure to establish the presence of enlarged para-aortic and pelvic nodes and enlarged nodes in the hilus on the liver and spleen (30,31). Lymph nodes that are larger than 1.5 cm are detected sonographically as elliptically shaped structures that are mildly to moderately echogenic (Fig. 4-11A). The character of echoes from enlarged nodes is not a reliable indicator of the cause of enlargement. Internal architecture should be assessed by contrast lymphography or biopsy under ultrasound guidance.

Normal Anatomy and Scanning Technique

Sonographic evaluation for lymphadenopathy should begin at the level of the diaphragm, using both longitudinal and transverse scans. The aorta and inferior

Figure 4-11. LYMPHADENOPATHY

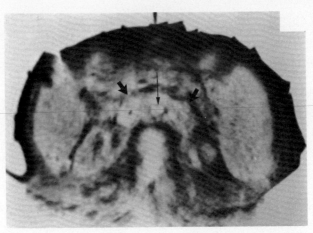

Figure 4-11A. Para-aortic lymphadenopathy (transverse, 8 cm below xiphoid). A lobulated, mildly echogenic mass (*large arrows*) to either side of the abdominal aorta (*small arrow*) is seen. The spleen is also markedly enlarged.

vena cava should be completely delineated since enlarged para-aortic nodes tend to obscure the outlines of these structures. A full bladder technique is necessary for evaluation of pelvic lymphadenopathy. A transverse sonogram obtained from the portal vein region allows evaluation of the liver hilus for lymphadenopathy. The spleen is more difficult to evaluate than the liver because of the spleen's location beneath the left costal margin. The splenic hilus can be visualized in some persons by using limited sector scans through the intercostal spaces. This technique involves performing a sector scan in a coronal fashion with the transducer placed in the appropriate intercostal space and the patient positioned with right side down. The area anterior to the iliopsoas muscle should be studied on longitudinal scans for detection of lymph node enlargement in the pelvis.

If lymphadenopathy is demonstrated, attention should then be directed to the evaluation of splenic, hepatic, and renal size and architecture. Lymphomatous processes will enlarge these organs and may cause diffuse or focal areas of decreased echogenicity in the parenchyma that can be detected by ultrasound.

Lymphadenopathy

Lymph nodes larger than 1.5 cm are seen as sonolucent masses with low-level echoes in characteristic locations (Figs. 4-11A,B,C). Nodal groups that can be readily identified include the para-aortic chain and those near the liver and splenic hilus. Lymph nodes within the pelvis are more difficult to evaluate. Sometimes it is difficult to differentiate lymph nodes from pelvic wall musculature or from fluid- and feces-filled bowel. Enlarged nodes can appear as isolated masses or in groups as conglomerate or matted complexes of echoes.

The ultrasound patterns that suggest lymphadenopathy range from a single enlarged, isolated node located centrally in the abdomen encountered in mesenteric lymphadenopathy, to the "mantle-shaped" mass overlying the aorta and

196

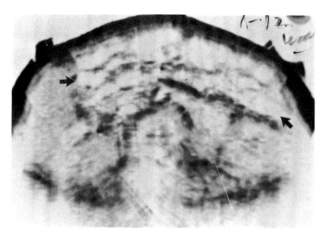

Figure 4-11B. Mesenteric lymphadenopathy (transverse, 12 cm below xiphoid). Numerous sonolucent rounded masses (*arrows*) are present in the center of the abdomen, representing mesenteric lymphadenopathy. The central location of the mass is helpful in distinguishing mesenteric from para-aortic lymphadenopathy, which tends to be located in the region of the prevertebral vessels.

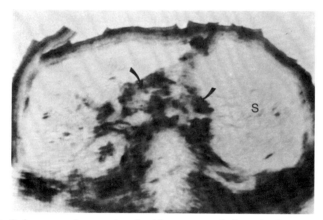

Figure 4-11C. Splenomegaly associated with para-aortic lymphadenopathy (transverse, 4 cm below xiphoid). The spleen (S) is markedly enlarged, causing extrinsic compression of the left kidney located posteriorly. Large nodes in the region of the splenic and hepatic hili are also present (*curved arrows*).

inferior vena cava indicating para-aortic lymphadenopathy (Fig. 4-11A). Para-aortic lymphadenopathy creates lobulated masses overlying the prevertebral vessels. The nodes in mesenteric lymphadenopathy tend to be more centrally located within the abdomen and usually appear distinct and mildly echogenic with marginal convexities. Rounded masses near the hilus of both the liver and spleen may indicate lymphadenopathy in these areas. Enlargement of the pelvic nodes is a most difficult determination to make sonographically, for enlarged nodes can simulate the appearance of normal pelvic organs, such as ovaries. However, when a group of pelvic nodes enlarge, they appear as nodular echogenic masses usually located medial and superior to the iliopsoas muscle groups.

One should be very familiar with the normal anatomical appearance of the pelvic organs on ultrasound before attempting to evaluate lymphadenopathy. The musculature and ligaments can be confused with enlarged nodes.

Efficacy Considerations

Because of the limitations of each diagnostic modality for the evaluation of lymphadenopathy, at least two modalities are often used for a complete evaluation. Although the multiple modality approach may not be necessary in every case, one should be aware of the advantages and limitations of each. For example, gallium-67 scanning is a sensitive but nonspecific indicator of lymphadenopathy. The information obtained by gallium-67 scanning should be combined with data from other modalities for specificity. Sonography is a noninvasive, easily performed examination that can detect most moderately enlarged nodes (over 1.5 cm). This examination can be significantly degraded by reason of the scattering properties of bowel gas lying anterior to node-bearing areas. CT is a reliable method for detection of lymphadenopathy, but enlarged nodes may be difficult to distinguish from fluid-filled bowel. Lymphangiography is the only modality that can reliably detect a normal-sized node that contains metastatic disease, but it requires technical skill, has some inherent morbidity, and is limited by nonvisualization of certain mesenteric node groups as well as node chains superior to the cisterna chyli. Evaluation of each patient suspected of lymphadenopathy requires careful clinical judgment to have the number and type of examinations tailored to the patient's particular problem.

THE GALLBLADDER

General Considerations

Since sonographic delineation of the gallbladder is independent of physiological function, such as the ability of the gallbladder to concentrate radiopaque contrast, ultrasound can be advantageously used when the gallbladder cannot be adequately visualized on oral cholecystography (OCG). Sonography can be used as a secondary procedure, after failure on OCG, but recent results of gallbladder sonography have shown it to be as accurate as routine OCG when used as a primary screening procedure (33). Sonography can also be employed to diagnose gallbladder carcinoma, polyps, chronic inflammation, cholesterosis, and septations within that organ (32) (Table 4-4).

Normal Anatomy and Scanning Technique

In order to visualize the gallbladder adequately, it must be distended with bile. This is accomplished by requesting patients to restrict their oral intake at least six hours before the study. The most important factor in establishing the presence or absence of cholelithiasis is obtaining a technically adequate study. Initially, the gallbladder can be located by real-time scanning. Once the longitudinal axis of the gallbladder is delineated, scans should be obtained in both the longitudinal

Table 4-4. Sonographic Features of Various Gallbladder Disorders

Entity	Sonographic Features
Cholelithiasis	Focal areas of high echogenicity with complete posterior acoustical shadowing
Bowel	Echogenic focus separate from gallbladder, especially when patient scanned in erect position
Septations	Thin echogenic linear interfaces that extend across entire lumen of gallbladder
Polyps	Echogenic intraluminal projections that do not change with patient position
Folding of gallbladder	Configuration change with deep inspiration and expiration
Hyperplastic cholecystoses and/or acute cholecystitis	Irregular, thickened wall
Viscid bile ("sludge")	Echogenic material layering material within gallbladder Sluggish movement when patient changes from supine to upright position
Empyema	Echogenic material within gallbladder similar to that seen with "sludge" Occasionally associated with thick gallbladder wall
Carcinoma	Irregular mass in wall of gallbladder Associated with calculi

and the transverse planes with the patient supine. Simple sector scans should be obtained with the patient in suspended inspiration. After the gallbladder is visualized in the supine position, scans in both the transverse and the longitudinal planes should be obtained with the patient in the left posterior oblique position; in this position the gallbladder is best visualized with transverse scans. Assuming the left posterior oblique position helps to displace the liver from under the right costal margin. The patient should be scanned in the longitudinal axis of the gallbladder while in the upright position, which allows the bowel to migrate caudally. Stones within the gallbladder should migrate toward the gallbladder fundus if they are not impacted.

In summary, the following procedure is advocated for sonographic evaluation of the gallbladder using real-time or static gray scale imaging:

1. Supine
    a. Longitudinal scans at 1-cm intervals from midline to 10 cm to right of midline
    b. Transverse scans from 2 cm to 10 cm below the xiphoid with particular emphasis on the right upper quadrant
    c. Modified longitudinal scan in the longitudinal axis of gallbladder

2. Left posterior oblique or left lateral decubitus position
   a. Transverse scan in region of gall bladder
   b. Longitudinal scan in region of gallbladder
3 Upright
   a. Modified longitudinal scan in longitudinal plane of gallbladder

The distended normal gallbladder appears as a pear-shaped organ located anterior to the right kidney and inferior to the right lobe of the liver on longitudinal scans. On transverse scans, the gallbladder has a rounded configuration lying inferior to the right lobe of the liver and lateral to the duodenum and pancreas (Figs. 4-12A,B). Since there is a wide range in the size of the gallbladder due to various states of contraction and distension, no definite clinical significance is placed on the actual size of the gallbladder. However, if it is greater than 10 cm in length and 6 cm in width and does not change with a fatty meal or other physiologic stimulation, it is probably pathologically enlarged.

Hydrops of the gallbladder is diagnosed by the large size of the organ and the presence of an impacted gallstone in the cystic duct. The calculus should produce shadowing. The spiral valves of Heister may also produce acoustical shadowing in the region of the neck of the gallbladder due to their fibrous content, but their shadowing will not be as great as that emanating from a stone in the cystic duct. The shadowing seen in the region of the gallbladder neck may also be explained by the refractive and reflective interactions that occur at curved surfaces.

Scans of the gallbladder should be obtained in both inspiration and expiration in order to distinguish echoes caused by a fold in the gallbladder from complex echoes created by stones or septa within the gallbladder (Figs. 4-12C,D). Similar patterns can be caused extrinsically by the transverse colon or gastric antrum

Figure 4-12. NORMAL GALLBLADDER

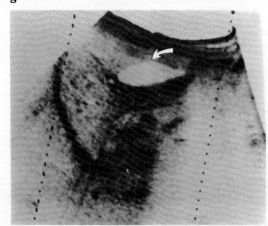

Figure 4-12A. Normal, distended gallbladder (longitudinal, 6 cm to right of midline). The gallbladder appears as a pear-shaped structure (*arrow*) inferior to the right lobe of the liver and superior to the right kidney.

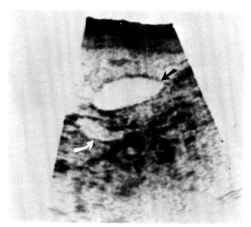

Figure 4-12B. Normal gallbladder with patient in left posterior oblique position (modified longitudinal, approximately 6 cm to right of midline). The gallbladder again appears as a fusiform sonolucent structure in the right upper quadrant (*black arrow*). The inferior vena cava is partially visualized posterior to the gallbladder (*white arrow*).

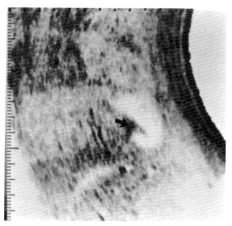

Figure 4-12C. Phrygian cap (upright, modified longitudinal). There is a series of linear echoes that have the pattern of a fold of the gallbladder (*arrow*), which appears as an echogenic projection into the lumen. On inspiration and expiration, the gallbladder was noted to change in configuration. Real-time imaging is very helpful in this regard.

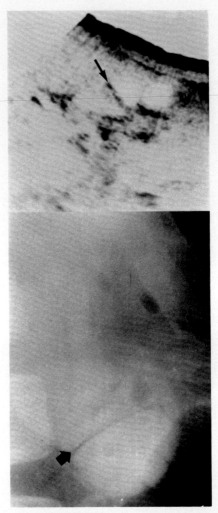

Figure 4-12D. Septated gallbladder (longitudinal, 6 cm to right of midline). There is an echogenic interface that extends across the lumen of the gallbladder (*arrow*) on the ultrasound study (*top*). This corresponds to the septum seen on oral cholecystography. (*bottom*) (*large arrow*).

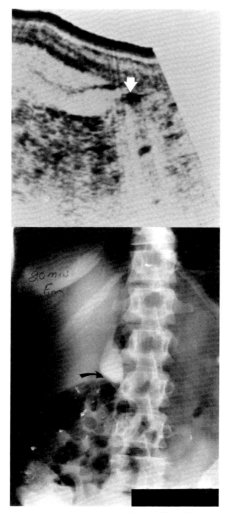

Figure 4-12E. Proximity of transverse colon to the gallbladder fundus (longitudinal, 6 cm to right of midline). There is an echogenic area with mottled distal acoustical shadowing in the region of the gallbladder fundus (*top*) (*arrow*). An oral cholecystogram (*OCG*) (*bottom*) in close proximity to the transverse colon and its indentation of the gallbladder fundus is seen (*curved arrow*).

in close proximity to the gallbladder fundus (Fig. 4-12E). One should be particularly aware of the close proximity of the gallbladder fundus to the transverse colon and not attribute echogenic areas and apparent shadowing produced by the colon to calculi within the gallbladder (Fig. 4-12E). Echo reflection due to bowel will cause a mottled rather than complete acoustical shadow due to scattering of the ultrasound beam as it passes through gas-filled bowel (2). As further differentiation of the effects of bowel from biliary calculi, the transverse colon should move in a caudal direction when the patient assumes an erect position. Real-time imaging can greatly assist in evaluation of acoustical shadowing in the area of the gallbladder.

Cholelithiasis and Cholecystitis

Cholelithiasis appears as focal areas of increased echoes within the gallbladder with distal (usually posterior) acoustical shadowing. As previously stated, it is important to establish that high-amplitude echos with acoustical shadowing are indeed within the gallbladder. The majority of calculi within the gallbladder are easily recognized because of their highly reflective interface and complete or "clean" distal acoustical shadowing (Figs. 4-13A,B,C,D). A maneuver that may make calculi within the gallbladder more apparent is to increase the amount of acoustical shadowing by scanning the patient with a transducer of higher frequency. Calculi as small as 2 mm can be seen sonographically if various maneuvers and real-time instrumentation are employed. Shadowing distal to calculi can also be optimized by using a transducer that has a focal length at a comparable depth to the stone.

Detection of calculi within the gallbladder depends primarily on the angle at which the interface between the calculi and the anterior abdominal wall is imaged. Failure to demonstrate acoustical shadowing is most likely due to technical factors rather than intrinsic properties of a calculus (Table 4-5). Studies of stone composition have shown that almost all are so highly reflective they will cause shadowing. Figure 4-13E illustrates the influence of transducer angle in relation to an interface on detection of returning echoes and production of acoustical shadowing. Distal acoustical shadowing becomes less apparent when the relative transducer angle is greater than 10 degrees from perpendicular.

The arrangement of gallstones in the gallbladder is also important in determining the amount of shadowing, for stones that tend to layer usually cast a more prominent shadow than those that do not (34). The size and number of stones also correlates with their shadowing properties.

The amount of acoustical shadowing is influenced slightly by the composition of the calculus. The pattern of shadowing has been correlated with the relative amount of crystalline structure within the stone. The greater amount of cholesterol crystals, the greater the echogenicity. It has also been observed that cholesterol stones tend to be more echogenic and float more often than stones of other types, such as mixed calcium bilirubinate stones.

The diagnosis of cholelithiasis can sometimes be made even when the gallbladder is not adequately visualized on the ultrasound study. In these cases, areas of marked echogenicity with acoustical shadowing can be seen in the gallbladder

Table 4-5. Sources of Diagnostic Errors in Sonographic Evaluation of the Gallbladder (32,37)

False-negative (5–10 %)	False-positive (2%)
Improper scanning technique	Confusion of bowel for calculus
Angle of transducer with respect to interface	Other intraluminal masses
	Polyps
Inadequately outlined gallbladder	Mucosal fold
	Carcinoma
All patient positions not used	

Figure 4-13. GALLBLADDER DISORDERS

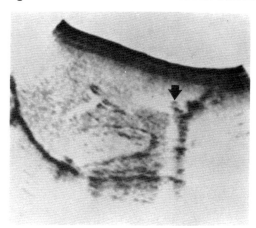

Figure 4-13A. Cholelithiasis (longitudinal, 6 cm to right of midline). Within the gallbladder, there is an echogenic focus that produces a complete or "clean" distal acoustical shadow (*arrow*).

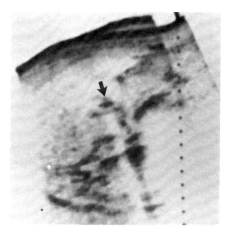

Figure 4-13B. Transverse scan of patient in Figure 4-13A. Again, dense focal echoes within the gallbladder are seen producing a complete acoustical shadow distally (*arrow*). This represented numerous small calculi within the gallbladder.

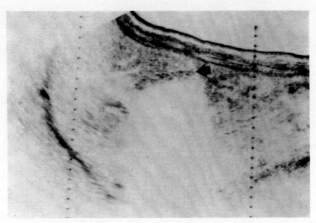

Figure 4-13C. Contracted gallbladder with calculi (longitudinal, 4 cm to right of midline). Even though the gallbladder could not be delineated, the diagnosis of cholelithiasis can be established due to the high-amplitude echoes (*arrow*) and complete acoustical shadowing of the calculi contained within the contracted gallbladder.

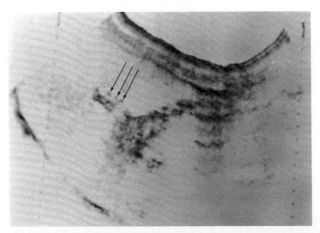

Figure 4-13D. Multiple small calculi within cystic duct (longitudinal, 5 cm to right of midline). There are three echogenic foci with distal acoustical shadowing in the region of the cystic duct (*arrows*).

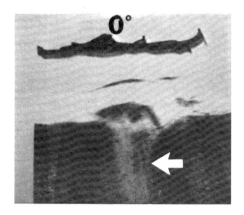

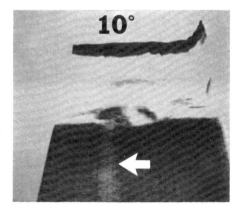

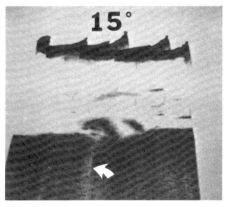

Figure 4-13E. Effect of transducer angle on posterior acoustical shadowing. Three gall-bladder calculi were placed in a surgical glove filled with water. This was mounted on top of a sponge and scanned at various degrees off "normal." When the transducer was perpendicular to the stones, a well-defined posterior acoustical shadow (*arrow*) was produced. When the transducer angle increased to 10 and 15 degrees, acoustical shadowing was not so apparent. This illustrates the importance of imaging gallbladder calculi perpendicular to their surface so that posterior acoustical shadowing can be demonstrated.

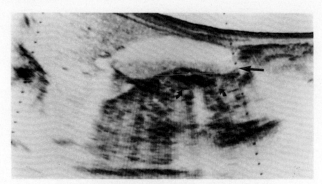

Figure 4-13F. Viscid bile or "sludge" (longitudinal, 4 cm to right of midline). Within the gallbladder, there is an echogenic layering of material in the posterior aspect of the gallbladder (*large arrow*). This represents viscid bile or "sludge." The transverse colon is posterior to the gallbladder and appears as a reniform structure (*small arrows*) containing a central echogenic core and a relatively sonolucent halo. (Courtesy of Karen Parker, R.D.M.S., and Clifton Greer, M.D., Baptist Hospital, Nashville, Tenn.)

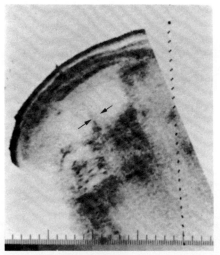

Figure 4-13G. Empyema of gallbladder (transverse, 6 cm below xiphoid). The gallbladder wall is thickened (*arrows*). This corresponded to gallbladder empyema in a diabetic patient. Gallbladder wall thickening may also be observed in acute cholecystitis. Its concentric distribution suggests a more diffuse process than a localized neoplastic tumor of the gallbladder wall.

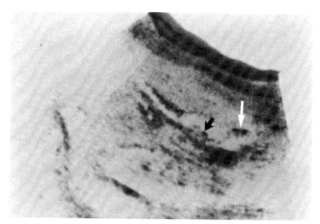

Figure 4-13H. Carcinoma of the gallbladder (longitudinal, 4 cm to right of midline). Within the gallbladder, there is a localized thickened area of the gallbladder wall (*black arrow*) associated with a gallbladder calculus (*white arrow*). The patient had carcinoma of the gallbladder associated with a calculus. Calculi are frequently associated with gallbladder carcinoma. The liver should be examined in these patients in order to exclude metastatic disease to the lymph nodes of the hepatic hilus or of the liver parenchyma.

area (36) (Fig. 4-13C). This appearance can be simulated by a gas-filled or collapsed gastric antrum or transverse colon, but shadowing posterior to gall-bladder calculi tends to be "complete" or "clean," as opposed to the incomplete shadowing associated with gastrointestinal structures (Fig. 4-13F). Again for emphasis, the echoes from bowel can be differentiated from calculi by scanning the patient in the upright position. This maneuver allows inferior displacement of bowel as opposed to collection of stones within the gallbladder fundus. If the echoes are not identified in the gallbladder area after the patient is placed upright, they are probably due to bowel. If the echogenic area remains within the gall-bladder, it is probably intrinsic.

Failure to delineate the gallbladder by ultrasound has clinical implications similar to those for nonvisualization with oral contrast media (37). If one finds a "contracted" gallbladder, the patient must be asked whether or not he or she has ingested food or smoked immediately prior to the examination. These ac-tivities will often result in physiological contraction of the gallbladder. Nonvi-sualization of the gallbladder may also be secondary to previous cholecystectomy. One must remember in obtaining the patient's history of surgery that the op-erative description is the only primary evidence. Oral testimony by patients and sometimes physicians may fail to differentiate a cholecystectomy from a chole-cystotomy. Again, one must obtain a complete clinical history at the time of examination.

Miscellaneous Gallbladder Conditions

Several other pathologic conditions of the gallbladder may be detected sono-graphically. These include intraluminal defects secondary to polyps, septations, and intraluminal defects secondary to carcinoma of the gallbladder. Ultrasound may be particularly helpful in establishing the diagnosis of gallbladder carcinoma (Fig. 4-13H); abnormal mucosa will often not provide concentration of oral contrast media adequate to visualize the mass. On OCG only nonvisualization will be noted; sonography may delineate the mass and possible metastatic disease. Carcinoma of the gallbladder usually appears as a mass that produces thickening and irregularity of the gallbladder wall. Calculi are frequently found within gallbladders that contain carcinoma. Enlarged lymph nodes in the region of the liver hilus are often the result of metastatic spread from a carcinoma of the gallbladder. Thus, the composite information obtained by ultrasound study may provide sufficient data for a definitive diagnosis.

Polyps of the gallbladder are seen as intraluminal echogenic projections that do not change in appearance with patient position. Polyps of the gallbladder should be differentiated from other intraluminal projections, such as prominent mucosal folds and septations. Folds of the gallbladder can be differentiated from intraluminal polyps by imaging in full inspiration and expiration and observing the difference in appearance. Folds should change in configuration. In addition, septations usually appear as thin echogenic interfaces that extend across the lumen of the gallbladder, whereas mucosal folds do not.

Frequently a linear, echogenic interface within the gallbladder is seen. This pattern may be due to viscid bile or "sludge." A bile-sludge layer is frequently observed in patients who have bile stasis. Sludge is commonly associated with intermittent obstruction of the cystic or common bile duct and can disappear after the cause of obstruction has been corrected. Sludge can be differentiated from layering stones by real-time scanning. Stones tend to move rapidly with changes in patient position, whereas it may take up to 20 minutes for sludge to layer. Sludge does not cause shadowing as commonly as do calculi. Pus within the gallbladder may also appear as an echogenic substance within the lumen, but the echoes are not as distinct as those of either calculi or sludge (Fig. 4-13G).

It is difficult to determine thickening of the gallbladder wall by sonography. Diffuse thickening can occasionally be demonstrated in patients with acute or chronic acalculous cholecystitis and emphysematous cholecystitis. In order to establish that there is thickening of the gallbladder wall, one should measure only when the gallbladder is distended with bile; contracted gallbladders may simulate a thickened wall. Because the gallbladder frequently becomes surrounded by ascitic fluid, the wall in patients with ascites may appear thickened due to acoustical enhancement. This "thickened" appearance may also be caused by fat around the gallbladder. Thickened gallbladder wall should be diagnosed in only the portion of the gallbladder where the transducer is perpendicular to the gallbladder wall, and the anterior wall measurement should be used. Because of the difficulty in determining the exact width of the wall, sonography appears to be less accurate than intravenous cholangiography or infusion tomography to measure gallbladder wall thickness.

Efficacy Considerations

At present oral cholecystography is probably the most reliable screening test for the presence of gallbladder calculi, but sonography with real-time imaging is also highly accurate (33). Guidelines for interpretation and implications of a nonvisualized gallbladder on an oral cholecystogram are better established than for nonvisualization on sonography. Sonography is particularly helpful in patients whose gallbladders cannot be adequately visualized on the first or second dose of an oral cholecystogram (32,37,38) and may even reduce cost and patient hospital stay. Sonography is the modality of choice in evaluating the gallbladder in pregnant patients, in whom exposure to radiation is a major concern. It is an excellent alternative in patients whose metabolic function or state of health prohibits adequate visualization of the gallbladder with radiographic contract methods.

OBSTRUCTIVE JAUNDICE

General Considerations

Sonography can accurately distinguish between obstructive and hepatocellular jaundice and is particularly useful in patients who present with jaundice. Even in patients with mild jaundice (bilirubin values of approximately 4 mg%), ultrasound can detect the dilated biliary ducts of an obstructed biliary system. The exact time period necessary to distend the ducts is not known but is thought to be approximately 48 hours. Distension of the intrahepatic bile ducts may be altered by the presence of preexisting hepatic disease. In cirrhosis, for example, intrahepatic bile duct distension may not be seen because of surrounding fibrosis, but the extrahepatic portion of the biliary tree may be markedly distended.

Normal Anatomy and Scanning Technique

When evaluating the liver for the presence of dilated ducts, it is important to distinguish ducts from normal intrahepatic vessels (Fig. 4-14A). The criteria outlined in Table 4-2 will allow a high degree of certainty. The origin, course, and branching pattern of these structures can be traced with real-time scanning. Another feature that distinguishes hepatic from and portal veins is the angle at which the branches point. Branching angles of hepatic veins have their apices pointing toward the inferior vena cava, whereas portal vein branches point toward the porta hepatis. Portal veins increase in caliber as they course towards the porta hepatis and have an echogenic "collar." This collar is thought to be due to a sheath of connective tissue and fat and the adjacent hepatic artery and ducts that are present in the portal triad. Hepatic veins, conversely, do not have an echogenic collar and enlarge as they course toward the inferior vena cava.

In contrast to portal and hepatic veins, dilated bile ducts are irregular or lobulated in their outline. The arborization of the biliary system is more extensive than that of the vascular system. Dilated biliary ducts ramify after a much shorter distance than vascular structures (Fig. 4-14B,C). Dilated bile ducts converge in the region of the porta hepatis giving a "stellate" appearance, also seen on radionuclide liver/spleen scans.

Obstructive Jaundice

Ultrasound studies are particularly useful and accurate in patients with obstructive jaundice. Several characteristic patterns have been described. The term

Figure 4-14. OBSTRUCTIVE JAUNDICE

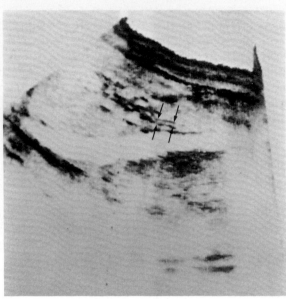

Figure 4-14A. Normal common bile duct (modified longitudinal, 4 cm to right of midline). The common bile duct (*arrows*) appears as a tubular structure whose caliber is approximately 6 mm. The course of the common bile duct runs anterior to the right portal vein and then posterior to the head of the pancreas. In normal persons who have not had cholecystectomy, the duct should measure no more than 6 mm. (Courtesy of M. Louis Weinstein, M.D.)

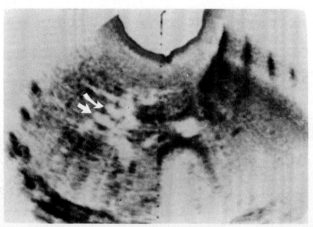

Figure 4-14B. Obstructive jaundice (transverse, 4 cm below xiphoid). Within the liver, there are numerous tubular structures that have a lobulated border and appear to converge in the region of the porta hepatis. The right portal vein appears as a linear structure only incompletely outlined (*straight arrow*). The dilated right hepatic duct lies immediately anterior to the right portal vein (*curved arrow*).

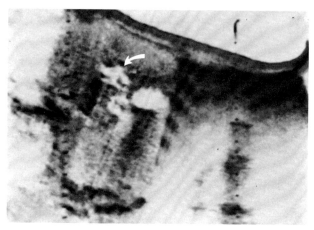

Figure 4-14C. Longitudinal in same patient as Figure 4-14B (longitudinal, 6 cm to right of midline). The dilated bile ducts appear as tubular structures that converge in the porta hepatis (*curved arrow*). This patient had recurrent carcinoma of the gastric antrum causing obstructive jaundice.

"parallel channel sign" refers to the presence of two parallel tubular structures in the region of the right portal vein on transverse scans. These two tubular structures represent the right portal vein and anterior to it a dilated right common hepatic duct. The "double-barrel" sign has been felt to be a sonographic manifestation of early bile duct distension (39,40).

The right hepatic artery shares a common course with the right portal vein and is seen as a tubular sonolucent structure anteriorly. Since the diameter of the right hepatic artery is usually less than 2 mm, it is infrequently delineated. When there is dilatation of the right common hepatic duct, its diameter approximates that of the right portal vein, resulting in the "parallel channel" sign on transverse scans (Fig. 4-14B). If these two structures are scanned in the longitudinal plane, the "double-barrel" or "shotgun" sign is seen, which represents the right portal vein and the right common hepatic duct depicted "end on." This sign is not always reliable, for the right portal vein after its bifurcation may also demonstrate what appears to be a "shotgun" sign. As biliary tract obstruction progresses, lobulated tubular structures converging in the region of the porta hepatis will be observed.

Preliminary scanning of the liver for bile duct distension should be performed in a longitudinal manner with the patient in suspended inspiration. The liver is even better delineated when it is displaced from under the right costal margin by gravity; this can be obtained with the patient in the left posterior oblique position. Oblique scans should also be performed to image the course of the right portal vein in the liver.

The common bile duct is best evaluated with the patient in the left posterior oblique position (43). On longitudinal scans, the common hepatic duct is seen crossing anteriorly over the right portal vein. The common bile duct, after receiving the cystic duct, courses inferiorly to the head of the pancreas (Figs. 4-14A,D). It will be seen to enter the medial wall of the descending duodenum.

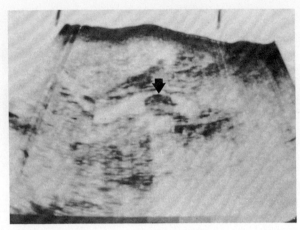

Figure 4-14D. Dilated common bile duct due to calculus (modified longitudinal, 4 cm to right of midline). The common bile duct appears as a tubular structure measuring approximately 1 cm in diameter. Within the distal aspect of the common bile duct is an echogenic focus that exhibits acoustical shadowing (*arrow*). This corresponded to a calculus within the common bile duct. (Courtesy of Marion Wier, M.D., Medical College of Georgia, Augusta, Ga.)

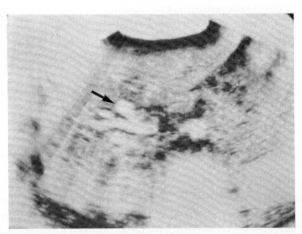

Figure 4-14E. Transverse scan of patient in Figure 4-14D (transverse, 4 cm below xiphoid). Dilated common bilt duct appears as a rounded structure anterior to the right portal vein (*arrow*).

On transverse scans, the common bile duct appears as a rounded fluid structure slightly anterior and lateral to the portal vein (Fig. 4-14E). The upper limit of normal for the common bile duct diameter is less on ultrasound than on intravenous cholangiography. This is because there is no magnification involved and the common bile duct is not distended with contrast media on sonography. In a postcholecystectomy patient, the common bile duct can measure up to 8 to 10 mm in diameter, whereas in patients who have not undergone surgery, the common bile duct should be no more than 6 mm in diameter.

An additional sign of obstruction of the biliary tree in the region of the ampulla of Vater is dilation of the pancreatic duct (9). A dilated pancreatic duct is seen as a fluid-filled tubular structure in the central portion of the pancreas. If pancreatic duct dilation is suspected on longitudinal scans, one should obtain a modified transverse study. This view includes most of the pancreas on a single study to trace the course of the duct to its insertion in the common bile duct. Dilatation of the pancreatic duct can only be proved when both margins of the dilated pancreatic duct are clearly seen. Dilatation implies inflammatory or neoplastic obstruction. Occasionally, the interface created by the posterior wall of the collapsed, mucus-containing gastic antrum can simulate the appearance of a pancreatic duct.

Other Conditions of the Biliary Tract

Neoplasms and inflammatory processes of the biliary tract do not have specific sonographic features. Cholangiosarcomas, if they infiltrate, can appear as irregular, rounded, echo-producing masses within the liver parenchyma, often associated with dilated biliary ducts proximal to the area on involvement. Ascending cholangitis does not have a specific sonographic pattern in our experience.

Efficacy Considerations

Of the several modalities for evaluation of the biliary tract, sonography is the least toxic and has a high degree of accuracy (43,44). CBT with contrast enhancement can also detect dilated ducts, but the flexibility of sonography allows more detailed evaluation of intrahepatic structures than nonenhanced CBT. Intravenous cholangiograms have limited effectiveness in the evaluation of jaundiced patients when the bilirubin is more than 4 mg% or when this level is increasing. Percutaneous transhepatic cholangiography (PTC) should be used if the results from the other noninvasive modalities are inconclusive or if decompression of the system is needed prior to surgery. Preliminary screening by sonography is still helpful prior to PTC. If dilated ducts are encountered, a needle of larger caliber can be selected to drain the distended bile ducts preoperatively.

BOWEL

Only recently have ultrasound studies been effectively applied to study of the bowel. The various patterns emanating from bowel should be distinguished from soft tissue lesions and other pathological abdominal or pelvic processes (Table 4-6). Abnormal bowel patterns can then direct further diagnostic studies to the gastrointestinal tract.

Normal Bowel

Since the bowel normally contains gas and variable amounts of fluid, its sonographic appearance has a wide spectrum. Gas and mucus within the bowel are highly reflective, causing mottled, distal acoustical shadowing (Fig. 4-15A). If

Figure 4-15. NORMAL BOWEL PATTERNS

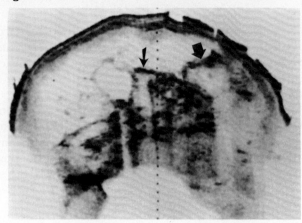

Figure 4-15A. Normal fluid-filled stomach and gas-filled duodenal bulb (transverse, 2 cm below xiphoid). Fluid-filled stomach appears as a partially sonolucent mass in the left upper quadrant (*large arrow*). Gas trapped within the duodenal bulb causes a mottled acoustical shadow posteriorly (*small arrow*). There is in contrast a complete shadow distal to the calculus within the gallbladder.

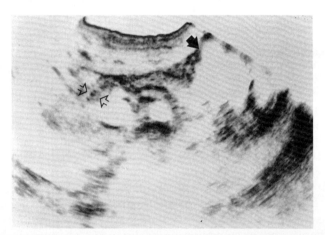

Figure 4-15B. Nondistended duodenal C-loop (transverse, 2 cm below xiphoid). The fluid-filled stomach appears as a sonolucent left upper quadrant mass (*solid arrow*). The mucus and gas trapped between and around the valvulae conniventes of the duodenal C-loop appear as rungs of a stepladder (*open arrows*).

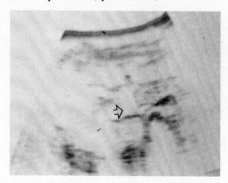

Figure 4-15C. Fluid-filled duodenum (modified transverse, 3 cm below xiphoid). The fluid-filled structure lateral to the pancreatic head is the duodenal C-loop (*arrow*).

216

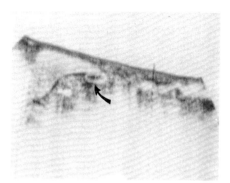

Figure 4-15D. Nondistended gastric antrum (longitudinal, 2 cm to left of midline). The nondistended gastric antrum containing mucus demonstrates a "bull's eye" pattern consisting of a central echogenicity and sonolucent halo (*arrow*). The wall of the gastric antrum is represented by the sonolucent halo, which should measure no more than 1 cm in thickness.

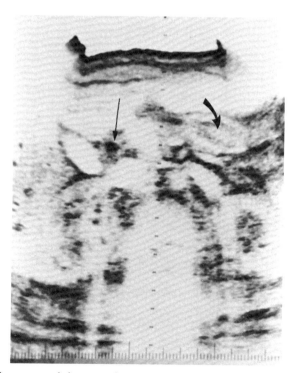

Figure 4-15E. Mucus-containing gastric antrum (transverse, 2 cm below xiphoid). The mucus-containing gastric antrum appears as an elliptically shaped mass in the left upper quadrant. The intraluminal echoes arise from mucus contained within the gastric antrum (*curved arrow*). Also note the gas-filled duodenal bulb (*straight arrow*).

Table 4-6. Sonographic Features of Normal and Abnormal Bowel

Bowel Segment	Sonographic Features
Normal nondistended (mucus and gas-filled)	
Gastric body	Echogenic, may cause reverberations
Gastric antrum, transverse colon	When imaged in transverse plane, "bull's eye" pattern Changes configuration with peristalsis
Duodenal bulb	Echogenic focus with posterior acoustical shadowing
Fluid-filled	
Duodenum	Tubular sonolucent structure adjacent to pancreatic head or caudal to pancreatic body
Jejunum	Periodic intraluminal projections corresponding to valvulae conniventes ("keyboard pattern")
Ileum	Smooth walls
Ascending, tranverse colon	Indentions of serosa at haustral sacculations
Descending, rectosigmoid colon	Echogenic borders, tubular
Rectum	Rectal valves
Tumors and related conditions	
Adenocarcinoma of stomach Adenocarcinoma of transverse colon	Bowel wall thickening as evidence by abnormal "bull's eye" or "target" pattern
Intussusception Bowel lymphoma Intramural hemorrhage Crohn's disease	Sonolucent halo greater than 2 cm in thickness
	Halo usually asymmetrical to echogenic core
	No demonstrable change in configuration with peristalsis

bowel is fluid-filled, certain distinctive anatomical structures of the bowel can occasionally be demonstrated (45) (Figs. 4-15B,C). In particular, the valvulae conniventes can frequently be seen in fluid-filled loops of proximal small bowel as lines of echoes that course across the bowel lumen or as intraluminal echogenic projections that produce a "keyboard" pattern (Figs. 4-16A,B). Distal small bowel, when fluid-filled, has smooth walls and is more tubular in shape than proximal small bowel. Valvulae conniventes are not as numerous in the distal

Figure 4-16. BOWEL DISORDERS

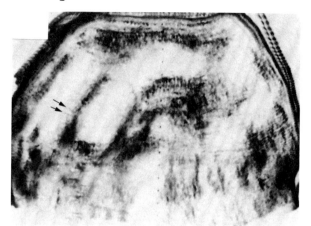

Figure 4-16A. Small bowel obstruction with dilated, fluid-filled jejunal loops (transverse, 6 cm below xiphoid). There are numerous tubular sonolucent structures in the right upper quadrant. Numerous fine echoes are seen emanating from the bowel wall (*small arrows*), representing valvulae conniventes ("keyboard sign").

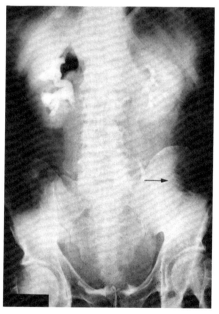

Figure 4-16B. Supine abdominal radiograph of same patient as in Figure 4-16A. There is only a single gas-filled loop of jejunum that appears nondistended (*arrow*). A "pseudotumor" effect of the fluid-filled bowel in the abdomen and pelvis is present. (Courtesy of Anthony Dowling, M.D.)

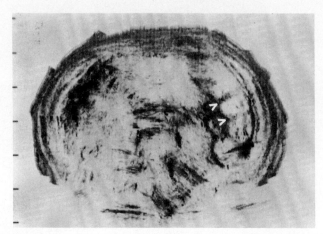

Figure 4-16C. Fluid-filled splenic flexure (transverse, 6 cm below xiphoid). The splenic flexure is fluid-filled. The colon can be differentiated from small bowel by its haustral indentations (*white arrowheads*).

small bowel as they are proximally. The ascending and transverse colon can be identified by its haustral indentations, which are periodic and involve the serosa (Fig. 4-16C). The rectum and rectosigmoid colon can be recognized by the rectal valves that can be demonstrated particularly well on water enema studies. The water enema technique can be used to assist in delineating structures in the pelvis. Tumor invasion into the bladder from uterine, adrenal, or colonic tumors can be documented using this method.

Another pattern associated with bowel is that produced by mucus. The mixture of mucus and gas trapped within the bowel causes multiple echoes. If the bowel contains only gas, the sound is reflected. Although mucus is moderately echogenic, it does not produce the shadowing that is observed distal to collections of gas (Figs. 4-15B,D,E).

Bowel Abnormalities

The "bull's-eye" or "target" patterns have been described with bowel tumors, but they have also been observed in collapsed bowel containing mucus or gas (47). These terms refer to an echo pattern consisting of central echogenic foci surrounded by a sonolucent halo. The collapsed gastric antrum and transverse colon may also produce this pattern, particularly in a location just caudal to the left lobe of the liver (Figs. 4-14A,B). The source of this pattern can usually be identified, and on real-time scanning normal bowel will change in configuration, whereas bowel tumors will not (Fig. 4-16D).

The bull's-eye pattern arises when a segment of bowel is imaged in transverse section. The bull's-eye pattern arising from a bowel tumor or inflammatory mass generally has a diameter greater than 3 cm and a sonolucent halo greater than 2 cm. These are helpful findings to distinguish tumor from normal bowel, as is peristalsis. The "bull's-eye" pattern has been associated with several neoplastic and inflammatory conditions of bowel including adenocarcinoma, intussusception, Crohn's disease, ischemia, and lymphoma. All these entities produce thick-

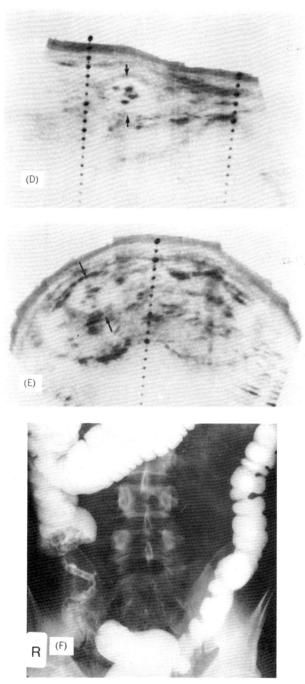

Figures 4-16D, E, F. Carcinoma of the cecum with ileocolic intussusception. In Figure 4-16D (longitudinal, 6 cm to right of midline) there is a "bull's eye" pattern in the right lower quadrant consisting of a central echogenic core and a sonolucent halo (*arrows*). A similar appearance is seen on the transverse scan (Fig. 4-16E) (*arrows*). This mass was found to correspond to an ileocolic intussusception on barium enema (Fig. 4-16F), which was secondary to adenocarcinoma of the cecum (R = right). This pattern can also be encountered in any condition that causes bowel wall thickening, such as Crohn's disease, lymphoma, or intramural hemorrhage.

221

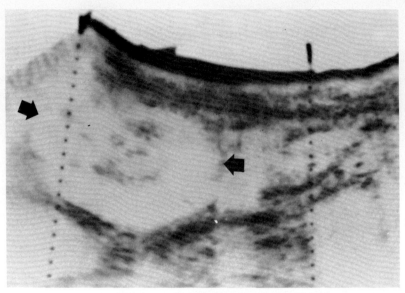

Figure 4-16G. Jejuno-jejunal intussusception (longitudinal, 4 cm to left of midline). There is a large left upper quadrant mass with a central echogenic core (*arrows*). This is an abnormal "target" pattern since the sonolucent halo is at least 5 cm thick. This represented jejuno-jejunal intussusception in a patient who had undergone a jejuno-ileal bypass. This was unsuspected clinically at the time of ultrasound examination.

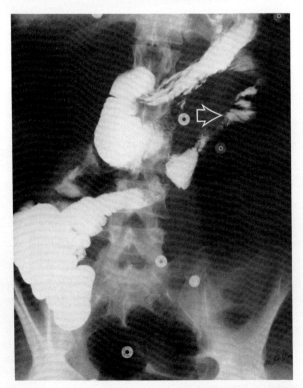

Figure 4-16H. Upper gastrointestinal series of patient in Figure 4-16G. There is partial filling of the proximal jejunum (*open arrow*). The intussusception was difficult to demonstrate radiographically.

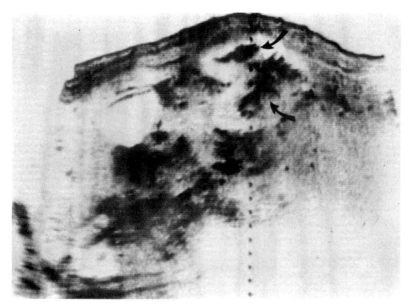

Figure 4-16I. Carcinoma of the transverse colon with fistula to stomach and small bowel (transverse, 3 cm below xiphoid). There are two masses in the left upper quadrant and epigastrium that demonstrate an abnormal "target" pattern (*curved arrows*). These masses corresponded to bowel wall thickening secondary to tumor infiltration of the transverse colon with a fistulous connection to the stomach and small bowel.

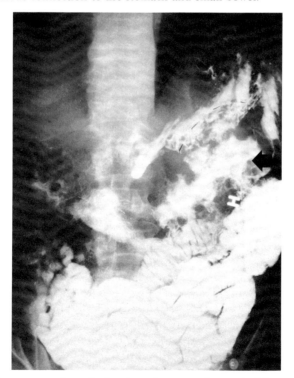

Figure 4-16J. Upper gastrointestinal series of same patient as in Figure 4-16I. There is marked destruction of the large bowel mucosa in the region of the splenic flexure (*arrow*). Fistulous connection between the stomach, transverse colon, and small bowel could be demonstrated. (Courtesy of Anthony Dowling, M.D.)

ening of the bowel wall. An elongated variant on the bull's eye pattern is observed when a bowel tumor is imaged in its longitudinal axis. Since some bowel tumors destroy their walls, they appear as isolated solid masses, especially if an insufficient amount of mucus is present within the bowel lumen.

Efficacy Considerations

At present, the most important aspect of recognizing the sonographic patterns of bowel is to differentiate bowel from pelvic or abdominal masses. In some cases where conventional radiographic evaluation is inconclusive, sonography can be diagnostic. For instance, an obstructed afferent loop can be recognized sonographically as a fluid-filled loop of bowel. Likewise, ultrasound can be employed to establish the diagnosis of an occult intussusception in the rare instance when it cannot be demonstrated radiographically. In the future, sonography may be helpful in detecting early invasion of bowel wall by tumor.

RETROPERITONEAL AND OTHER ABDOMINAL MASSES

Because of the soft tissue planes and constant position of organs in the retroperitoneum, CT is probably better suited for evaluation in this area than ultrasound; nevertheless, ultrasound can establish distortion of retroperitoneal structures with some reliability. This subject will be considered again in discussions in Chapter 5.

Sonographic evaluation of the retroperitoneum can be accomplished with the patient in either the supine or prone position. The major organs of the retroperitoneum—the kidneys, the pancreas, the great vessels—can be studied in the supine position. The major muscle groups of the retroperitoneum are best evaluated by longitudinal scans made in the prone position (Fig. 4-17A).

A knowledge of the retroperitoneal compartments is necessary to understand their sonographic and radiographic features. The anterior pararenal space includes the pancreas, the ascending and descending colon, and the great vessels. Inflammatory or neoplastic processes in that compartment may easily affect all of these major structures. The perirenal space envelops both kidneys, but is not continuous across the midline. Perirenal abscesses are contained in the perirenal spaces. The posterior pararenal space contains no organs but can be affected by hemorrhage—especially in hemophilia.

The most common abnormality in the retroperitoneum is abdominal aortic aneurysm, the second being lymphadenopathy. The most frequently recognized tumor of the retroperitoneum is liposarcoma, which can be recognized sonographically as an asymmetrical enlargement of the retroperitoneal outline. Liposarcomas tend to outgrow their blood supply resulting in central necrosis (Fig. 4-17B) (49). Iliopsoas abscess can be suggested by unilateral enlargement on the iliopsoas and paraspinal muscle configuration at sonography (Fig. 4-17C). Occasionally, pus can be identified as a sonolucency located between the iliac and psoas muscle groups (48,49). Bleeding into an iliopsoas muscle is another cause of unilateral enlargement and may be found in hemophiliacs who have no other visible signs of hemorrhage.

Figure 4-17. RETROPERITONEAL MASSES

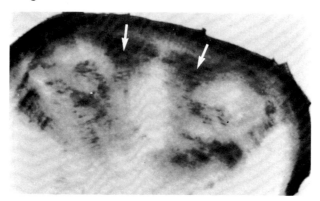

Figure 4-17A. Normal retroperitoneal structures (prone, transverse, 8 cm above iliac crests). The paraspinal and iliopsoas muscle groups (*white arrows*) are symmetrical and lie to either side of the spine. Their appearance can be differentiated from kidneys since they do not contain a central echogenic interface representing the renal pelvis.

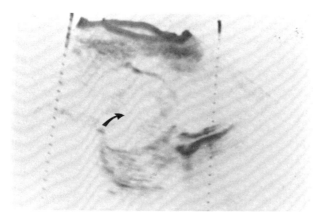

Figure 4-17B. Necrotic rhabdomyosarcoma (longitudinal, pelvic sonogram at midline with distended bladder). There is a rounded mass posterior to the urinary bladder. The central area of sonolucency (*curved arrow*) corresponds to an area of necrosis within the mass.

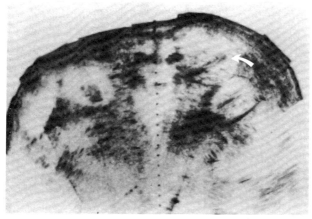

Figure 4-17C. Iliopsoas abscess (transverse prone, 5 cm above iliac crest). There is asymmetrical enlargement (*arrow*) of the paraspinal and iliopsoas muscles that resulted from an abscess in these structures. A similar appearance can be encountered in an iliopsoas hematoma in hemophiliacs.

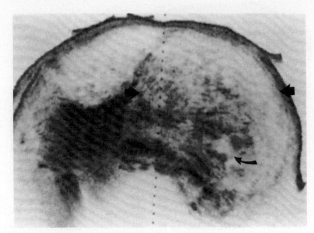

Figure 4-17D. Retroperitoneal neurofibroma (transverse, 15 cm below xiphoid). There is a large nonhomogeneous mass arising from the retroperitoneum (*large arrow*). The mass contains a central area of necrosis (*curved arrow*). This mass simulated the sonographic features of an intra-abdominal mass. At surgery, a 30-pound neurofibroma originating from the retroperitoneum was found.

Other less common abdominal masses include a variety of mesenchymal sarcomas. These tumors may go unnoticed by the patient, until they have attained large sizes. Mesenchymal sarcomas also tend to proliferate rapidly, outgrowing their blood supplies and exhibiting central necrosis (50).

SUMMARY

Thus, there are several clinical applications of sonography for the evaluation of pathological processes within the abdomen. The noninvasive, atraumatic quality of sonography contributes to its utility as a screening procedure. The availability of numerous other imaging modalities for use in the abdomen necessitates consideration of the relative efficacy of each diagnostic modality according to the clinical problem to be investigated. The availability of high-resolution real-time scanning devices allows a more flexible approach for evaluation of abdominal disorders and should be used in a manner similar to fluoroscopy in the evaluation of the abdomen.

REFERENCES

Normal Anatomy

1. Sample, W.: Techniques for improved delineation of normal anatomy of upper abdomen and high retroperitoneum with gray scale ultrasound. *Radiology* 124:197–202, 1977.
2. Sample, W., Sarti, D.: Computerized body tomography and gray scale ultrasonography: Anatomic correlations and pitfalls in upper abdomen. *Gastrointest. Radiol.* 3:243–249, 1978.

Abdominal Aorta

3. Wheeler, W., Beachley, M., Ranniger, K.: Angiography and ultrasonography: A comparative study of abdominal aorta aneurysm. *Am. J. Roentgenol.* 126(1):95–100, 1976.

4. Gooding, G., Herzog, K., Hedgecock, M, Eisenberg, R.: B-mode ultrasonography of prosthetic vascular grafts. *Radiology* 127:763–766, 1978.

Pancreas

5. Levitt, R., Grisseo, G., Sagal, S., Stanley, R., Evens, R., Koehler, J., Jost, R.: Complementary use of ultrasound and CT in studying the pancreas and kidneys. *Radiology* 126:149–152, 1978.

6. Johnson, M., Mack, L.: Sonographic evaluation of the pancreas. *Gastrointest. Radiol.* 3:257–266, 1978.

7. Crade, M., Taylor, K., Rosenfeld, A.: Water distension of the gut in evaluation of the pancreas by ultrasound. *Am. J. Roentgenol.* 131:348–349, 1978.

8. DeGraff, C., Taylor, K., Simmonds, B., Rosenfeld, A.: Gray scale echography of the pancreas: Re-evaluation of normal size. *Radiology* 129:157–161, 1978.

9. Gosink, B., Leopold, G.: The dilated pancreatic duct: Ultrasonic evaluation. *Radiology* 126:475–478, 1978.

10. Doust, B., Pearce, J.: Gray scale ultrasonographic properties of normal and inflamed pancreas. *Radiology* 120:653–647, 1976.

11. Sarti, D.: Rapid development and spontaneous regression of pancreatic pseudocysts documented by ultrasound. *Radiology* 125:789–793, 1977.

12. Weinstein. D., Weinstein, B.: Ultrasonic demonstration of the pancreatic duct: An analysis of 41 cases. *Radiology* 130:729–734, 1979.

13. Goldstein, H., Katragadda, C.: Prone view ultrasonography for pancreatic tail neoplasms. *Am. J. Roentgenol.* 131:231–234, 1978.

Liver

14. Pertertek, L., Mack, L., Johnson, M.: Ultrasonographic evaluation of the liver. *Appl. Radiol.* 139:150, 1978.

15. Sample, W., Gray, R., Hoe, N., Graham, L., Bennett, C.: Nuclear imaging, tomographic nuclear imaging, and gray scale ultrasound in the evaluation of porta hepatis. *Radiology* 122:773, 1977.

16. Taylor, K., Carpenter, D., Hill, C., McCready, V.: Gray scale ultrasonic imaging: The anatomy and pathology of the liver. *Radiology* 229:415–423, 1976.

17. Weaver, R., Goldstein, H., Greenberg, B., Perkins, C.: Gray scale evaluation of hepatic cystic disease. *Am. J. Roentgenol.* 130:849–852, 1978.

18. Scheible, W., Goldstein, B., Leopold, G.: Gray scale echographic patterns of hepatic metastatic disease. *Am. J. Roentgenol.* 129:983–987, 1977.

19. Green, G., Bree, R., Goldstein, H., Stanley, C.: Gray scale ultrasound evaluation for hepatic neoplasms: Patterns and correlations. *Radiology* 124:203, 298, 1977.

20. Sullivan, D., Taylor, K., Gottschalk, A.: The use of ultrasound to enhance the diagnostic utility of the equivocal liver scintigraph. *Radiology* 128: 1978.

21. Bryan, P., Dunn, W., Grossman, Z., Winstow, B., McAfee, J., Kieffer, J.: Correlation of CT, gray scale ultrasound and radionuclide imaging of liver in detecting space-occupying processes. *Radiology* 124:387–393, 1977.

Abscess

22. Doust, B., Quiroz, F., Stewart, J.: Ultrasonic distinction of abscess from other intraabdominal fluid collections. *Radiology* 125:213–218, 1977.

23. Kressel, H., Filly, R.: Ultrasonic appearance of gas-containing abscesses in abdomen. *Am. J. Roentgenol.* 130:71–73, 1978.

24. Meyers, M.: Intraperitoneal spread of infection, in *Dynamic Radiology of the Abdomen: Normal and Abnormal Anatomy.* New York: Springer-Verlag, 1976, pp. 1–34.

25. Taylor, K., Sullivan, D., Lawson, J., Rosenfeld, A.: Ultrasound and gallium for diagnosis of abdominal and pelvic abscess. *Gastrointest. Radiol.* 3:281–286, 1978.

26. Korobkin, M., Callen, P., Filly, R., Hoffer, P., Shinshak, R., Kressel, H.: Comparison of computerized tomography, ultrasonography, gallium-67 scanning in evaluation of suspected abdominal abscesses. *Radiology* 129:89–93, 1978.

Ascites

27. Yeh, H., Wolf, B.: Ultrasonography in ascites. *Radiology* 124:783–790, 1977.

28. Myers, M.: Pathways of ascitic flow, in *Dynamic Radiology of the Abdomen: Normal and Abnormal Anatomy.* New York: Springer-Verlag, 1976, p. 56.

29. Hall, D., Hann, L., Ferrucci, J., et al.: Sonographic morphology of the normal menstrual cycle. *Radiology* 133:185–188, 1979.

Lymph Nodes

30. Rochester, D., Bowie, J., Kunzmann, A., Lester, E.: Ultrasound in staging lymphomas. *Radiology* 124:483–487, 1977.

Gallbladder

32. Lawson, T.: Gray scale cholecystosonography: Diagnostic accuracy. *Radiology* 122:247–251, 1977.

33. Wolson, A., Goldberg, B.: Gray scale sonographic cholecystography: A primary screening procedure. *J.A.M.A.* 240 (19):2073–2075, 1978.

34. Grossman, M.: Cholelithiasis and acoustic shadowing. *J. Clin. Ultrasound* 6:182–184, 1978.

35. Carroll, B.: In vitro comparison of physical properties of gallstones. *Am. J. Roentgenol.* 131:223–226, 1978.

36. Purdom, R., Thomas, S., Krugh, K., Spitz, H., Kereiaches, J.: Ultrasonic properties of biliary calculi. Presented at Radiological Society of North America meeting, November 25–December 1, 1978, Chicago, Illinois.

37. Leopold, G., Amberg, J., Gossink, B., Mittelstaedt, C.: Gray scale ultrasonic cholecystography: A comparison with conventional radiographic techniques. *Radiology* 121:445–448, 1976.

38. Arnon, S., Rosenquist, C.: Gray scale cholecystosonography: An evaluation of accuracy. *Am. J. Roentgenol.* 127:817–818, 1976.

Jaundice

39. Conrad, M., Landay, M., James, J.: Sonographic "parallel channel" sign of biliary tree enlargement in mild to moderate obstructive jaundice. *Am. J. Roentgenol.* 130:270–286, 1978.

40. Malini, S., Sabel, J.: Ultrasonography in obstructive jaundice. *Radiology* 123:429–433, 1977.

41. Weill, F., Eisencher, A., Zeltner, F.: Ultrasonic study of the normal and dilated biliary tree. *Radiology* 127:221–224, 1978.

42. Lee, T., Henderson, S., Ehrlich, R.: Ultrasound diagnosis of common bile duct dilatation. *Radiology* 124:783–787, 1977.

43. Behan, M., Kazam, E.: Sonography of the common bile duct: Value of the right anterior oblique view. *Am. J. Roentgenol.* 130:701–709, 1978.

44. Sample, W., Sarti, D., Goldstein, L., Weiner, M., Kadell, B.: Gray scale ultrasonography of jaundiced patient. *Radiology* 128:719–725, 1978.

45. Raskin, M.: Hepatobiliary disease: A comparative evaluation by ultrasound and computerized tomography. *Gastrointest. Radiol.* 3:267–271, 1978.

Bowel

46. Fleischer, A., Dowling. A., Weinstein, M., James, A.: Sonographic patterns of distended fluid-filled small and large bowel: Anatomic and radiographic correlation. *Radiology* 133, 1979, in press.
47. Fleischer, A., Muhletaler, C., James, A.: Sonographic patterns arising from normal and abnormal bowel. *Rad. Clin. N.A.* 18(2), 1980, in press.

Retroperitoneal Masses

48. McCullogh, D., Leopold, G.: Diagnosis of retroperitoneal fluid collections by ultrasonogtaphy: A series of surgically proven cases. *J. Urol.* 115:656–658, 1976.
49. Laing, F., Jacobs, R.: Value of ultrasonography in detection of retroperitoneal inflammatory masses. *Radiology* 123:169–172, 1977.

Miscellaneous

50. Bree, R., Green, B.: Gray scale sonographic appearance of intraabdominal mesenchymal sarcomas. *Radiology* 128:193–197, 1978.
51. Meyers, M.: Intraperitoneal spread of malignancy, in *Dynamic Radiology of the Abdomen: Normal and Abnormal Anatomy*. New York: Springer-Verlag, 1976, pp. 37–80.
52. Taylor, K., Atkinson, P., deGraff, C., Dember, A., Rosenfield, A.: Clinical evaluation of pulse-Doppler device linked to gray scale B-scan equipment. *Radiology* 129:745–749, 1978.

5
Urological
Sonography

INDICATIONS

The application of sonography to the study of urologic disorders has undergone significant change in response to improvements in image resolution. The first application of ultrasound in this area was in the evaluation of renal masses that were often detected by routine excretory urography. This remains one of the most common indications for renal ultrasound studies. With the recent improvement in scanning resolution afforded by gray scale imaging, excellent delineation of intrarenal structures can routinely be obtained. This has resulted in the detection not only of anatomic derangements such as hydronephrosis but also of parenchymal disorders that may affect focal areas or an entire kidney.

At present, sonography is most helpful in the evaluation and detection of the following urologic disorders or problems:

1. Poorly functioning kidneys (hydronephrotic versus parenchymal lesions such as end-stage kidney)
2. Differentiation of cystic from complex and solid renal masses
3. Renal transplant
   a. Cystic masses
   b. Rejection
4. Congenital renal anomalies
5. Scrotal disorders
   a. Epididymitis versus neoplasm
   b. Abscesses
6. Perirenal abscesses and adenopathy
7. Confirmation of presence or absence of kidney

One can sometimes evaluate adrenal masses and bladder tumors by sonography. Sonography also has potential application in the evaluation of prostatic masses.

It should be emphasized that sonography depicts the anatomy of the kidney rather than its function. Radionuclide renograms can be used in combination with renal sonograms for combined evaluation of the anatomical and physiologic status of the kidney. Computerized body tomography (CBT) demonstrates anatomical data similar to that obtained by sonography and can be used as an alternative method for evaluation of renal masses when the sonographic examination is not diagnostic (26). The arterial supply of a renal mass can only be depicted specifically by arteriography, although overall blood flow is qualitatively assessed by dynamic radionuclide renograms. Therefore, ultrasound is but one of many alternative imaging modalities to evaluate the kidney—it has certain advantages that will be emphasized in this chapter. Table 5-1 lists the sonographic features of various renal disorders.

TECHNIQUE AND ANATOMY

Since the kidneys are retroperitoneal organs, they are best imaged with the patient in the prone position. Because of the excursion of the kidney with respiration, scans should be performed with the patient in suspended respiration. Insiiration is preferred to expiration since the kidney is displaced farther away from the ribs. Images of the kidneys are obtained by sweeping the transducer in a slightly oblique fashion from the upper portion of the kidney to the lower (Fig. 5-1). On transverse scans, the renal pelvis is identified as a central echogenic interface oriented obliquely in the anterior-posterior plane (Fig.

Table 5-1. Sonographic Features of Various Adult Renal Disorders

Entity	Sonographic Features
Masses	
Cysts	Sonolucent, smooth, well-defined borders; posterior acoustical enhancement
Renal cell tumor	Echogenic, intrarenal mass; complex texture if necrotic; may have tumor extension into renal vein and inferior vena cava
Polycystic disease	Bilaterally enlarged kidneys that contain numerous cysts of various sizes; may have liver involvement
Angiomyolipoma	Echogenic masses; associated with tuberous sclerosis in approximately 70% of cases
Obstruction	
Hydronephrosis	Various degrees of pelvocaliceal system distension; separation of normally closely opposed interfaces arising from renal pelvis
Upper pole or segmental obstruction	Only portion of pelvocaliceal system distended
Parenchymal disease	
End-stage kidney	Small kidney with echogenic, thinned renal cortex
Other	
Perirenal abscess	Complex collection surrounding kidney confined to perirenal space

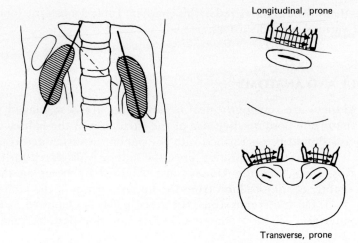

Longitudinal, prone

Transverse, prone

Figure 5-1. Scanning planes for prone renal scans. The long axes of the kidneys are oblique with respect to the spine. The axis of the left kidney is usually slightly more oblique than that of the right. In addition, the right kidney is usually lower than the left. For prone scans of the kidneys, a single sweep scan in 1- to 2-cm intervals, with the patient in suspended respiration, along the longitudinal and transverse axes of the kidney is performed. Single-sweep prone transverse scans are marked by their distance above the iliac crests.

5-2B). Because of adequate transmission through the liver, the right kidney can also be evaluated with the patient in the supine position (Fig. 5-2C).

If the routine views do not adequately demonstrate the region of interest, additional scans can be obtained of the kidneys with the patient in the decubitus position. In this position the kidney that is elevated away from the table can be scanned in a transverse plane (4). Other views that may be employed in the evaluation of the kidney include a coronal scan for the delineation of the left kidney. In this technique, a simple sector scan is obtained between the ribs of the lower hemithorax with the transducer aimed at the midabdomen.

In summary, the following patient positions are recommended for sonographic examination of the kidneys:

1. Prone
   a. Modified longitudinal scan along the axis of the kidney
   b. Transverse scan over kidneys
2. Supine (for right kidney)
   a. Longitudinal scan in suspended inspiration

If necessary,

3. Decubitus
   a. Transverse
4. Coronal
   a. Through 9th or 10th interspace; aim transducer through center of body

The normal adult kidneys measure 10 to 12 cm in length, 5 to 6 cm in width, and 3 to 4 cm in anterior-posterior dimension (26). On renal sonograms with

Figure 5-2. NORMAL KIDNEYS

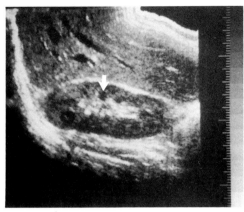

Figure 5-2A. Normal right kidney (supine, longitudinal, 5 cm to right of midline, white-on-black image). Since the liver overlies the right kidney, this kidney can usually be adequately delineated with the patient in the supine position. The nondistended pelvis (*arrows*) appears as a linear echogenic interface in the center of the kidney. The echogenicity of the renal pelvis probably arises from fat, vessels, and fibrous tissue. A renal pyramid (*white arrow*) appears as a wedge-shaped sonolucency within the parenchyma of the kidney.

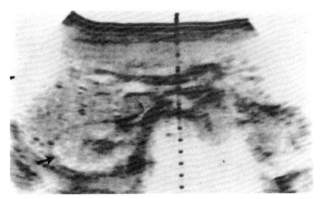

Figure 5-2B. Normal right kidney (supine, transverse, 4 cm below xiphoid). The right kidney (*large arrow*) appears as an ovoid structure with central linear echoes representing the renal pelvis. The right renal artery can be delineated in this image as it originates from the aorta (*small arrow*).

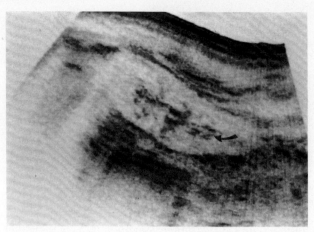

Figure 5-2C. Normal left kidney (prone, longitudinal, 4 cm to left of midline). The left kidney is best visualized in the prone position. The renal pelvis appears as a central echogenic interface (*curved arrow*).

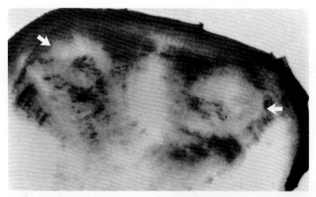

Figure 5-2D. Normal kidneys (prone, 8 cm above iliac crest). Both kidneys are visualized (*arrows*). The spine between the kidneys causes an acoustical shadow. A 1- to 2-cm discrepancy in the transverse width of the kidneys is often due to the difference in the transverse anatomical level through which the kidneys are imaged.

high-frequency transducers (5-MHz) and high-gain settings, the renal pyramids can be distinguished from the renal cortex (5). The renal pyramids appear as triangular areas of diminished echogenicity within the renal parenchyma. The apex of the triangle represents the renal papillae and is pointed toward the renal pelvis. The columns of Bertin are seen as echogenic extensions of the cortex between the pyramids. Occasionally, a small cluster of echoes in the middle of the base of the pyramid at the corticomedullary junction can be recognized. This is thought to represent the arcuate arteries. These structures can only be consistently delineated with scans in vitro at present, but may be consistently seen with improved resolution (5).

The linear series of echoes emanating from the renal pelvis serves as a landmark for the center of the kidney. The central linear echogenic interface arises from the renal pelvis and surrounding renal vessels and fat. When mildly distended, the calices appear as small, rounded sonolucencies located centrally in the renal pelvis (Fig. 5-3A).

When nondistended, the ureters are difficult to evaluate. These are seen in some normals and not in others. However, when they become dilated, they are recognized as tubular structures that have a longitudinal course (Fig. 2-16B). The diameter of a ureter can measure up to 1 cm normally.

Abnormal renal parenchymal texture can be detected when the echogenicity of the liver parenchyma is compared to that of the renal cortex. Normally, since the portal triads of the liver contain fibrotic tissue, the liver is more echogenic

Figure 5-3. OBSTRUCTIVE UROPATHY

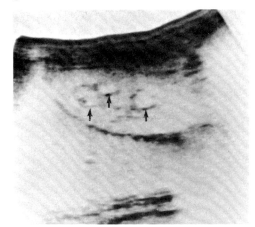

Figure 5-3A. Mild hydronephrosis (prone, modified longitudinal, 6 cm to left of midline). There are numerous sonolucent areas in the region of the renal collecting systems representing dilated calices (*arrows*).

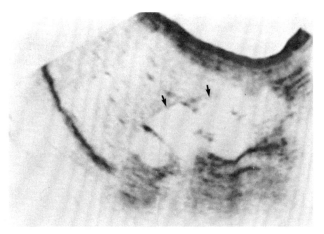

Figure 5-3B. Marked hydronephrosis (supine, modified longitudinal, 6 cm to left of midline). Numerous fluid-filled sacs representing a distended collecting system are seen (*arrows*).

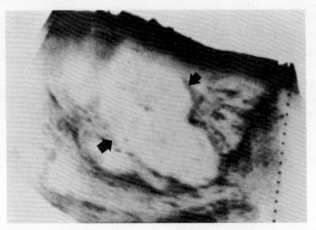

Figure 5-3C. Pyohydronephrosis (prone, modified longitudinal, 4 cm to right of midline). The right renal pelvis is markedly distended (*arrows*) and contains echogenic material representing cellular debris.

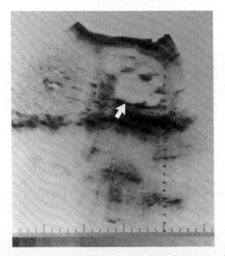

Figure 5-3D. Marked hydronephrosis (prone, modified longitudinal, 3 cm to right of midline). The distended renal pelvis (*white arrow*) and calices are apparent on this single image.

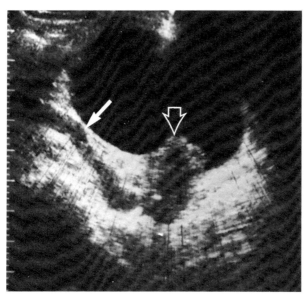

Figure 5-3E. Carcinoma of the cervix with ureteric obstruction (longitudinal, 2 cm to right of midline, white-on-black image). There is an irregular solid mass (*open white arrow*) in the region of the uterine cervix. The distended distal ureter is also noted (*white arrow*). The echoes recorded within the ureter are artifactual due to excessively high gain setting.

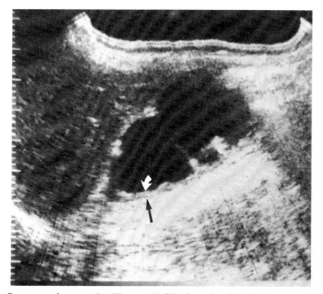

Figure 5-3F. Same patient as in Figure 5-3E (longitudinal, 4 cm to right of midline, white-on-black image). Since a pelvic mass and distended distal ureter was found, the kidneys were evaluated for obstructive uropathy. Marked hydronephrosis was found in the right kidney. Only a thin sliver of renal cortex (*arrows*) remained. (Courtesy of M. Louis Weinstein, M.D.)

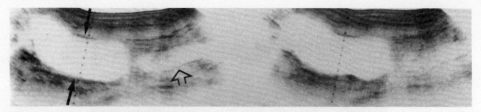

Figure 5-3G. Hydronephrotic upper collecting system with hydroureter (prone, longitudinal, 5 cm to left of midline). The obstructed upper pole collecting system appears as an elliptical sonolucent structure in the region of the left kidney (*arrow*). The distended ureter is also seen (*open arrow*). The nondistended right kidney depicted in Figure 5-9B also has a duplex collecting system. (Courtesy of Karen Parker, R.D.M.S., and Clifton Greer, M.D.)

than the renal cortex. However, when the renal cortex contains abnormal amounts of fibrous tissue, the echogenicity of the renal cortex can approximate or be greater than that of the liver. Evaluation of the texture of solid organs appears to be an area of great future for ultrasound.

RENAL MASSES

One of the most frequent requests for renal sonography is to further characterize a renal mass that is initially discovered during excretory urography. By using this method, cystic masses can be differentiated from complex and soft tissue equivalent (solid) masses. Masses smaller than 2 cm may be difficult to delineate sonographically because of the limits of instrument resolution.

Cystic Masses

Cystic masses reveal three major sonographic characteristics:

1. Echo-free, even at high-gain settings
2. Posterior acoustical enhancement
3. Smooth, well-defined walls

In order to diagnose a renal mass as a cyst, these three characteristics must be documented in at least two scanning planes (6).

Solitary renal cysts are found frequently in asymptomatic patients at the time of initial urography, CT, or sonography. It has been estimated that one-third of the adult population has renal cysts (28). Cystic masses appear as sonolucent areas within the renal cortex, have a well-defined border, and exhibit distal acoustical enhancement. They may be located within the renal cortex or in the peripelvic area. For complete evaluation of a cystic renal mass, many advocate aspiration and analysis of the cyst fluid. Whether or not this is performed should depend upon the intended use of the data. If one decides to operate upon a mass if it is a neoplasm, then cyst puncture is indicated. A technique using ultrasound for cyst aspiration is described in another section of this chapter (Figs. 5-4A,B).

Figure 5-4. CYSTIC RENAL MASSES

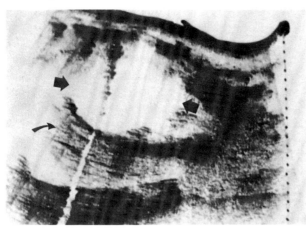

Figure 5-4A. Simple renal cyst (prone, modified longitudinal, 4 cm to right of midline). There is an 8-cm rounded, sonolucent mass in the upper pole of right kidney (*large arrows*). The walls of the mass are well defined, and there is posterior acoustical enhancement (*curved arrow*). In addition, there is a reverberation artifact with complete posterior acoustical shadowing along the midportion of the cyst caused by a rib.

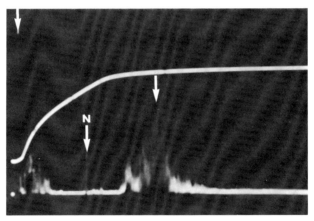

Figure 5-4B. Ultrasonically guided cyst aspiration (A-mode trace directed through posterior-anterior dimension of cyst, aspiration needle inserted). This A-mode trace depicts the cyst as an echo-free space with high-amplitude posterior wall echoes. The tip of the aspiration needle is identified as an echo peak (N) within the echo-free space representing the cyst. The arrow to the left of the image represents the peak created by the main bang of of the transducer. The arrow distal to the needle demarcates the echo peak arising from the posterior wall of the cyst.

Solitary cystic masses in the kidney include peripelvic cysts and more rarely cysts created by obstructed upper collecting tract associated with a duplicated collecting system (Fig. 5-3G). In both cases, a cystic mass is delineated in the region of the renal pelvis. The round contour of the peripelvic cyst aids in its differentiation from a septated cystic mass representing an obstructed upper tract system. If polycystic kidneys are encountered, the liver should also be examined, since approximately 30% of patients with polycystic kidney disease will also have liver cysts. The spleen and pancreas may also contain cysts—all can be evaluated by single ultrasound study. Multiple cystic masses within the kidney are most commonly encountered in polycystic kidney disease (10). In this disorder both kidneys appear enlarged and contain cysts of various sizes (Fig. 5-7A). The kidneys appear to be diffusely affected, whereas in multiple congenital cysts, only a portion of the kidney usually contains cysts.

In an obstructed upper pole system, the sonolucency in the region of the renal pelvis is usually pie-shaped with the apex directed medially (Fig. 5-3G). Frequently, septations can be recognized in a hydronephrotic upper pole collecting system. Thus, the appearance of a peripelvic cyst can mimic the appearance of a hydronephrotic renal pelvis. The borders of a peripelvic cyst are usually rounded, whereas an obstructed pelvis is most often triangular.

Complex Masses

Complex masses of the kidney may represent necrotic renal cell tumors, cysts that contain clotted blood and cellular debris, or intrarenal abscesses (Figs. 5-5A,B). If a renal mass has a complex pattern, a necrotic renal cell tumor should

Figure 5-5. COMPLEX RENAL MASSES

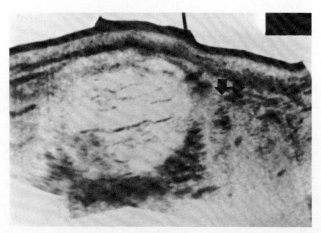

Figure 5-5A. Necrotic renal cell tumor (supine, longitudinal, 4 cm to left of midline). There is a large, complex mass in the left upper quadrant containing septations and solid components. The relation of the mass to the kidney could not be identified. Bowel is displaced along the inferior aspect of the mass (*arrows*) and is recognized by its high echogenicity and mottled distal acoustical shadow. Recognition of the location of the displaced bowel implies that the mass arose from within the abdomen or retroperitoneum, as opposed to masses that arise from the pelvis which frequently displace bowel along their superior aspect.

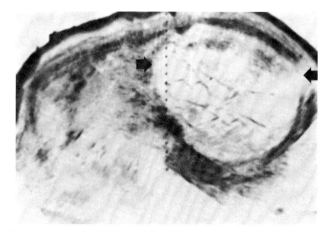

Figure 5-5B. Necrotic renal cell tumor (supine, transverse, 8 cm below xiphoid). The complex internal contents of this mass (*arrows*) represented marked internal necrosis. This appearance is similar to that encountered in cystic ovarian tumors. However, the displacement of bowel along its inferior border suggested its abdominal or retroperitoneal origin. (Courtesy of M. Louis Weinstein, M.D.)

be considered as a diagnostic possibility. When a complex mass is encountered, angiography is frequently performed in an attempt to assess the origin, extent, and vascularity of the mass.

Solid Masses

The most common solid renal mass is renal cell carcinoma. These tumors appear as moderately echogenic masses within the outline of the kidney (Figs. 5-6 A,B,C). Frequently, their sonographic texture is more inhomogeneous than that of the

Figure 5-6. SOLID RENAL MASSES

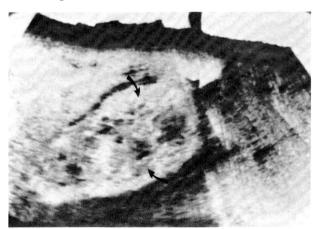

Figure 5-6A. Renal cell tumor (supine, longitudinal, 6 cm to right of midline). An echogenic mass is seen in the right lower pole (*curved arrows*).

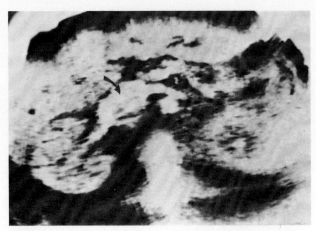

Figure 5-6B. Renal cell tumor (supine, transverse, 5 cm below xiphoid of same patient as in Fig. 5-6A). The right renal vein is distended, and there is evidence of echogenic material within the inferior vena cava (*curved arrow*). This represented tumor embolus into the right renal vein from the renal cell tumor.

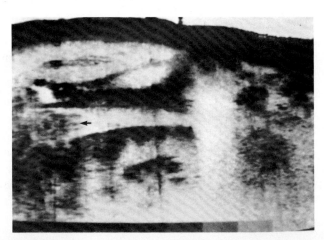

Figure 5-6C. Renal cell tumor with tumor embolus (supine, longitudinal, 2 cm to right of midline, same patient as in Figs. 5-6A,B). Within the inferior vena cava, there is an echogenic focus representing a tumor embolus from a renal cell tumor (*arrow*). This illustrates the importance of evaluating the renal veins and inferior vena cava when a solid renal mass is encountered. (Courtesy of Marion Wier, M.D.)

renal cortex. The texture of a renal cell tumor tends to have a variety of echo amplitudes when compared to the homogeneous echo pattern of normal renal parenchyma.

The echogenicity of a renal mass is related to its vascularity and the presence or absence of central necrosis (7). Tumors that contain numerous vessels appear to be more echogenic than those that are relatively avascular. The echogenicity of vascular tumors might be explained on the basis that the numerous vessels create multiple interfaces for the production of echoes. Masses that contain central necrosis usually appear as sonolucent to complex masses because of their predominantly cystic internal texture. Occasionally, the extension of a renal cell tumor into a renal vein and inferior vena cava can be documented (Figs. 5-6A,B,C). Tumor emboli within the vessel appear as intraluminal echoes that are usually outlined by sonolucent blood.

Another, less common, solid renal tumor that appears to have a relatively consistent sonographic appearance is the angiomyolipoma (9). These fatty tumors exhibit a very echogenic texture and may be associated with tuberous sclerosis.

POORLY FUNCTIONING KIDNEYS

Since sonographic imaging of the kidneys is independent of renal function, ultrasound evaluation of the kidney is particularly useful in patients with markedly diminished renal function. Sonographic evaluation of the kidney is particularly helpful in patients whose renal function does not allow adequate radiographic opacification (17). Sonography can often differentiate the major causes of poorly functioning kidneys, namely, obstructive uropathy versus small contracted end-stage kidney resulting from multiple causes. In addition, ultrasound is used to detect certain parenchymal abnormalities such as polycystic renal disease that can result in poor renal function (Figs. 5-7A,B). Conversely, some conditions that cause renal failure, such as infantile polycystic and medullary cystic disease, demonstrate only very subtle parenchymal changes and may be difficult to detect on a routine examination.

Hydronephrotic Kidney

As previously stated, the hydronephrotic kidney is recognized by variable degrees of separation of the fluid-filled renal collecting system (13). Various degrees of hydronephrosis can be documented. Mildly dilated calices appear as small, rounded sonolucent masses that are best demonstrated on longitudinal sonograms (Fig. 5-3A). The small sonolucencies representing dilated calices can be

Figure 5-7. POORLY FUNCTIONING KIDNEYS

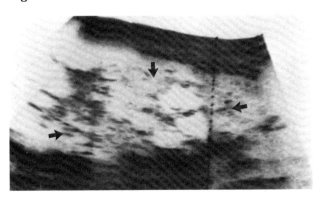

Figure 5-7A. Polycystic kidney (supine, longitudinal, 4 cm to right of midline). The kidney is enlarged and contains numerous cysts of various sizes (*arrows*).

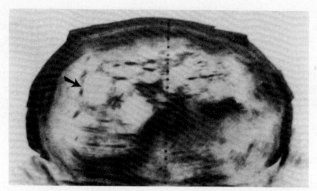

Figure 5-7B. Polycystic liver disease associated with polycystic kidney disease (supine, transverse, 4 cm below xiphoid, same patient as in Fig. 5-7A). The liver is enlarged and also contains numerous cysts (*arrow*). Approximately 30% of patients with polycystic kidney disease will also have a polycystic liver.

differentiated from the renal pyramids. The renal pyramids are slightly more echogenic than the urine-filled calices but are less echogenic than the cortex of the kidney. Moderate hydronephrosis can be detected by 0.5- to 1-cm separation of the normally closely opposed renal pelvic echoes (Fig. 5-3B). Severe hydronephrosis is diagnosed by marked separation of the renal pelvis (Fig. 5-3C). The renal pelvis may assume a "dumbbell" appearance on longitudinal scans indicating distension of both intra- and extrarenal portions of the renal pelvis (Figs. 5-3D,E,F,G).

End-Stage Kidney

The end-stage kidney is seen as an elliptical structure of small size (Fig. 5-7C). The renal cortex in these kidneys is markedly echogenic compared to the renal pyramids, with the echogenicity of the renal cortex equal to or greater than that of the liver parenchyma. As stated previously, this finding indicates that the renal cortex contains abnormal amounts of collagen and fibrotic tissue (1) (Fig. 5-7D).

RENAL TRANSPLANTS

Ultrasound is an excellent imaging technique for anatomical detail of the transplanted kidney as well as abnormalities that occur in the area that may cause decreased renal function. In particular, sonography is most useful in establishing the presence or absence of a mass within the transplant bed that may cause obstruction to the excretion of urine, resulting in decreased renal function after transplantation. Here one is most concerned with hematoma, urinoma, lymphocele, or abscess. At present, radionuclide renograms are more sensitive for the detection of diminished renal function and early rejection after renal transplantation than renal sonography. There are subtle sonographic textural signs that occur in rejection, but in general they are less specific than the data obtained in radionuclide renography (18). However, the anatomical information obtained by

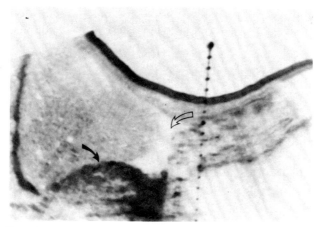

Figure 5-7C. Chronic glomerulonephritis (supine, longitudinal, 6 cm to right of midline). The kidney is small (*solid arrow*), and the echogenicity of its parenchyma is greater than that of the liver. The patient also has ascites, (*open arrow*), as depicted by a collection of fluid in the hepatorenal or Morrison's pouch. In this patient, the ascites was attributed to concomitant hepatic cirrhosis.

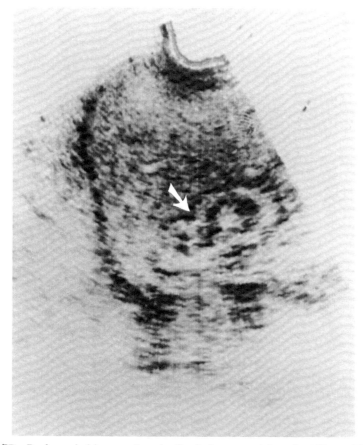

Figure 5-7D. Pyelonephritic scar (longitudinal, 6 cm to right of midline). There is an impression of the renal cortex (*arrow*) representing a parenchymal scar. A fetal lobulation has a similar appearance.

sonography should be combined with the physiologic data portrayed by the radionuclide renogram to detect early signs of rejection.

Technique for Renal Transplant Study

Sonographic examination for the renal transplant should begin with longitudinal scans oriented along the axis of the transplanted kidney, followed by a series of scans perpendicular to the long axis of the transplanted kidney. Following these routine scans, one should perform scans along the expected course of the ureter. The course of the ureter can be approximated by a plane extending from the renal pelvis to the inferior lateral aspect of the bladder. A series of scans should be performed both with a distended full bladder and with a postvoid bladder since a lymphocele can mimic the sonographic findings of an enlarged bladder.

In summary, the scanning routine employed for the evaluation of renal transplants should include:

1. Scan made longitudinally and transversely to renal transplanted kidney with patient's bladder distended
2. Scans obtained along plane of ureter
3. Repeat the above measures after patient voids

Since the transplanted kidney is superficial in location, a high-frequency transducer with short internal focus should be employed for delineation of the transplanted kidney (Fig. 5-8A). In most cases, a 5-MHz transducer with 3- to 7-cm

Figure 5-8. RENAL TRANSPLANT SONOGRAMS

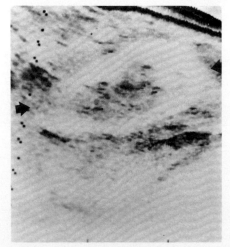

Figure 5-8A. Normal renal transplant (modified longitudinal, directed along longitudinal axis of renal transplant). The transplanted kidney lies immediately beneath the subcutaneous tissue and is oriented obliquely within the iliac fossa. Its superficial location allows good resolution since a high-frequency transducer with short internal focus can be used. A moderate degree of pelvic distension may be encountered in an uncomplicated renal transplant due to the denervation of the renal pelvis and ureter that occurs during the initial resection of the kidney.

focus allows excellent resolution of the transplant area and intrarenal structures. The time gain compensation (TGC) should be adjusted so that it slopes back to base line posterior to the renal transplant. If the TGC slope is too steep, the anterior aspect of the transplant may appear to have a more sonolucent texture than the posterior aspect of the kidney. This may result in misinterpretation of the appearance of a subtle parenchymal change of the kidney as hematoma, edema, or rejection, when it really is an artifact.

The pelvis of the transplanted kidney may appear somewhat distended when compared to the closely opposed interfaces seen in a normal kidney. Apparent widening of the renal pelvis of the transplanted kidney is thought to be secondary to denervation of the renal pelvis of the transplanted kidney. Distension of the renal pelvis may also be observed when the patient undergoes diuresis and is commonly observed in transplanted kidneys, as evidenced by the bladder being fully distended. This may be a simple "back pressure" phenomenon from a short ureter that should not be interpreted as abnormal in most cases. This is another reason why scans should be obtained pre- and postvoid in order to evaluate any changes in the configuration of the renal pelvis secondary to distension of the bladder.

Masses Associated with Transplants

In the first few days after transplantation, an area of relative sonolucency posterior to and surrounding the kidney will be present due to hematoma and edema. These should regress in four to five days. The most common mass that occurs two to six weeks after transplantation and causes diminished renal function is the lymphocele. These masses result from continual escape of lymph secondary to surgical transection of the lymphatic channels in the renal transplant bed. Lymphoceles are readily detected by sonography as sonolucent masses in the region of the transplant area. Lymphoceles can range from only a few centimeters up to 10 to 15 cm (Figs. 5-8B,C). They occasionally contain internal septations.

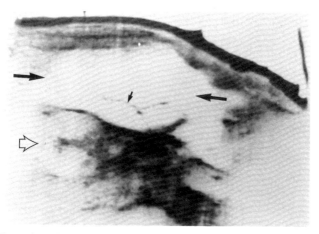

Figure 5-8B. Lymphocele (supine, longitudinal, 6 cm to right of midline). A predominantly cystic mass (*large arrows*) with septations (*small arrow*) is seen superior to the transplanted kidney (*open arrow*).

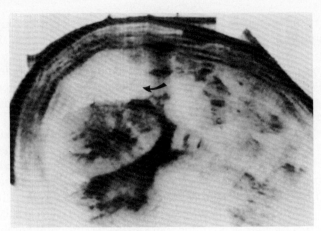

Figure 5-8C. Lymphocele (supine, transverse, 16 cm below xiphoid, same patient as in Figure 5-8B). Superior to the transplanted kidney is a cystic mass representing a lymphocele (*curved arrow*).

Lymphoceles cannot be distinguished from other fluid-filled masses, such as seromas, abscesses, urinomas, or hematomas with unclotted blood, by their sonographic appearance alone.

Seromas, urinomas, and fresh hematomas appear as sonolucent masses in the transplant bed (Fig. 5-8D). When the blood in the hematoma organizes, multiple

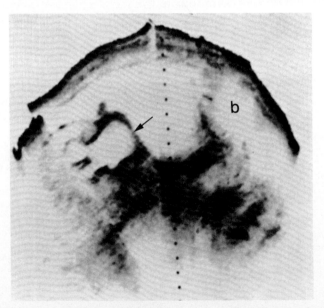

Figure 5-8D. Urinoma with obstruction (transverse, 6 cm above symphysis pubis). Marked distension of the renal pelvis of the transplanted kidney (*arrow*) resulted from obstruction of antegrade flow into the bladder (b). An irregularly shaped cystic mass was present between the renal pelvis and bladder representing a urinoma. The urinoma had a sonographic appearance similar to a bladder. At surgery, a laceration in the posterior aspect of the renal pelvis was found as the cause of urine extravasation.

echoes can be seen within it. The synechiae within the clot may appear as internal interfaces after the clot has organized. Abscesses around the renal pelvis will also often be sonolucent. However, if they contain a significant amount of pus and cellular debris, they may appear as complex masses that contain an internal interface arising from a fluid-pus layer. Clinical symptomatology and correlation with the data obtained on the renogram is very helpful.

Rejection

Subtle textural changes in the renal parenchyma occur with rejection. In cases of acute rejection, the renal pyramids swell and the cortico-medullary junction are less distinct. Focal areas of sonolucency have also been found in the cortex and are thought to represent focal areas of infarction. In chronic rejection, the kidney is small and the overall consistency of the cortex is more echogenic than in well-functioning transplants. The sonographic features of acute and chronic rejection are summarized in Table 5-2 (Fig. 5-8E).

CONGENITAL ANOMALIES

Congenital anomalies of the kidney, such as horseshoe and ectopic kidney, can be demonstrated as incidental findings or further evaluated when detected at excretory urography. Therefore, ultrasound can be used as a primary screening test or secondary diagnostic modality for the detection of certain congenital anomalies of the kidney. The congenital anomalies of the kidney that can be detected sonographically include ectopic, polycystic, multicystic, and horseshoe kidneys, as well as kidneys with a duplicated collecting system. Occasionally, an ectopic or horseshoe kidney will be first discovered on sonography and later confirmed on excretory urography. Ultrasound is very useful in that the soft tissue fusion can be directly demonstrated. In case of ectopic kidney, it is important to recognize these abnormally located kidneys so that they are not confused with other abdominal or pelvic masses.

Table 5-2. Sonographic Signs of Rejection

Acute
    Enlargement and decreased echogenicity of pyramids
    Hyperechogenic cortex
    Focal areas of decreased echogenicity
    Distortion of renal outline
    Patchy sonolucent areas of cortex and medulla which may exhibit coalescence
Long-standing
    Normal sized renal transplant with very little differentiation between parenchymal
      and renal sinus echoes
    Small kidney with irregular margins

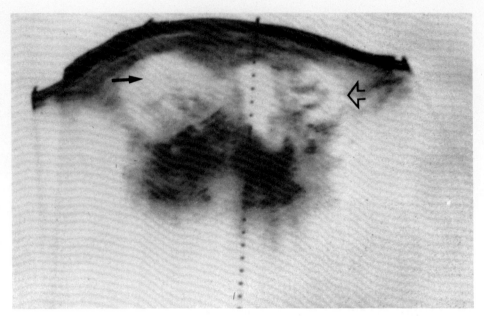

Figure 5-8E. Acute and chronic rejection (transverse, 6 cm above symphysis pubis). This individual had two transplanted kidneys; the one on the left (*open arrow*) had undergone chronic rejection, the one on the right (*arrow*) had been recently transplanted. The cortex of the recently transplanted kidney demonstrated focal areas of sonolucency and overall loss of the normally distinct cortico-medullary junction. Arteriography showed stretched intrarenal vessels and slow flow indicative of acute rejection in the recently transplanted kidney.

Ectopic Kidneys

Ectopic kidneys can present as a mass in the pelvis (Fig. 5-9A). If they have adequate function, ectopic kidneys can be readily identified on excretory urography. In these cases, sonography can confirm that the mass is indeed a kidney by documenting the characteristic reniform shape. Crossed renal ectopic kidneys are most often seen in the pediatric age group. Ectopic kidneys can also be encountered in pregnant patients. In these cases, a C-section may be advised because of the likelihood of damaging the kidney during labor (Fig. 5-9A).

Polycystic Kidneys

As previously mentioned, polycystic kidneys appear as enlarged kidneys with multiple cysts of various sizes comprising the major portion of the kidneys. Sonography is useful in polycystic kidney disease in evaluation of other organs such as the liver, spleen, and pancreas for the presence of other cystic masses (Fig. 5-7A).

Horseshoe Kidneys

Because of the renal tissue or fibrotic strand that crosses the midline, a horseshoe kidney may be confused with para-aortic nodes based on its sonographic ap-

Figure 5-9. CONGENITAL RENAL ANOMALIES

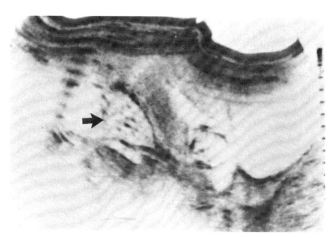

Figure 5-9A. Ectopic kidney with early second trimester intrauterine pregnancy (supine, longitudinal, midline). Posterior to the gravid uterus is an ectopic kidney (*arrow*). (Courtesy of Dean Birdwell, R.D.M.S.)

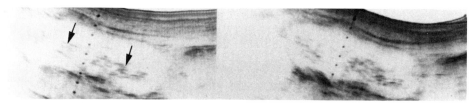

Figure 5-9B. Duplex collecting system (prone, modified longitudinal, 4 cm to right of midine). The presence of a duplex collecting system was suggested by discontinuity of the central echogenic interface representing the separate renal pelves. This configuration can be created by shadowing of an overlying rib which might produce artifactual discontinuity in the central echogenic structure arising from the renal pelvis. Real-time scanning of the patient without breath-holding may be helpful in distinguishing between these entities. (Courtesy of Clifton Greer, M.D., Baptist Hospital, Nashville, Tenn.)

pearance. However, the malrotated renal pelvis can be demonstrated sonographically, for the pelvic echoes are oriented in a more vertical direction than in the normal pelvic structure (Fig. 5-9C).

Kidneys with Duplicated Collecting System

Duplication of the renal collecting system is seen as two lines of echoes representing the renal collecting system with a separation between them. Frequently, the upper pole collecting system in a duplication is obstructed due to extrinsic compression of the lower pole ureter. A hydronephrotic upper pole collecting system appears as a triangular sonolucent sac in the upper aspect of the kidney. The hydronephrotic sac can also have septations due to the fibrotic structures around the renal pelvis (Fig. 5-3B).

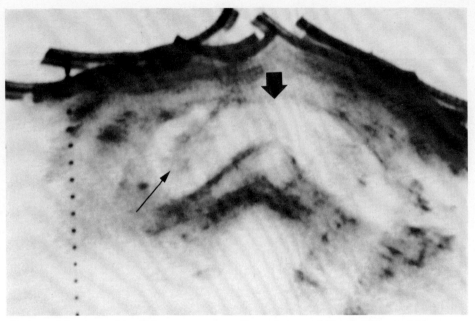

Figure 5-9C. Horseshoe kidney (transverse, 5 cm above umbilicus). The two kidneys are seen to be connected in the midline by moderately echogenic renal tissue (*large arrow*). Also note the unusual orientation of the renal pelves (*small arrow*). (Courtesy of Karen Parker, R.D.M.S., and Henry Howerton, M.D., Baptist Hospital, Nashville, Tenn.)

RENAL CYST ASPIRATION AND RENAL BIOPSY

Because of the frequency of renal cysts in asymptomatic persons, there is some controversy as to whether or not to aspirate a renal cyst once it is delineated on ultrasound. With cyst aspiration and analysis of the fluid and cells, one can attain above 95% accuracy in differentiating benign from malignant lesions. Imaging studies are about 90% accurate. Thus, the decision to aspirate a potential renal cyst is most often a clinical one.

If aspiration of a cystic lesion is desired, it can be performed using ultrasound guidance. The advantages of performing cyst aspiration and/or biopsy under ultrasound are that the patient is not exposed to ionizing radiation and no contrast material need be injected.

Cyst aspiration and/or renal biopsy can be performed using A-mode techniques or real-time B-mode scanning. When compared to the limited sampling area of A-mode scanning, B-mode scanning has advantages for aspiration and/or biopsy of the kidney because it affords a larger field of view. Aspiration using fluoroscopy may still be preferred since fluoroscopy allows delineation of the bony landmarks.

A specialized transducer with a hollow lumen is used for A-mode aspiration. The cystic area is identified by its A-mode pattern and a needle directed toward the region of interest (Figs. 5-4A,B). During introduction the tip of the needle can be followed as a distinct echo peak. The volume of the cyst can be estimated and approximately one-half aspirated and replaced with radiopaque contrast and air for subsequent evaluation of the cyst wall. The needle should be introduced with the patient in suspended expiration. This is done so that the likelihood of puncturing the posterior costophrenic sulcus is less than if the patient were in suspended inspiration.

It may be preferable to perform cyst aspiration using real-time sonography. In this procedure, the kidney itself can be visualized. When the needle is within the area of the body that the beam width covers, it is well visualized. However, if the needle is not entirely within this plane, only a portion of the needle will be visualized. Since many different views can be obtained, this is not usually a problem. One should be aware of the potential complication of a pneumothorax that is most often encountered in aspiration of upper pole lesions. For this reason, a chest radiograph may be obtained after the aspiration so that a pneumothorax can be documented (27).

The technique for renal biopsy is similar to that for cyst aspiration. For the purpose of renal biopsy, a portion of the renal cortex usually in the lower pole is localized and sampled by a special biopsy needle. The reader, if interested, is encouraged to refer to the detailed descriptions of aspiration and biopsy before attempting these procedures (3).

MISCELLANEOUS RENAL DISORDERS

Sonography may be useful in evaluating a variety of renal disorders, including perirenal abscess, nonopaque renal calculi, and pyohydronephrosis, and establishing the presence of renal sinus lipomatosis. Perirenal abscesses appear as sonolucent or complex collections of echoes surrounding the kidney. Echogenic areas emanate from pockets of pus and gas within the abscess. If the diagnosis cannot be established by sonography or radiography, CT may be indicated, since it can detect small pockets of air in masses around the kidney (26). Pyohydronephrosis presents sonographically as multiple echoes within a distended renal pelvis (Fig. 5-3C).

Nonopaque Renal Calculi

Sonography has also been used in the detection of nonopaque renal calculi (16). Since calculi have a different acoustical impedance from the renal parenchyma and peripelvic fat, the majority produce posterior acoustical shadowing regardless of their calcium content.

Renal Sinus Lipomatosis

Excessive fat in the region of the renal pelvis can be established radiographically. However, in some cases when an excretory urogram is contraindicated, renal sinus lipomatosis will be detected on renal sonograms as a thick band of dense echoes from an area conforming to the renal pelvis.

ADRENAL MASSES

Although normal adrenals may be difficult to delineate sonographically, adrenal masses greater than 2 cm can usually be detected. CBT is a reliable means for delineation of the normal as well as abnormal adrenals; sonography has only a secondary role in the evaluation of adrenal masses. The technique advocated for sonographic delineation of the adrenals is somewhat difficult to perform and only occasionally results in adequate delineation of the adrenals with present instrumentation (Figs. 5-10A,B,C,D).

The technique for delineation of the adrenals using a modified coronal approach has been described (20). In this procedure, the adrenals appear as comma-shaped or triangular structures that reflect low-to-medium gray scale shade echoes (Fig. 5-10A). The relationship of the adrenal location to the inferior vena cava and aorta is more constant than their relationship to the upper pole of the kidneys.

Metastatic Tumor

The most commonly encountered adrenal mass is metastatic adrenal tumor. Usually, the primary is from the lung. Metastases within the adrenals enlarge the glands and alter the echogenicity of the texture (Fig. 5-10B). Adrenal masses can be differentiated from pancreatic lesions, for masses arising from the adrenals displace the splenic vein anteriorly, as opposed to pancreatic lesions, which displace the splenic vein posteriorly. The sonographic appearances of adrenal carcinomas, adenomas, and metastases are similar; thus, differentiation by ultrasound alone is difficult. Other soft tissue lesions that occur in this area include the pheochromocytoma and neuroblastoma.

Figure 5-10. ADRENAL SONOGRAMS

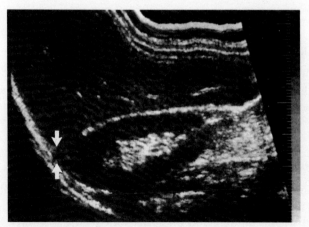

Figure 5-10A. Normal adrenal (supine, modified longitudinal). The normal adrenal can occasionally be identified as a triangular structure superior to the kidney (*arrow*).

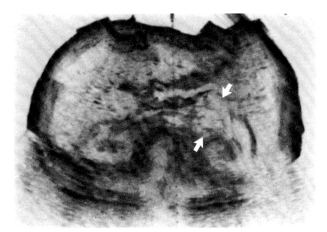

Figure 5-10B. Metastatic melanoma to left adrenal (supine, transverse, 6 cm below xiphoid). There is a mildly echogenic mass located along the superior and medial aspect of the upper pole of the left kidney. The mass (*arrows*) displaces the splenic vein anteriorly which implies that it arises from the adrenal. Masses arising from the adrenal gland can be distinguished from those arising from the pancreatic tail by their direction of displacement of the splenic vein. Since the normal adrenals are very rarely delineated on routine renal or abdominal sonograms, masses that are superior to the kidneys imply pathological enlargement of these glands. This mass represented metastatic melanoma to the left adrenal.

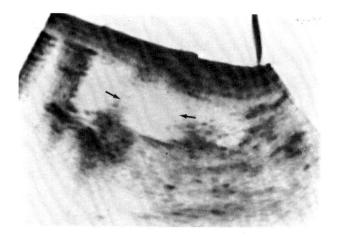

Figure 5-10C. "Pseudotumor" effect simulating enlarged adrenal (prone, longitudinal, 5 cm to left of midline). There is suggestion of an ill-defined mass (*arrows*) in the region of the upper pole of the left kidney. The medial lobe of the spleen frequently produces this "pseudotumor" effect because of its proximity to the upper pole of the left kidney.

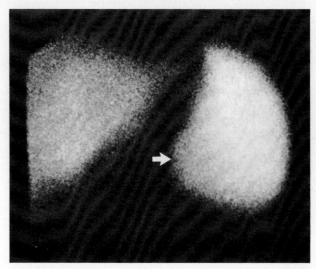

Figure 5-10D. "Pseudotumor" effect (liver/spleen scan). The enlarged medial lobe of the spleen is shown, which accounts for the "pseudotumor" effect on the prone renal sonogram. A liver/spleen scan is useful in evaluating apparent masses in the region of the left upper pole.

Adrenal Hemorrhagic Cyst

Another mass in the adrenal that can be evaluated by ultrasound is the adrenal cyst. These are uncommon lesions in the adrenal that are often secondary to adrenal hemorrhage in childhood. Enlarged adrenals that contain internal hemorrhage may simulate the appearance of a solid adrenal mass since both cause enlargement.

Other Adrenal Masses

In the case of some adrenal masses such as the aldosteronomas and adenomas, neither sonography nor CT can adequately detect these small masses. Adrenal venography with hormonal sampling seems to be the most efficacious procedure in these cases.

PROSTATE AND BLADDER

Sonographic evaluation of the prostate has been a subject of investigation for a number of years. Scanners that have been devised for evaluation of the prostate have a transducer mounted in a transrectal probe (25). Although the results from investigations using these scanners appear promising, the information obtained from them cannot reliably differentiate between malignant and benign conditions. Both prostatic tumors and hyperplastic nodules appear as nodular masses of decreased echogenicity. Benign masses tend to be circumscribed with a definable capsule around them. Patient acceptance of the transrectal scanning method has also been a rather formidable problem. With further technical development, images of the prostate obtained from an anterior approach may become practical, thereby increasing the value of this procedure.

Sonography can be occasionally used in the evaluation of bladder tumors, particularly in the evaluation of their extravesicular extension (24). Neoplasms involving the bladder produce marked thickening of the bladder wall. Evaluation of a bladder tumor should be performed using a single sweep since artifactual thickening can be produced by compound motion. Tumors involving the distal ureter may cause hydronephrosis and a distended ureter. Tumor extension into the bladder from ovarian carcinoma is demonstrated by the pattern as seen in Figure 5-11. This patient presented for evaluation of hypertension. Obstruction at the lower urinary tract was suspected because of the detection of bilateral hydronephrosis. The value of ultrasound studies in these lesions will probably increase.

SCROTAL DISORDERS

Sonographic examination of the scrotum is particularly helpful in patients who present with a painful and/or enlarged scrotum. The entire scrotal contents can be evaluated by sonography when a tumor is suspected. Ultrasound studies have been shown to be a useful adjunct to evaluation by direct palpation and trans-illumination (23,24). Most important, sonographic examination can be used to distinguish masses or processes affecting the testicles from extratesticular masses.

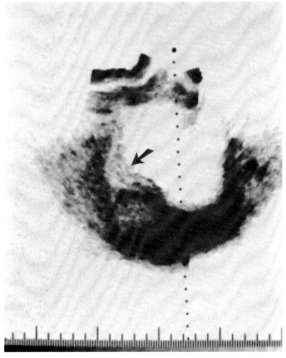

Figure 5-11. Tumor invasion of bladder from ovarian carcinoma (transverse, 6 cm above symphysis pubis). There is irregular thickening of the right posterior wall of the bladder representing tumor invasion from an ovarian carcinoma (*arrow*).

Technique

The scrotal contents can be examined either by a contact gray scale scanner using a 5- or 7-MHz transducer or by a "small parts" scanner that uses a 10-MHz transducer housed with a water bath. If available, a small parts scanner is the preferred device for scrotal scanning because of high resolution capabilities. In most cases, the scrotal contents are imaged adequately using a contact gray scale scanner with a high-frequency, short internal focus transducer. Examination of the scrotum with a contact scanner involves manual support of the scrotum as the organ is scanned in a transverse manner. Longitudinal scans are preferred when the small parts scanner is used because the relation of a mass to the head of the epididymis can be readily identified.

Normal

The normal testicle exhibits a homogeneous medium-level echogenicity (Fig. 5-12A). A few focal areas of high reflectivity may be identified, the significance of which is unknown. The body and tail of the epididymis appear as a linear area of coarse echoes posterior and medial to the testicle. A small amount of fluid may be present between the tunica vaginalis surrounding the testicle in normal men. The head of the epididymis produces a cluster of high-amplitude, coarse echoes in the superior aspect of the testicle. This structure serves as a landmark for the evaluation of the testes by the small parts scanner.

Figure 5-12. SCROTAL SONOGRAMS

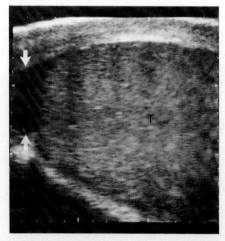

Figure 5-12A. Normal testicle with small hydrocele. (longitudinal, centered over head of epididymis, 3 × 3 cm fields, white-on-black image). The testicle appears as a moderately echogenic structure with a relatively homogeneous texture. There is a sonolucent collection superior to the testicle representing a small hydrocele (*arrows*). Hydroceles usually result from testicular trauma or infection. (Courtesy of George Leopold, M.D. University of California, San Diego, Cal.)

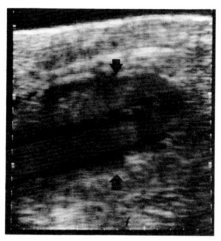

Figure 5-12B. Testicular abscess (longitudinal, centered over head of epididymis, 3 × 4 cm field). There is a complex collection superior to the testicle representing a testicular abscess (*arrows*). Abscesses usually result from previous epididymal infection. (Courtesy of George Leopold, M.D., University of California, San Diego, Cal.)

Extratesticular Masses

As stated previously, sonography is an accurate means of differentiating testicular masses from those that are extratesticular. Extratesticular masses, in general, do not disrupt the homogeneous texture of the testicle, whereas intratesticular masses distort the internal texture (Fig. 5-12B).

Cystic masses that can be identified extrinsic to the testicle include a spermatocele and varicocele. Both of the lesions appear as well-defined, sonolucent masses usually located along the superior aspect of the testes. A varicocele can occasionally be differentiated from a spermatocele by its tendency to be left-sided and its frequent association with the left spermatic vein.

Hydrocele

Hydroceles appear as sonolucent collections around the testes (Fig. 5-12B). They may occur as a sequela to trauma or intratesticular inflammation. When hydroceles contain pus and cellular debris, these abscesses around the testicle appear as complex collections. Abscesses within the scrotal sac most commonly occur as a sequela to epididymitis and usually spread to involve the testicle, producing epididymal orchitis.

Epididymitis

Although the sonographic findings may be subtle, epididymitis usually appears as swelling and decreased echogenicity of the organ. A similar sonographic appearance may be produced by testicular torsion, except that with torsion, the normally diffusely fine echogenicity of the testes becomes coarse and irregular. Doppler examination and radionuclide flow studies are also useful in establishing the presence of testicular torsion (24).

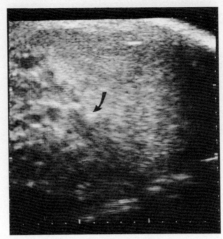

Figure 5-12C. Testicular tumor (longitudinal, centered over head of epididymis 3×3 cm field). The patient was thought to have a testicular abscess. However, this scrotal sonogram demonstrates a markedly disorganized and inhomogeneous texture (*arrow*) at the testicle, suggesting the presence of an intratesticular tumor. (Courtesy of George Leopold, M.D., University of California, San Diego, Cal.)

Tumors

The majority of intratesticular tumors appear as focal areas of decreased echoes within the testes. In addition, the textural pattern in the area of diminished echogenicity is inhomogeneous and disorganized (Fig. 5-12C). Testicular tumors that demonstrate this sonographic appearance include seminomas, embryonal cell tumors, and histiocystic lymphomas (23). The only entity that has been observed to produce a focal area of increased echogenicity is testicular infarction. Additional clinical experience with the sonographic evaluation of testicular masses is needed before the specificity of these patterns is known (Fig. 5-12C).

SUMMARY

Ultrasonic imaging can be used effectively in many disorders of the urogenital system. In particular, ultrasound has a major role in the establishment of benign cystic masses of the kidney. Since sonography is an anatomic study, poorly functioning kidneys can be evaluated and the presence or absence of obstructive uropathy documented. Sonography plays a major role in the detection of perirenal collections around a transplanted kidney and affords detailed textural analysis of the scrotal contents.

REFERENCES

General

1. Rosenfield, A., Taylor, K., Crade, M., DeGraaf, C.: Anatomy and pathology of the kidney by gray-scale ultrasonography. *Radiology* 128: 737–744, 1978.

Technique and Anatomy

2. Bartrum, J., Crow, H.: Examination of the kidney, in *Gray Scale Ultrasound: A Manual for Technicians and Physicians*. Philadelphia: Saunders, 1977, pp. 132–142.
3. Goldberg, B., Pollach, H.: Ultrasonic aspiration biopsy techniques. *J. Clin. Ultrasound* 4:141–151, 1976.
4. Albarelli, J., Lawson, T.: Renal ultrasonography: Advantage of the decubitus position. *J. Clin. Ultrasound* 6:115–116, 1978.
5. Cook, J., Rosenfield, A., Taylor, K.: Ultrasonic demonstration of intrarenal anatomy. *Am. J. Roentgenol.* 129:831–835, 1977.

Renal Disorders

6. Green, W., King, D., Casarella, W.: A reappraisal of sonolucent renal masses. *Radiology* 121:163–171, 1976.
7. Maklad, N., Chuang, V., Doust, B., Cho, K., Curran, J.: Ultrasonic characterization of solid renal lesions: Echographic, angiographic and pathologic correlation. *Radiology* 123:733–739, 1977.
8. Lee, T., Henderson, S., Freeny, P., Askin, M., Benson, E., Pearse, H.: Ultrasound findings of renal angiomyolipoma. *J. Clin. Ultrasound* 63:150–155, 1978.
9. Scheible, W., Ellenbogen, P., Leopold, G., Siso, N.: Lipomatous tumors of the kidney and adrenal: Apparent echographic specificity. *Radiology* 129:153–156, 1978.

Congenital Anomalies

10. Kelsey, J., Bowie, J.: Gray scale ultrasonography in the diagnosis of polycystic kidney disease. *Radiology* 122:791–795, 1977.
11. Mindell, H., Kubic, E.: Horseshoe kidney: Ultrasonic demonstration. *Am. J. Roentgenol.* 129:526–527, 1977.
12. Muscatello, V., Smith, E., Carera, F., Burger, M., Teele, R.: Ultrasonic evaluation of obstructive duplex kidney. *Am. J. Roentgenol.* 125:113–120, 1977.
13. Ellenbogen, P., Schieble, F., Talner, L., Leopold, G.: Sensitivity of gray scale ultrasound in detecting urinary tract obstruction. *Am. J. Roentgenol.* 130:731–733, 1978.
14. Yeh, H., Mitty, H., Wolf, B.: Ultrasonography of the renal sinus lipomatosis. *Radiology* 124:799–801, 1977.
15. Schneider, M., Becker, J., Staiano, S., Campos, E.: Sonographic-radio-graphic correlation of renal and perirenal infections. *Am. J. Roentgenol.* 127:1007–1014, 1976.
16. Pollach, H., Arger, P., Goldberg, B., Mulholland, S.: Ultrasonic detection of nonopaque renal calculi. *Radiology* 127:233–237, 1978.
17. Sanders, R.: The place of diagnostic ultrasound in the examination of kidneys not seen on excretory urography. *J. Urol.* 114:813–821, 1975.

Renal Transplants

18. Conrad, M., Dickerson, R., Love, J., Curry, T., Peters, P., Hull, A., Lerman, G., Helderman, H.: New observations in renal transplants using ultrasound. *Am. J. Roentgenol.* 131:851–855, 1978.
19. Bartrum, R., Smith, E., D'Orsi, L., Teirey, N., Dantaris, J.: Evaluation of renal transplants with ultrasound. *Radiology* 118:405–410, 1976

Adrenal Masses

20. Sample, W.: Adrenal ultrasonography. *Radiology* 127:461–466, 1978.
21. Bernardino, M., Goldstein, H., Green, B.: Gray scale ultrasonography of adrenal neoplasms. *Am. J. Roentgenol.* 130:741–744, 1978.

Prostate

22. Sukof, R., Scardino, P., Sample, W., Weiner, J., Confer, D.: Computed tomography and trans-abdominal ultrasound in evaluation of the prostate. *J. Computed Assisted Tomography* 1(3):281–288, 1977.

Scrotal Masses

23. Sample, W., Gottesman, J., Skinner, G., Erlic,R.: Gray scale ultrasound of the scrotum. *Radiology* 127:225–228, 1978.
24. Winston, M., Handler, S., Pritchard, J.: Ultrasonography of the testes—correlation with radio-tracer perfusion. *J. Nucl. Med.* 19(6):615–618, 1978.

Bladder Disorders

25. Resnick, M., Willard, J., Boyce, W.: Recent progress in ultrasonography of bladder and prostate disorders. *J. Urol.* 117:444, 1977.

Miscellaneous

26. Levitt, R., Geisse, G., Sagel, S., Stanley, R., Evens, R., Koehler, R., Jost, R.,: Complementary use of ultrasound and CT in studies of the pancreas and kidney. *Radiology* 126:149–152, 1978.
27. *Gray's Anatomy.* Warwick, R., Williams, p., eds. Thirty-fifth ed. Philadalphia: Saunders, 1973, p. 1316.
28. Lang. E.: Renal cyst puncture and aspiration: A survey of complications. *Am. J. Roentgenol* 128:723–727, 1977.

6
Pediatric Sonography

INTRODUCTORY REMARKS

The considerations that lead to the decision to use a particular diagnostic imaging modality in the pediatric age group are somewhat different from those that pertain to adults. The requirements of resolution, constraints regarding biological burden, and emphasis upon patient and user acceptance tend to favor certain characteristics. This chapter will discuss some of these characteristics and their relation to those of diagnostic sonography. A few of the common alternative decisions that can be made in selecting the most suitable diagnostic imaging modality will be emphasized. Often the choices involve considerations of risk versus gain for any particular procedure, and thus they are so complex as to require a thorough understanding of the virtues and limitations of each imaging modality.

We hope that after the general discussion of diagnostic sonography in pediatrics and emphasis upon particular clinical problems for illustration, the reader will have a better appreciation of the role of this diagnostic modality in the pediatric age group.

INDICATIONS

Because of its noninvasive quality and lack of significant biological risk to the patient, sonography is an excellent diagnostic modality for the evaluation of a variety of pediatric disorders. The high-frequency transducers (3.5, 5 and 7 MHz) with a small diameter (6 mm) that have recently become available allow improved resolution and better sonographic imaging of pediatric patients than was previously possible with the larger transducers used for adults. The improved resolution with real-time and mechanical sector scanners has increased our flexibility in examining infants and children.

At present, sonography is most commonly used in pediatrics as an adjunctive diagnostic modality, more conventional radiographic studies being chosen for the primary role. Sonographic imaging has been commonly employed for the evaluation of abdominal and renal masses in children, and is becoming advantageously employed in other areas (1). The anatomical information acquired by sonography can be coupled with data obtained by radionuclide imaging for physiologic as well as anatomical evaluation. Because of the paucity of perivisceral fat in children, sonography may have some advantages in visualizing pediatric disorders when compared with computed body tomography (CBT). Imaging flexibility, biological burden considerations, and costs are also features favoring sonography.

As discussed in Chapter 2, the resolution of sonography occasionally allows recognition of anatomical malformations of the fetus in utero (2). At present, certain anomalies of the central nervous system, genitourinary tract, and gastrointestinal tract can be detected antenatally. In fact, it has been suggested that surgical correction of certain malformations detected by ultrasound can be performed prior to delivery. For example, it may be possible to detect and treat hydrocephalus in utero before irreversible neurological changes occur.

This chapter will emphasize those disorders that can be evaluated by sonography and are specific to patients of the pediatric age group. Disease entities such as cholelithiasis that are also encountered in adults are discussed in other chapters. In general, sonographic imaging can be used in evaluating the following conditions:

1. Abdominal, hepatic, or pelvic masses
2. Abdominal, hepatic, or pelvic abscesses
3. Poorly functioning kidneys, obstructive uropathy, and selected congenital genitourinary anomalies
4. Suspected intrauterine pregnancy
5. Obstructive versus hepatocellular jaundice
6. Pancreatitis secondary to trauma or chemotherapy
7. Chest masses
8. Ambiguous genitalia, genital trauma, and related developmental disorders
9. Hydrocephalus and intracranial cystic masses

NORMAL ANATOMY AND SCANNING TECHNIQUE IN PEDIATRIC PATIENTS

Except for the smaller size of most of the abdominal organs of children, the anatomical features as depicted by sonography are similar to those in the adult. Children may be initially more difficult to scan because of their lack of cooperation during the examination. However, if they are handled with an appropriate blend of patience and firmness, most infants and children will cooperate long enough to allow completion of the ultrasound study.

The acoustical coupling medium should be warmed to body temperature before it is applied to the body. Neonates may cooperate to a greater degree if they are placed on their stomach and kept warm by a heat lamp. A 5.0-MHz, 13-mm diameter transducer with short internal focus (5 to 7 cm) or a 3.5-MHz, 19-mm transducer with short internal focus is used for scanning children. The transducer should be warmed before being gently applied to the skin. Patient positioning is comparable to that used for adults. Because the infant or child may cooperate for only a short period of time, simple sector scans covering a specific area of interest are frequently used.

Smaller organ size in children poses some resolution problems. The kidneys in normal neonates measure approximately 5 cm in length and 2 to 3 cm in anterior-posterior and transverse dimensions. The uterus is tubular in shape in neonates, with the cervical portion larger than the fundus, contrary to the anatomy in adults (Fig. 6-1B). The diameter of the uterine fundus compared to that of the cervix increases as puberty is approached (17). Due to the small size and

Figure 6-1. NORMAL PEDIATRIC ORGANS

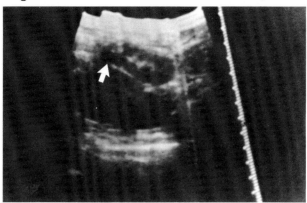

Figure 6-1A. Normal adrenal (prone, 6 cm to left of midline). The adrenal gland (*arrow*) in neonates may simulate the configuration and appear up to one-half the size of the kidney. However, the adrenals do not have a central echogenic interface representing the renal pelvis of the kidney.

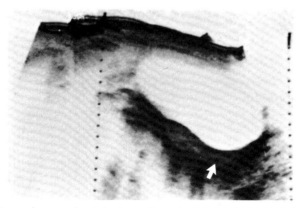

Figure 6-1B. Normal, prepubertal uterus (longitudinal, midline). Before puberty, the uterus is more tubular in shape, with the cervix (*arrow*) equal to or greater than the thickness of the uterine fundus. As puberty is approached, the fundus becomes larger than the cervix.

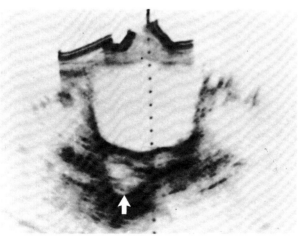

Figure 6-1C. Enlarged ovary at the menarche (transverse, 4 cm above symphysis pubis). The ovary (*arrow*) in this girl is enlarged prior to ovulation. In most prepubertal females, the ovaries are small and not demonstrable on routine pelvic sonograms.

variable location, the ovaries of infants are only infrequently visualized. The same statement could have been made several years ago about adults, but improved gray scale resolution allows reliable delineation of normal-size adult ovaries. Ovaries can become prominent at the menarche and reach as much as 3 cm in length. The size of the internal genital organs according to the pubertal status of the girl has been documented, but this is the type of information that is only useful on a comparative basis (17).

The adrenal glands and the liver in neonates constitute obvious exception included in the remark that most pediatric organs are similiar to the adult organs except for size (Fig. 6-1A). In the neonate, the adrenals may be two to three times larger than in the adult and may approximate the size of the infant kidney. The adrenals do not contain the central echogenic interface that arises from the renal pelvis and can be differentiated from the kidneys. The liver in a neonate may extend well below the right costal margin and will fill more of the abdomen and is a more midline structure than in the adult.

EVALUATION OF RENAL MASSES AND RELATED DISORDERS

Sonographic imaging is very helpful in the evaluation of renal masses in children. Hydronephrosis and certain congenital anomalies of the kidney can also be detected by ultrasound (3–10). Sonographic evaluation of renal disorders is especially important when one considers the relative frequency of masses related to the kidney that are encountered in the pediatric age group.

Excretory urography in neonates and young children is often unsatisfactory because of patient motion, overlying bowel gas, and the relatively poor excretory function. When compared to other imaging techniques, sonography, of the kidney has many advantages. Since, for example, the ability to visualize the kidneys with ultrasound is independent of renal function, poorly functioning kidneys can be evaluated by this modality.

Table 6-1 lists the sonographic features of some of the common pediatric renal and adrenal disorders. This list is not meant to be complete but does offer an overview of salient considerations.

In the neonate, unilateral nonvisualization of a kidney on excretory urography is most commonly due to a multicystic or dysplastic kidney (Fig. 6-2A). Sonographically, multicystic kidneys appear as reniform masses that contain multiple cysts. In some instances, the atrophic renal pelvis can be identified. Multicystic kidney is usually unilateral, as opposed to renal agenesis or Potter's syndrome, which is frequently bilateral. Potter's syndrome is characterized by bilateral agenesis of the kidneys. In these patients, the adrenals, due to their large size during infancy, may sonographically mimic atrophic kidneys (9). The mothers of infants affected by Potter's syndrome may have an obstetrical history of oligohydramnios because of diminished production of amniotic fluid by the kidney. Infants affected by Potter's syndrome lie in a low position in the uterus as a reflection of a diminished amount of amniotic fluid.

A common cause of a nonvisualized kidney on urography is hydronephrosis secondary to obstructive uropathy. Ultrasound studies are very important here. Sonography can be used to assess accurately the degree of hydronephrosis by

Figure 6-2. RENAL DISORDERS

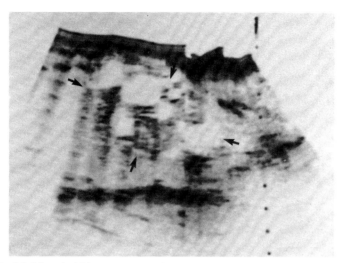

Figure 6-2A. Multicystic kidney (prone, 4 cm to right of midline). Numerous cysts are contained within the renal outline (*arrows*). This kidney had poor function, although the contralateral kidney was normal. This ultrasound pattern is characteristic of multicystic kidney.

Table 6-1. Sonographic Features of Common Pediatric Disorders Related to the Kidney and Adrenals

Condition	Sonographic Features
Wilms' tumor, mesoblastic nephroma	Solid mass within renal outline causing distortion of pelvocaliceal system
Multicystic or dysplastic kidney	Unilaterally poorly functioning kidney that contains multiple cysts within parenchyma
Neuroblastoma	Solid extrarenal mass in region of adrenal, sympathetic chain, or pelvis
	May exhibit focal areas of echogenicity corresponding to areas of calcification
Adrenal hyperplasia, adrenal hemorrhage	Bilaterally enlarged adrenals; hemorrhage appears as sonolucent to mildly echogenic area
Hydronephrosis	Separated pelvocaliceal echoes
Infantile polycystic disease	Bilaterally enlarged kidneys with punctate sonolucencies in parenchyma

detecting the amount of distension of the renal collecting system (Fig. 6-2B), (see Chapter 5). Mild caliectasis appears as multiple, small rounded masses in the region of the renal pelvis. Marked hydronephrosis can result in a "dumbbell" configuration of the renal pelvis, which indicates distension of both the intra- and extrarenal pelvis. Similarly, obstruction to the upper portion of a duplicated collecting system can be identified (Fig. 6-2B) (5). In these cases, the echoes emanating from the renal pelvis of the upper pole are widely separated. A septated configuration of the upper portion of the kidney arises from the massively distended hydronephrotic sac.

Other, less common, causes of poor renal function in neonates that can be detected by ultrasound include infantile polycystic kidney disease and renal tubular ectasia. In infantile polycystic kidney disease, the kidneys are usually enlarged. Small ectatic renal tubules can occasionally be identified along the periphery of the cortex which appear as punctate sonolucencies located along the periphery of the renal outline (8). Sonographically, renal tubular ectasia can have an appearance similar to that of infantile polycystic kidney disease, but the sonolucent structures are located more centrally than those seen in patients who have infantile polycystic kidney disease. In addition, renal tubular ectasia may be associated with hepatic fibrosis, which can be detected on the same ultrasound study. As stated previously, hepatic fibrosis appears as an unusually echogenic texture of the liver (7).

Wilms' tumor is the most common solid renal mass encountered in children (Fig. 6-2C). These tumors appear as echogenic masses that can be delineated within the renal outline. Sonography can be helpful in evaluating the size and extent of the tumor in these patients and in identifying a Wilms' tumor in the

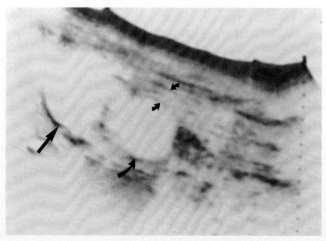

Figure 6-2B. Hydronephrosis (prone, modified longitudinal, 4 cm to right of midline). There are two ovoid cystic masses in the region of the right kidney. The upper one (*large arrow*) represents a totally hydronephrotic upper collecting system. The more spherical sonolucent mass represents a moderately hydronephrotic lower pole collecting system (*large curved arrow*). Only a small amount of renal parenchyma remains in the lower half of the kidney (*small curved arrows*).

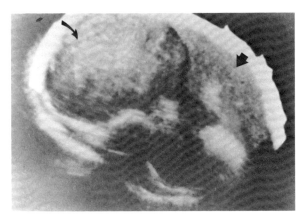

Figure 6-2C. Wilms' tumor (supine, 6 cm below xiphoid, white-on-black image). There is a large echogenic mass in the region of the upper pole of the right kidney (*curved arrow*). The liver is displaced to the left (*large arrow*). Angiography demonstrated contralateral tumor, thus emphasizing the importance of scanning both kidneys in the presence of a Wilms' tumor.

opposite kidney. Therefore, when evaluating a patient with a known Wilms' tumor, the opposite kidney should be carefully studied.

Neuroblastomas can sonographically mimic Wilms' tumor, except that neuroblastomas are observed to displace the kidney rather than to be intrarenal in location. With large lesions it is often difficult to differentiate the origin of the lesion by ultrasound. Angiography may be the procedure of choice in this instance.

Ultrasound studies are useful in evaluating pelvic lesions in pediatric patients. Retrovesical masses such as rhabdomyosarcoma and retroperitoneal tumors can be identified by using the full bladder technique. These lesions appear as echogenic, ill-defined masses posterior to the bladder wall, The bladder may also be asymmetrically displaced in this instance (1). In older girls, one must be constantly aware of the possibility of an intrauterine pregnancy.

Sonography can be used in other renal disorders such as focal pyelonephritis, chronic glomerulonephritis, and renal vein thrombosis. Acute pyelonephritis may be identified sonographically by focal enlargement of the renal outline. This may be difficult to detect since the changes in this condition are subtle and may mimic those found in fetal lobulations which are an anatomic variant. Chronic glomerulonephritis can be identified as a kidney that is small but exhibits high-level echogenicity compared to the moderate echogenicity of the normal renal cortex (Fig. 5-7C). By establishing a discrepancy in renal size, sonography may be helpful in the diagnosis of renal vein thrombosis. Visualization of the thrombus in the inferior vena cava has been reported with the resolution capabilities of modern instrumentation, but this is a rare occurrence. This condition is usually associated with dehydration, septicemia, hypercoagulability, and/or prematurity. Since the sonographic manifestations in the above diseases may be minimal, ultrasound is often employed in conjunction with other modalities for establishing these diagnoses.

EVALUATION OF INTRA-ABDOMINAL
(EXTRAHEPATIC, EXTRARENAL) MASSES

Sonography can be used to determine the size, location, and internal consistency of an abdominal mass. This will often assist in the differential diagnosis. By completely delineating the borders of a mass, one can differentiate lesions related to the liver from renal, intra-abdominal extrahepatic, or pelvic masses (Table 6-2).

Occasionally, a mass that originates in the pelvis will be difficult to distinguish from a mass located in the abdomen on the basis of physical examination alone. As in the adult, the pelvic origin of a mass can be sonographically identified by its displacement of bowel. Masses that originate in the pelvis and enlarge in a cephalic direction displace the bowel superiorly, whereas those that originate in the abdomen and grow caudally displace the bowel inferiorly. Displaced loops

Table 6-2. Sonographic Differential Diagnosis of Masses in Children

INTRA-ABDOMINAL (EXTRAHEPATIC, EXTRARENAL)

Cystic	Complex	Solid
Ovarian cyst	Abscess	Neuroblastoma
Dermoid cyst	Intussusception	
Choledochal cyst	Enlarged lymph nodes	
Pancreatic pseudocyst	Fluid-filled bowel	
Mesenteric cyst		
Omental cyst		
Gastrointestinal duplication cyst		

HEPATIC

Cystic	Complex	Solid
Simple cyst	Abscess	Hepatoblastoma
Polycystic liver and kidney disease	Hematoma	Hepatoma
	Hemangioma	Adenoma
	Necrotic liver tumor (hepatoblastoma)	

PELVIC

Extrauterine

Cystic	Complex	Solid
Physiological ovarian cyst	Dermoid cyst	Dermoid cyst
Dermoid cyst	Teratomas	Teratocarcinoma
Paraovarian cyst	Dysgerminoma	Pelvic neuroblastoma
	Tubo-ovarian abscess	Rhabdomyosarcoma

Intrauterine

Cystic	Complex	Solid
Hydrometrocolpos	Intrauterine pregnancy	Bicornuate uterus
	Hematometrocolpos	

of bowel can be identified as a group of high-level echoes that have a mottled acoustical shadow (Fig. 5-5A).

When an abdominal mass is discovered by ultrasound, the patency and course of the inferior vena cava should be evaluated during the same imaging study. As in the adult, the inferior vena (IVC) appears as a tubular sonolucent structure that has a horizontal course and widens as it approaches the diaphragm. The IVC is delineated on longitudinal sonograms made 1 to 3 cm to the right of midline (Fig. 4-1D). If the sonographic examination does not localize the inferior vena cava in relation to an abdominal mass, or if there is any question concerning its patency, an inferior vena cavagram can be performed as part of an excretory urogram. Given the current instrumentation and diligent scanning technique, some ultrasound assessment of the IVC can usually be made.

Sonography is very helpful in the evaluation of pediatric patients who present with abdominal pain of unknown etiology. Cholelithiasis and pancreatitis can be detected sonographically in children. Although the cause of pancreatitis is frequently unknown in the pediatric population, it may be encountered secondary to trauma or as a sequela to chemotherapy. By identifying an enlarged and edematous gland, sonography can confirm the clinical suspicion of pancreatitis (Fig. 6-3A). We believe that this entity is much more common than previously recognized. Sonography can also be used to detect pancreatic pseudocysts that occur as a sequela to trauma or pancreatitis. As in adults, pseudocysts appear as sonolucent masses located in the abdomen, pelvis, or even in the mediastinum (Fig. 6-3B). These must be differentiated from other cysts that can produce pain. Detection of a cystic mass in a patient who presents with acute abdominal pain may imply that torsion of the cystic mass about its pedicle has occurred or that there has been superimposed hemorrhage or infection.

Figure 6-3. ABDOMINAL DISORDERS

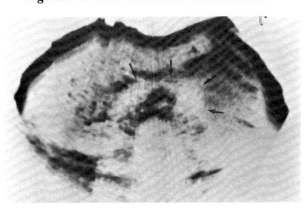

Figure 6-3A. Acute pancreatitis (transverse, 1 cm below xiphoid). The pancreas (*arrows*) is enlarged, and its echogenicity is less than that of the surrounding liver. This patient had acute abdominal pain. The pancreas returned to normal configuration and texture after the clinical symptoms subsided.

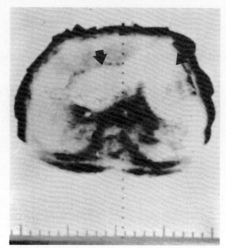

Figure 6-3B. Pancreatic pseudocyst (transverse, 6 cm below xiphoid). The child sustained blunt trauma to her abdomen. There is a large cystic mass (*arrow*) in the epigastrium representing a pancreatic pseudocyst.

Although cholelithiasis is more common in adults, this condition may be encountered in children as a result of a metabolic or hematologic disorder or as a sequela to intra-abdominal inflammation or biliary tract obstruction. As in the adult, gallbladder calculi appear as echogenic foci within the gallbladder that cast a distal acoustical shadow (Fig. 4-13A).

The first portion of Table 6-2 deals with the sonographic classification of the major intra-abdominal masses that are located separate from the liver and kidney. The most commonly encountered mass in this category is neuroblastoma, which is usually located in the region of the adrenal gland, but can be located anywhere in the abdomen along the course of the sympathetic nerve chain. These masses become evident when they cause displacement of one or both kidneys and may sometimes contain the fine calcifications that can be identified radiographically in almost half of the tumors. Metastases from a neuroblastoma may extend into and involve the para-aortic lymph nodes (Fig. 6-3C). When this occurs, the enlarged nodes that contain metastatic tumor appear as lobulated, mildly echogenic structures that straddle the prevertebral vessels.

Abdominal masses created by enlarged para-aortic or mesenteric lymph nodes can also present sonographically as a complex or solid, lobulated, intra-abdominal mass (Fig. 6-3C). The location of enlarged lymph nodes on ultrasound studies may be used to select the appropriate treatment portals for radiation therapy. Enlarged nodes demonstrate a series of convexities in outline. They can assume several configurations ranging from isolated, elliptical, relatively sonolucent masses to an enlarged, lobulated mass of conglomerate or matted nodes. Enlarged para-aortic nodes frequently appear as a lobulated, mildly echogenic mass that straddles the prevertebral vessels and silhouettes them. As opposed to enlarged para-aortic nodes, enlarged mesenteric nodes tend to be central in location. Even when a full bladder technique is used, enlarged pelvic nodes less than 2.0 cm may be difficult to delineate due to location and relative angle in

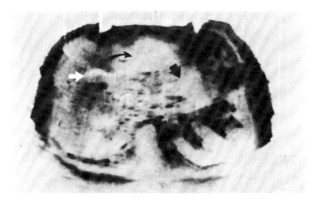

Figure 6-3C. Neuroblastoma and lymphadenopathy (transverse, 2 cm below xiphoid). There is a lobulated, mildly echogenic midline mass representing enlarged nodes (*curved arrow*). In addition, there is an ill-defined mildly echogenic mass in the left suprarenal area which corresponded to a neuroblastoma (*large arrow*). The enlarged para-aortic lymph nodes resulted in biliary tract obstruction, as evidenced by "sludge" within the gallbladder (*white arrow*).

relation to the transducer. Sonographic establishment of splenic enlargement in the presence of enlarged nodes suggests diffuse reticuloendothelial involvement such as that encountered in leukemia and lymphomas.

Abdominal masses in children that exhibit a complex sonographic appearance include abscesses and solid tumors that undergo cystic degeneration or cystic masses that contain clot, cellular debris, or fatty material. For example, appendiceal abscesses than contain pus and cellular debris exhibit a complex sonographic texture (Fig. 6-3D). As is true in most abscesses, pus and cellular debris

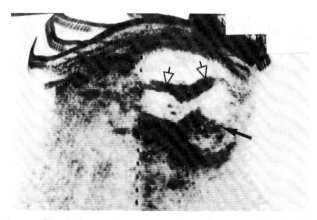

Figure 6-3D. Appendiceal abscess (transverse, 6 cm above symphysis pubis with distended bladder). There are multiple fluid-filled masses posterior to the bladder (*open arrows*). In addition, echogenic material is demonstrated within this mass (*solid arrow*). The mass representing a large appendiceal abscess secondary to appendiceal rupture may be totally sonolucent or complex depending on whether cellular debris and inflammatory fluid are present.

are gravity-dependent, and they layer within the mass. The boundary between lighter serous fluid and pus frequently creates a recognizable interface within the mass. The orientation of the interface within the mass can be shown to be gravity-dependent by scanning the child in the right and left posterior oblique positions and right and left lateral decubitus positions.

In general, the use of sonography as a screening procedure for detection of an appendiceal abscess is limited, for overlying bowel gas in adynamic loops tends to prevent adequate penetration and visualization of masses that are deep in the abdomen. However, if radiographic signs are suggestive of an intra-abdominal abscess, sonography can be used to confirm this diagnosis.

Although intussusceptions of the small and/or large bowel are usually diagnosed by physical examination or barium enema, occult intussusceptions may be discovered initially during abdominal sonography. Intussuscepted bowel appears as a rounded intra-abdominal mass that consists of an echogenic core and sonolucent rim ("bull's eye" or "target" configuration) (Fig. 4-16D). The central echoes represent the intussusceptum, and the sonolucent rim represents edematous bowel wall and fluid (16). Many gastrointestinal tract tumors as well as normal bowel containing mucus and gas that are collapsed may exhibit this configuration. However, the bull's eye pattern emanating from bowel tumors and intussusceptions can be differentiated from the bull's eye patterns seen in normal bowel, because the sonolucent rim is usually more than 2 to 3 cm in thickness (16). In addition, this configuration does not change as one might expect if normal peristalsis is present.

Another sonographically complex or cystic intra-abdominal mass that can be encountered in girls is a dermoid cyst. Because of their variable internal consistency, dermoid cysts have a wide variety of sonographic appearances in the pediatric as well as the adult population; these cysts range from completely sonolucent lesions in a pelvoabdominal location to complex, predominantly solid pelvoabdominal masses. Similarly, they range in size between 3 to 5 cm and 15 to 20 cm. Totally cystic dermoids are frequently encountered in teenage girls and tend to be lined by neuroectoderm that secrete a cerebrospinal fluid-like fluid (Fig. 6-5D). Dermoid cysts that appear as sonographically complex masses usually contain a large amount of sebaceous component. Due to the "tip of the iceberg" effect, these masses are sometimes difficult to delineate, although they can be in part palpated. This effect may be manifest in the difficulty one encounters in delineating the posterior aspect of a dermoid cyst sonographically because of the echogenic properties of the sebaceous material contained within these masses. Sonographically, dermoid cysts that contain sebaceous material can be misinterpreted as gas-filled bowel because of their echogenic properties. Dermoid cysts can produce pain when torsion along the pedicle of the mass occurs.

Cystic abdominal masses in the pediatric patient are readily identified by sonography. Because an enlarged bladder may simulate the physical findings of an enlarged cystic abdominal mass, the child should void or be catheterized before the examination. This will exclude the possibility that the enlarged cystic mass represents a massively distended bladder. Masses that present as large cysts in the abdomen of children include mesenteric and omental, choledochal, and dermoid cysts, as well as pseudocysts secondary to pancreatic trauma.

Choledochal cysts present as fluid-filled masses in the right upper quadrant. Depending on the type, such a cyst may look like a cystic diverticulum branching

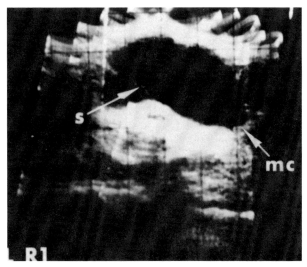

Figure 6-3E. Mesenteric cyst (longitudinal, 1 cm to right of midline, white-on-black image). This patient was thought to have a distended bladder as the cause of her abdominal enlargement. However, after voiding, there was no change in the size of the mass. This image demonstrates a large cystic mass occupying the majority of the lower abdomen (mc). Within the mass, there is a linear interface that probably represents a septum (s).

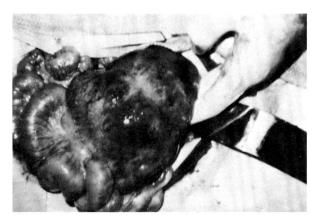

Figure 6-3F. Mesenteric cyst at surgery. The mass depicted in Figure 6-3E was found to represent a mesenteric cyst. Note the relationship of the mass to the bowel.

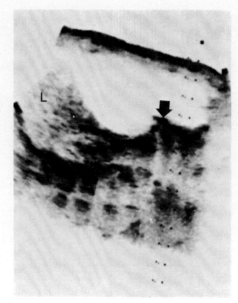

Figure 6-3G. Ileocecal duplication cyst (longitudinal, 3 cm to right of midline). There is a large multilobulated cystic mass inferior to the liver (L) and right kidney. An echogenic area is seen along the posterior aspect of this mass corresponding to the terminal ileum. At surgery, a large duplication cyst arising from, but not in communication with, the terminal ileum was found.

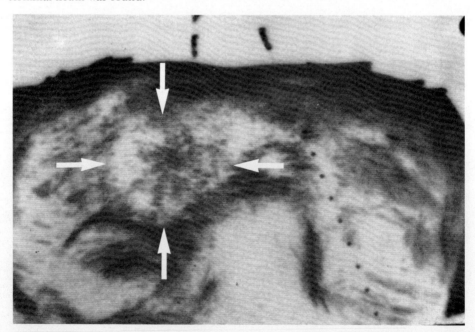

Figure 6-3H. Duodenal hematoma (transverse, 4 cm below xiphoid). This child had sustained trauma to the upper abdomen. The echogenic mass anterior and medial to the right kidney represented a duodenal hematoma (*arrows*). (Courtesy of Steven S. Dumond R.D.M.S., Valley General Hospital, Renton, Wash.)

off the common bile duct or diffuse cystic enlargement of the entire common bile duct. Occasionally, the continuity of these cysts with the common bile duct can be established by ultrasound (15). Radionuclide examinations utilizing hepatobiliary agents may be used in combination with ultrasound to evaluate children suspected of having choledochal cysts.

Other intra-abdominal cystic masses that may have an appearance similar to that of choledochal cysts include a mesenteric or gastrointestinal duplication cyst (Fig. 6-3E). Duplication cysts of the gastrointestinal tract may escape identification on barium enema X-ray contrast studies because these duplications lack communication with the true lumen of the bowel and will not fill with the contrast media. Mesenteric cysts appear as cystic abdominal masses that are usually centrally located and displace the bowel to either side of the abdomen. Pseudocysts of the pancreas may also appear as cystic abdominal masses. These masses are suspected because of a history of trauma to the pancreatic area or history of previous pancreatitis. Cystic masses in patients with malfunctioning ventriculoperitoneal shunts may be identified as sonolucent intra-abdominal masses. The distal tip of the ventriculoperitoneal shunts may be identified as a linear echogenicity within the cystic mass.

EVALUATION OF HEPATIC MASSES

Ultrasound is useful in the evaluation of masses within and associated with the liver of infants and children. Sonography is more efficaciously employed if combined with radionuclide studies of the liver for further characterization of hepatic lesions (11). Most hepatic tumors are first detected as space-occupying, photon-deficient areas on liver/spleen reticuloendothelial scans. Additional information concerning differential diagnosis of hepatic lesions may be gained by correlating the sonographic appearance of the mass with the vascularity as revealed by dynamic radionuclide studies (11). The echoes within the mass probably arise from the numerous interfaces that are present at the surface of vessels. In general, the more vascular a hepatic tumor is, the more echogenic it appears.

The most common liver tumor in children is the heptoblastoma. These hepatic tumors appear on ultrasound studies as moderately echogenic, ill-defined masses that may contain central necrosis, depicted as irregular sonolucent areas within the lesion (Figs. 6-4C,D). A similar sonographic appearance is encountered in a most uncommon tumor referred to as a hepatic hemangioepithelioma (Fig. 6-4B). Again, the echoes observed emanating from these masses probably arise from the numerous vessels that comprise the mass. If the border of the mass is well delineated, it may be displacing normal liver parenchyma. Diffuse infiltration will often be seen as an ill-defined perimeter of the lesion, as is noted in adults.

Intrahepatic hematomas and abscesses reveal a complex sonographic appearance that is frequently indistinguishable from focal necrosis or tumors of the liver. Hepatic abscesses tend to be more irregular in contour than cysts or hematomas. Because of the frequent involvement of the liver, spleen, and duodenum in children who experience abdominal trauma, the evaluation of the liver for laceration or hematoma is of great clinical importance. The sonographic

Figure 6-4. LIVER MASSES

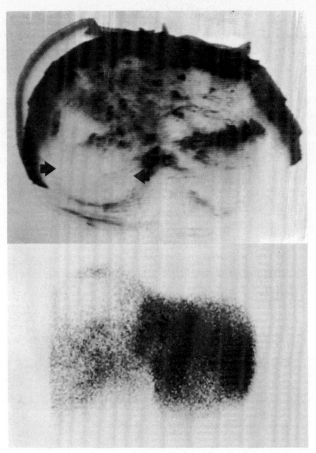

Figure 6-4A. Hematoma (transverse, 2 cm below xiphoid). This seven-year-old boy sustained blunt upper abdominal trauma one week prior to admission. A liver/spleen scan was performed to exclude liver laceration (*bottom*). An infected hematoma was clinically suspected. There is an irregular area of diminished echogenicity in the posterior aspect of the right hepatic lobe representing a hepatic hematoma (*top*) (*arrows*), which corresponds to the area of decreased activity on the liver/spleen scan. The appearance of a hematoma varies according to its age and presence of organized clot. Hematomas that are one to two weeks old usually appear as sonolucent masses. As the clot organizes, the hematoma appears echogenic. Chronic hematomas (over one month old) may show only a few internal echoes. This probably occurs as a result of liquefaction of the hematoma.

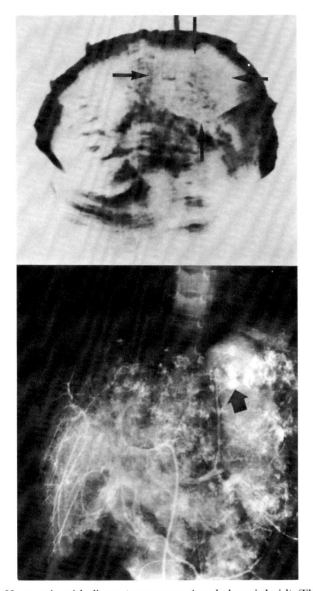

Figure 6-4B. Hemangioepithelioma (transverse, 4 cm below xiphoid). There is a complex mass in the left lobe of the liver (*top*) (*arrows*). Angiography demonstrated multiple neoplastic vessels and venous lakes (*arrows*) suggesting the diagnosis of hemangioepithelioma (*bottom*).

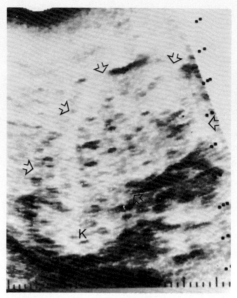

Figure 6-4C. Hepatoblastoma (transverse, magnified image, 4 cm below xiphoid). There is a solid, irregularly shaped mass (*open arrows*) within the liver and extrinsic to the kidneys (K). It was difficult to distinguish this from a neuroblastoma.

appearance of hematoma depends on the amount of its internal organization. Immediately after bleeding occurs, the hematoma appears sonolucent, but with further organization of the clot, it becomes echogenic (Fig. 6-4A). Trauma to the liver may also cause disruption of the bile ducts, and irregular sonolucent areas are seen within the liver resulting from extravasated bile. An advantage of ultrasound is that the renal structures and spleen can be examined at the same time. Duodenal hematomas appear as mildly echogenic masses in the right upper quadrant (Fig. 6-3H).

The multiple cysts seen in the liver and kidney in the adult form of polycystic liver and kidney disease can be readily identified by sonography. Polycystic liver disease appears as multiple rounded cystic areas, of various sizes within the liver (Fig. 5-7A). Occasionally, hepatic fibrosis will be associated with the infantile type of polycystic disease and/or renal tubular ectasia. Hepatic fibrosis can be identified sonographically because of its unusually high echogenicity compared to that of the normal texture of the liver parenchyma (7).

As in adult patients, ultrasound is very useful in the detection of dilated bile ducts secondary to biliary tract obstruction. As stated in the subsection in Chapter 4, the sonographic appearance of metastatic disease is variable and does not appear to be a reliable indicator of the primary tumor. Metastatic foci in the liver of children vary from markedly echogenic, which is usually secondary to adenocarcinoma, to totally sonolucent metastases, which can be seen with lymphorma or sarcomas.

EVALUATION OF PELVIC MASSES

Sonography can be useful in determining the size, location, origin, and internal consistency of pelvic masses in pediatric patients (18). In general, sonography of the pelvis may also be helpful in patients in whom an adequate pelvic examination cannot be performed. The relative frequency of the various types of pelvic masses in children differs from that in adults. For example, dysgerminomas are almost exclusively found in pediatric patients. The age of the patient is an important factor in the differential diagnosis of pelvic masses, for certain pelvic masses are most common in certain age groups. For example, when one encounters a cystic pelvic mass, one can predict that from infancy to 2 years of age it most likely is a physiologic ovarian cyst, whereas from 5 to 15 years of age the most common cystic pelvic mass is a germ cell tumor, such as a dermoid cyst or dysgerminoma (21).

Physiological or functional ovarian cysts may cause acute abdominal pain as a result of torsion on the pedicle of the mass. They may also become clinically manifest if they cause difficulty in urination or defecation. As in adults, cystic pelvic masses in children appear as sonolucent masses with well-defined walls and enhanced through transmission (Fig. 6-5A). When cystic masses contain hemorrhage, pus, or organized clot, an echogenic interface can be demonstrated within the mass. Occasionally, thickening of the cyst wall can be identified in some cystic pelvic masses that have undergone torsion. The thickening of the cyst wall is most commonly due to edema resulting from vascular occlusion by the torsion along the pedicle of the mass.

Sonography can be useful in establishing the diagnosis of hydrometrocolpos (Fig. 6-5B) (20). Sonographically, the massively distended vagina and uterus can be identified as a large pear-shaped cystic mass occupying the pelvis and lower

Figure 6-5.   PELVIC MASSES

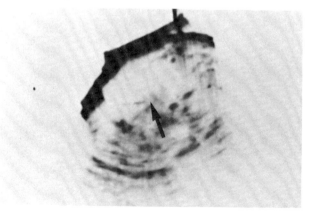

Figure 6-5A. Ovarian cyst (transverse, 2 cm above symphysis pubis). This limited scan reveals a cystic mass in the right lower quadrant. The mass was shown to be relatively hypovascular, showing a radiolucent area on total body opacification effect during excretory urography. This was a cystic mass representing a physiologic ovarian cyst that had undergone torsion.

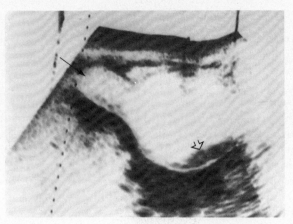

Figure 6-5B. Hydrometrocolpos (longitudinal, 2 cm to right of midline). There is a large globular cystic mass inferior to the uterus (*solid arrow*). The mass contains an echogenic collection (*open arrow*) along its dependent portion. This patient was found to have a bicornuate uterus, but only involving the vagina and lower uterine segment. The echogenic material corresponded to clotted blood. (Courtesy of Thomas Lawson, M.D.)

abdomen. Hydrocolpos can be seen in neonates as a result of collection of vaginal and uterine secretions within these structures secondary to an imperforate hymen or stenosis of the vagina or cervix. In these conditions, the normal uterine and vaginal secretions collect within the distended uterus and vagina. If a patient is postpubertal, blood may collect within the distended uterus and vagina. Clotted blood within a distended uterus and vagina can be identified due to its echogenic appearance (Fig. 6-5B). Atresia of the vagina may be associated with an imperforate anus. In these cases, a fecal-filled or fluid-filled rectum may simulate a pelvic mass. Hydrometrocolpos is associated with renal anomalies (such as unilateral agenesis), as well as skeletal anomalies (20) (Fig. 6-5C).

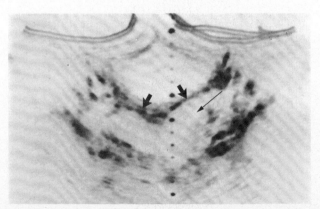

Figure 6-5C. Bicornuate uterus with obstructed horn (transverse, 3 cm above symphysis pubis). There is a binodular appearance to the uterine outline (*large arrows*) with the left horn greater than the right. The uterine lumen in the left horn is distended (*small arrow*). This patient also had unilateral renal agenesis. At surgery, an obstructed left uterine horn of a bicornuate uterus was found. There is an association between congenital anomalies of the uterus, renal agenesis, and vertebral anomalies.

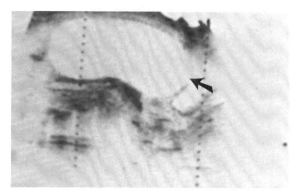

Figure 6-5D. Dermoid cyst (longitudinal, 3 cm to right of midline). This 13-year-old patient had an enlarging abdomen. The sonogram reveals a cystic pelvoabdominal mass (*arrow*). A mass representing a dermoid cyst that was lined by neuroectoderm and secreted cerebrospinal fluid was found at surgery.

Like ovarian cysts, germ cell tumors may appear as cystic masses in children. Dermoid cysts encountered in this age group tend to be lined by neuroectoderm that secrete a cerebrospinal fluid-like fluid (Fig. 6-5D). Therefore, these masses appear as totally sonolucent, and they may attain pelvoabdominal dimensions. Teratomas are important considerations in this differential. Ovarian teratomas may also contain septations (Fig. 6-5E). Other cystic masses that can be encountered in children include paraovarian cysts and mesenteric cysts. Paraovarian cysts present as abdominal or adnexal masses that occur as the result of cystic enlargement of the remnant of Gartner's duct (5). Mesenteric cysts are congenital cysts within the mesentery that usually present as abdominal rather than pelvoabdominal masses (13).

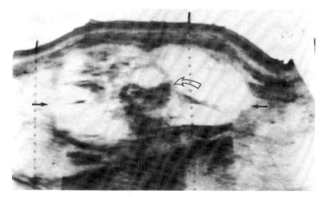

Figure 6-5E. Teratocarcinoma (longitudinal, 2 cm to left of midline). This 8-year-old girl presented with a history of blunt abdominal trauma and a large palpable pelvoabdominal mass. The sonogram reveals a predominantly cystic pelvoabdominal mass (*solid arrows*) that contains solid internal components (*open arrow*). Because of its complex internal consistency, a dermoid cyst or hematoma with organized clot was considered. At surgery, a large pelvoabdomonal mass that contained tissue arising from all three embryonal cell layers was noted. A portion of this mass revealed malignant degeneration microscopically.

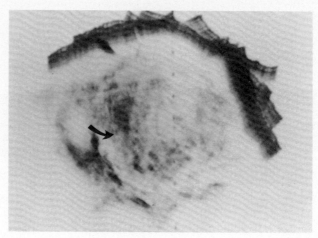

Figure 6-5F. Pelvic neuroblastoma (longitudinal, midline). The large ill-defined solid mass represents a pelvic neuroblastoma (*curved arrow*).

Complex pelvic masses in children include cystic masses that contain either hemorrhage, clot, or pus, or solid masses such as dysgerminomas. Germ cell tumors and dysgerminomas frequently undergo cystic degeneration when they are large. They can be hormonally active, producing precocious puberty (21). As stated previously, dermoid cysts have a large spectrum of sonographic appearances, ranging from totally sonolucent to echogenic depending on the distribution of internal components. Dermoid cysts that contain sebaceous material and/or calcification are the most common type of complex mass. As in the adult, the sebaceous component of dermoid cysts can be very echogenic, resulting in an inability to delineate the posterior wall and confusion of this mass with a gas-filled loop of bowel. Fat is much more echogenic than one would suspect and appears to vary in this property.

Ectopic pregnancies and tubo-ovarian abscesses, although most frequently encountered in adult women, can also be encountered in postpubertal girls. On ultrasound, these conditions exhibit an appearance similar to that seen in adults. Occasionally, the diagnosis of intrauterine pregnancy will be established in a pediatric patient in whom this condition is clinically unsuspected. This is mentioned again for emphasis.

In children, solid pelvic masses are less common than other pelvic masses. Fecal-filled colon may mimic the sonographic appearance of a solid mass. These pseudomasses will usually disappear after evacuation. Pelvic neuroblastomas (Fig. 6-5F) and solid teratomas are rare soft tissue (solid) tumors that may present as pelvic masses.

OTHER APPLICATIONS OF ULTRASOUND IN PEDIATRIC PATIENTS

As in adults, cystic thoracic masses and loculated pleural effusions in children can be identified and distinguished from solid masses. Fluid-filled bowel may occasionally be recognized within the chest in foramen of Morgagni and Bochdalek hernias. Sonography can also be used for guidance and localization in procedures for aspiration of pleural fluid in pediatric patients. Diaphragmatic abnormalities and mediastinal masses can be evaluated by ultrasound, but no large series of these disorders is presently available.

One of the important applications of sonography in pediatrics is in the evaluation of hydrocephalus and other intracranial cysts (22). The neonatal skull is not as densely reflective as the adult skull; therefore, ultrasound can be employed for intracranial evaluations in children. Criteria for establishing ventricular enlargement have been established. Hydrocephalus appears as a sonolucent enlargement of the lateral ventricles due to an increased amount of cerebrospinal fluid (Fig. 6-6B). Porencephalic cysts, posterior fossa cysts, and ventricular dilatation may also be evaluated sonographically (23). They appear as sonolucent areas within the skull which can correspond to the ventricular system. CT is probably more reliable than ultrasound for detection of intracranial hemorrhage. Therefore, a child with macrocrania is probably best evaluated by serial ultrasound study after an initial CT scan is obtained (Figs. 6-6A,B,C).

Sonography can be used to evaluate the scrotum in young boys who present with an enlarged and/or painful scrotum. Hydroceles that may result from trauma to the scrotum appear as fluid collections, displacing the testicle. Torsion of the testes can be depicted as an increased coarseness of the testicular texture. The scrotal anomalies that can be evaluated sonographically are discussed in detail in Chapter 5.

Figure 6-6. CRANIAL SCANNING

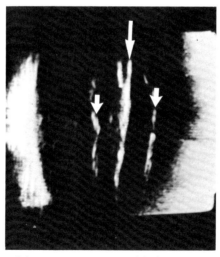

Figure 6-6A. Normal cranial scan (transverse, at 20-degree cephalic tilt in relation to the canthomeateal line). The falx cerebri appears as a linear echogenic structure between the cerebral hemispheres. The normal lateral ventricles appear as linear echogenic interfaces (*arrows*) to either side of the falx cerebri (*large arrow*). (Courtesty of Carlisle Morgan, Ph.D., M.D., Duke University, Durham, N.C.)

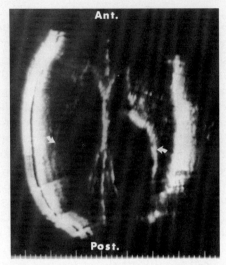

Figure 6-6B. Hydrocephalus (transverse, at 20-degree angle to canthomeateal line). This 8-day-old infant had a meningomyelocele and an associated hydrocephalus. The markedly distended occipital horns of the lateral ventricles (*arrow*) appear as sonolucent fusiform structures to either side of the falx cerebri. (Courtesy of Carlisle Morgan, Ph.D., M.D., Duke University, Durham, N.C.)

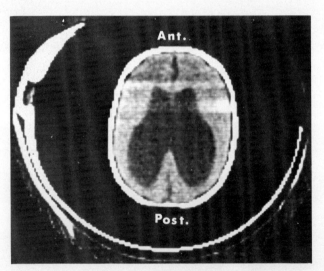

Figure 6-6C. Corresponding CT scan of patient in Figure 6-6B demonstrating marked distension of lateral ventricles as seen in the cephalic sonogram. The intracranial contents in infants up to one year of age can usually be visualized by sonography. Compared to CT scanning, sonographic scanning of the cranium appears in very specific instances to be equally accurate, less costly, and less traumatic to the patient. (Courtesy of Carlisle Morgan, Ph.D., M.D., Duke University, Durham, N.C.)

SUMMARY

Because of some of the advantages of ultrasound, we predict that it will be employed much more commonly in the future to evaluate pediatric disorders. As both the flexibility of the instrumentation and the resolution improve, certain conventional radiographic techniques may be replaced by sonographic studies.

REFERENCES

General

1. Gates, G.: *Atlas of Abdominal Ultrasonography in Children*. New York: Churchill-Livingston, 1978.

Antepartum Detection of Fetal Anomalies

2. Garrett, W.: Use of ultrasonography in selecting neonate for immediate neonatal surgery. *Aust. Pediat. J.* 12:313–318, 1977.

Renal Masses

3. Sample, W., Gypes, M., Ehrlich, R.: Gray scale ultrasound in pediatric urology. *J. Urol.* 117:518–526, 1977.
4. Shkolnik, A.: B-mode ultrasound and non-visualizing kidney in pediatrics. *Am. J. Roentgenol.* 128:121–125, 1977.
5. Mascatelo, V., Smith, E., Carera, F., Burger, M., Teele, R.: Ultrasonic evaluation of obstructive duplex kidney. *Am. J. Roentgenol.* 129:113–120, 1977.
6. Kangarloo, H., Suhov, R., Sample, W., Lipson, M., Sanito, L.: Sonographic evaluation of juxtadiaphragmatic masses in children. *Radiology* 125:785–788, 1977.
7. Rosenfield, A., Siegel, N., Kappelman, N., Taylor, K.: Gray-scale ultrasonographic findings in medullary cystic disease of the kidney and congenital hepatic fibrosis with tubular ectasia: New observations. *Am. J. Roentgenol.* 129:297–303, 1977.
8. Thomas, J., Summer, T., Crowe, J.: Neonatal detection and evaluation of infantile polycystic disease by gray scale echography. *J. Clin. Ultrasound* 6 (5):343–344, 1978.
9. Toomey, F., Fritzsche, P., Carlsen, E., Caggriano, H., Vynmeister, N., Kullman, V.: Applications of aortography and ultrasonography in evaluation of renal agenesis. *Pediat. Radiol.* 6:168–171, 1977.
10. Wietzel, D., Troger, J., Staub, E.: Renal sonography in pediatric patients: A comparative study between sonography and urography. *Pediat. Radiol.* 6:226–232, 1977.

Abdominal Masses

11. Gates, G., Miller, J.: Radionuclide and ultrasonic assessment of upper abdominal masses in children. *Am. J. Roentgenol.* 128:773–780, 1977.
12. Wicks, J., Silver, T., Bree, R.: Giant cystic abdominal masses in children and adolescents: Sonographic differential diagnosis. *Am. J. Roentgenol.* 130:853, 1978.
13. Haller, J., Schneider, M., Cassner, G., Slovis, T., Perl, L.: Sonographic evaluation of mesenteric and omental masses in children. *Am. J. Roentgenol.* 130:269–272, 1978.
14. Mittlestaedt, C.: Ultrasonic diagnosis of omental cyst. *Radiology* 117:673–676, 1975.
15. Filly, R., Carlsen, E.: Choledochal cysts: Report of a case with specific sonographic findings. *J. Clin. Ultrasound* 4 (1):7–10, 1976.
16. Fleischer, A., Muhletaler, C., James, A.: Sonographic patterns arising from normal and abnormal bowel. *Rad. Clin. N.A.* 18(2), 1980. (In press.)

Pelvic Masses

17. Sample, W., Lippe, B., Gypes, M.: Gray scale ultrasonography of normal female pelvis. *Radiology* 125:473–477, 1977.
18. Haller, J., Schneider, M., Kassner, E., Staino, S., Noyes, M., Campos, E., McPherson, H.: Ultrasonography in pediatric gynecology and obstetrics. *Am. J. Roentgenol.* 128:423–429, 1977.
19. Wilson, D., Stacy, T., Smith, E.: Ultrasonic diagnosis of hydrocolpos and hydrometrocolpos. *Radiology* 128:451–454, 1978.
20. White, J., Lawson, T.: Congenital uterine anomaly with unilateral renal agenesis: A case report. *J. Clin. Ultrasound* 6:117–118, 1978.
21. Towne, B.: Mahour, H., Woodley, M., Isaacs, H.: Ovarian cysts and tumors in infancy and childhood. *J. Pediat. Surg.* 10 (3):311–320, 1978.

Intracranial Disorders

22. Johnson, M., Mack, L., Rumack, C., et al.: B-mode echoencephalography in the normal and high risk infant. *Am. J. Roentgenol.* 133:375–381, 1979.
23. Lees, R., Harrison, B., Teates, C., Williamson, R.: Ultrasonic demonstration of a cyst of the velum interposition. *So. Med. J.* 71 (4):401–402, 1978.

7
Cardiac Sonography

One of the first clinical applications of ultrasonic imaging was in the evaluation of cardiac disorders. Edler, the recipient of the 1977 Lasker Award, pioneered development of ultrasonic imaging of the heart in the mid-1950s. Since then, the techniques of M-mode (M = motion) and two-dimensional real-time echography, abbreviated as 2D-RT, have found widespread clinical applications in a number of cardiac disorders.

Ultrasound evaluation of the heart differs from sonographic imaging of abdominal structures in that the motion of structures in relation to time is displayed. The motion of an echogenic point toward or away from the transducer is displayed along the Y-axis in relation to time which is recorded along the X-axis. This M-mode tracing is recorded on a strip chart recorder in a manner similar to that used for ECG recording. Real-time imaging of the heart employs either a phased array linear multicrystal transducer or a mechanical sector scan arrangement (described in Chapter 1). Dynamic images of the cardiac structures are recorded on video tape or multi-image hard copy.

In general, M-mode echocardiography or, as it is frequently called, M-mode "echo" has its greatest application in the evaluation of the motion of the mitral and aortic valves. In comparison with real-time scanning, M-mode echocardiography is limited as to the size of the area interrogated. This is due to the fact that with M-mode echocardiography the heart is adequately imaged only through the left fourth or fifth intercostal space. On the other hand, 2D-RT echocardiography employs a variety of approaches (Table 7-1).

The following is a list of clinical conditions that can be evaluated with conventional M-mode echocardiography and 2D-RT scanning.

M-Mode:
1. Evaluation of abnormal valvular motion (mitral stenosis, aortic stenosis, mitral valve prolapse)
2. Evaluation of pericardial effusion
3. Evaluation of left ventricular hypertrophy, right ventricular hypertrophy, left atrial enlargement
4. Evaluation of patients with suspected idiopathic hypertrophic subaortic stenosis (IHSS)
5. Detection of left atrial myxoma

2D-RT:
1. Examining segmental ventricular wall motion
2. Evaluation of ventricular size, shape, and function
3. Evaluation of complex congenital heart disease
4. Quantitating valvular orifice size

Table 7-1. Normal M-Mode Values for the Heart in Adults[a] (1)

	Mean (cm)	Range (cm)
Right ventricular diameter	1.6	0.7–2.6
Left ventricular diameter	4.6	3.5–5.6
Left ventricular wall thickness	0.9	0.7–1.1
Interventricular wall thickness	0.9	0.7–1.1
Left atrial dimension	2.9	1.9–4.0
Aortic root dimension	2.7	2.0–3.7
Aortic valve opening	1.9	1.6–2.6

[a] Mean body surface area, 1.79m².

Because the M-mode echo reveals motion of a certain point of the heart rather than anatomical structures, it may be initially difficult for a physician who deals primarily with images that portray specific anatomical structures to become accustomed to the data displayed by M-mode echocardiography. However, after becoming accustomed to normal patterns of heart motion, one will be able to distinguish normal from abnormal patterns. Similarly, one should be aware of the various projections of 2D-RT imaging of heart so that structures can be optimally displayed (5).

There are several modalities available for study of cardiac disorders. The relative efficacy of each examination should be considered with respect to the problems to be assessed. In general, echocardiography is noninvasive and is probably most effectively employed as a screening device for specific cardiac disorders such as cardiac valve abnormalities and pericardial effusion. Although cardiac angiography affords the best resolution of the patency of the major cardiac arteries and heart wall motion, it is an invasive method and carries a definite risk. Radioisotopic studies of ventricular wall motion are clinically informative but are somewhat limited because of limited resolution. However, isotopic scanning is very important clinically for the detection of ischemic and hypokinetic areas of the heart wall.

IMPORTANT M-MODE ECHOCARDIOGRAPHIC LANDMARKS, PATTERNS, AND SCANNING TECHNIQUES

M-mode scanning can be considered as a B-mode scan in which the motion of the echo points is constantly displayed in a horizontal manner with regard to time (Fig. 7-1A). The principle of M-mode scanning has been described in the subsection of the different display modes in Chapter 1. For M-mode echocardiograms, the patient is scanned in either the supine or left posterior oblique position. The posterior oblique position brings the heart closer to the thoracic wall. A nonfocused 2.25-MHz transducer or one with medium internal focus is held in the fourth left intercostal space. TGC or depth compensation curves

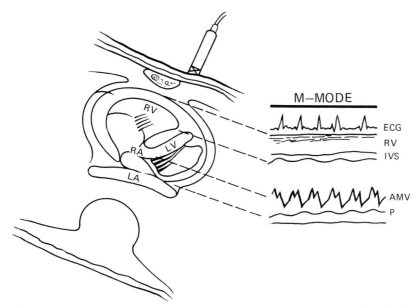

Figure 7-1A. Scanning position for M-mode echocardiography. The patient is placed in the left posterior oblique position, and the transducer is held in the medial aspect of the left fourth intercostal space and aimed in the various positions diagrammed in Figure 7-1B. (IVS = interventricular septum; RV = right ventricle; LV = left ventricle; RA = right atrium; LA = left atrium; P = pericardium; AMV = anterior leaflet of mitral valve.)

should be set to optimize the area of interest. For example, maximum depth compensation should be used for imaging the left ventricle since it is a distant structure; strong near field echoes would decrease the amount of the incident beam that reaches deep structures. The gain and reject controls should also be set so that the best resolution is achieved without degradation of the image by artifactual echoes or "noise."

Once the optimal settings are calculated, the patient is placed in the left posterior oblique position and the transducer held at the medial aspect of the left fourth intercostal space. Initially, the mitral and aortic valves are located by their characteristic motions. The motion of the mitral valve appears as a wavy line that has two components. Anterior mitral valve leaflet motion is in the shape of an *M*, whereas the posterior mitral valve leaflet pattern is similar to a *W*. Motion towards the transducer is depicted by points that extend toward the top of the recording paper. The aortic valve motion has a box-like configuration. The patterns formed by the aortic and mitral valves are discussed in more detail in the following subsection. A sweep of the transducer from either the apex to the aortic root or arch to the apex is performed (Fig. 7-1B). This sweep may be performed in any order, depending on which structures are identified first. The transducer is moved in a reverse S pattern when the sweep is obtained from the apex to the aortic root.

The angle of the transducer is the main determinant of the quality of the image and the diagnostic information obtained from the study (3). Patients with protruding chests or chronic obstructive pulmonary disease are difficult to ex-

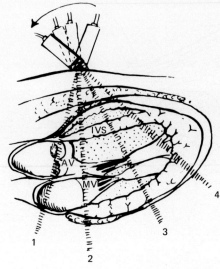

Figure 7-1B. Scanning positions used in echocardiography. The first pattern that is usually delineated is that arising from the mitral valves (MV) corresponding to the position marked 2. After adequate images of the mitral valves are obtained, the transducer is usually aimed in a caudal direction to position 3 or 4, which images the left ventricle and chordae tendineae. Alternatively, the transducer can be aimed in a cephalic and medial direction for demonstration of the aortic valve (AV) motion.

amine but may be successfully imaged with 2D-RT using the subxiphoid approach. Because the tricuspid and pulmonary valves are located beneath the sternum, M-mode images of these valves may be difficult to obtain. Another approach used in M-mode echocardiography is the suprasternal, which may be used to evaluate portions of the aortic arch.

Position 1

In position 1, the beam is directed toward the aortic valve. Strong echoes emanate from the anterior and posterior walls of the aortic root; the diameter of the aortic root should measure no more than 38 mm (Fig. 7-2). To keep the measurement of the aortic root consistent, it is measured at the level of the aortic valve during systole. The aortic valve can be recognized by its box-shaped motion. Although it is usually difficult to image all three aortic valve cusps, the right aortic and noncoronary cusps can usually be visualized. The left atrium is measured from the posterior aortic root wall to the posterior left atrial wall, and the distance should be no greater than 4.0 cm or 1.3 times the aortic root size.

Position 2

When the transducer is directed inferiolaterally from position 1, the M-shaped motion of the anterior leaflet can be recognized (Fig. 7-2). When the transducer is moved slightly cranial, the M-motion of the anterior mitral leaflet can be seen

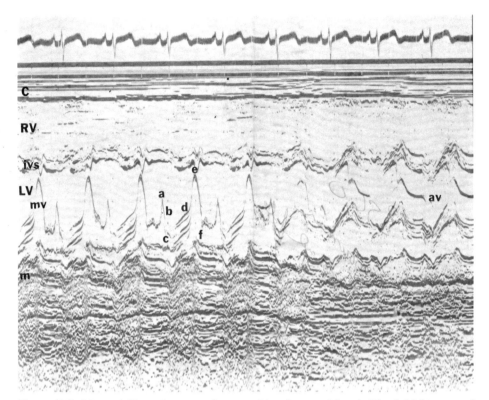

Figure 7-2. Normal M-mode sweep from position 2 to position 1. The initial group of linear stationary echoes arises from the chest wall (c). The right ventricle (RV) appears as a sonolucent area between the stationary echoes of the chest wall and the band of echoes representing the interventricular septum (ivs). Between the interventricular septum and the myocardium (m) is the left ventricle (LV). Within the left ventricle, the leaflets of the mitral valve (mv) are demonstrated. The reference points of the anterior leaflet of the mitral valve are depicted as points a, b, c, d, e, and f. As the transducer is aimed superiorly and medially, the echoes emanating from the aortic valve can be delineated (av). The closed aortic leaflets appear as a linear interface in the center of the echoes arising from the aortic root.

as a mirror image of the *W*-shaped motion of the posterior mitral leaflet. These two echogenic structures should meet during systole to form a single line that gradually slopes anteriorly. The left ventricular wall can be identified posterior to the posterior mitral leaflet. During systole the interventricular septum and posterior left ventricular wall approach each other. Occasionally, the chordae tendineae are seen as a single echo or a cluster of echoes that move with the mitral valve echoes in systole. The normal values for left ventricular dimensions are given in Table 7-1 (1).

The size of the left ventricle can be approximated by the distance between the leading edge of the interventricular septum to the posterior aspect of the left ventricle during end diastole. This measurement should be no more than 5.6 cm in adults.

Position 3

In position 3, the anterior and posterior mitral leaflets are demonstrated (Fig. 7-2). The motion of the anterior leaflet of the mitral valve has a characteristic M shape. During diastole, there is rapid anterior motion and partial closure of the anterior mitral leaflet. In systole, the anterior and posterior mitral leaflets move together with a slow anterior motion.

Points of the path of the anterior mitral leaflet motion have been labeled, by convention, a through f (Fig. 7-2). At point a the atrial contraction is greatest; at point b the ventricular systole begins. Point c denotes mitral valve closure, and point d, the beginning of mitral valve opening. The maximum anterior position of the anterior mitral leaflet is depicted by point e. Following initial rapid left ventricular filling, the leaflet is partially closed at point f.

The slope between points e and f can be used to quantitate mitral valve excursion and may be used to diagnose mitral stenosis. However, the functional severity of mitral stenosis does not correspond well with the e to f slope. Slopes of e to f greater than 60 mm/sec essentially exclude mitral stenosis, whereas slopes less than 35 mm/sec are strongly indicative of mitral stenosis.

Position 4

When the transducer is aimed inferiolaterally from position 3, the left ventricle can be delineated (Fig. 7-2). Since the anterior chest wall is a stationary structure, echoes arising from it appear as a group of linear echoes located immediately beneath the skin. The lumen of the right ventricle appears as an echo-free space between the immobile echoes of the anterior chest wall and the moving band of echoes representing the interventricular septum. The interventricular septum is identified as a band of echoes that undergo rhythmic shortening. Changes in the thickness of this band can be recognized during systole and diastole. Papillary muscles appear as echogenic bands posterior to the interventricular septum in a sonolucent area representing the blood-filled left ventricle, which extends to the next dense line, the endocardium. The myocardium can be recognized as a band of echoes that moves in the direction opposite to the interventricular septum. Contractions of the myocardium can be correlated with the ECG. The most distal strong echo that can be delineated emanates from the epicardial-pericardial interface. There should be no separation of the echoes between the epicardium and pericardium. M-mode measurements of the upper limits of normal for the different cardiac chambers are summarized in Table 7-1.

As mentioned previously, a major limitation to the study of the heart, using M-mode echocardiography, is its small sampling area. In addition, certain portions of the heart may be difficult to visualize, such as the tricuspid and pulmonary valves and the right ventricle and atrium. However, these structures are adequately visualized by using 2D-RT. Emphysematous patients may be difficult to evaluate sonographically because air-filled bullae, which reflect the incident beam, may be interposed between the chest wall and heart.

ABNORMAL VALVE MOTION

Mitral Stenosis

The motion of the mitral valve can be quantitated by the e to f slope. Although the severity of mitral stenosis is not directly correlated with a decrease in the e to f slope, an e to f slope of less than 35 mm/sec is highly suggestive of mitral stenosis (Fig. 7-3). High-amplitude echoes can be recorded from a calcified mitral valve.

Aortic Stenosis

Since the opening of the aortic valve leaflets depends upon flow, the amount of aortic valve opening cannot be routinely used as an indication of aortic stenosis. However, an aortic valve opening of less than 1.6 cm suggests a hemodynamically significant diminution of the aortic valve opening. High-amplitude echoes may be recorded from calcific areas within the aortic valve (Fig. 7-5). Like mitral stenosis the 2D-RT scanning may be more accurate in evaluating the physiologic severity of stenosis by calculating the orifice size at its greatest opening. This is described in more detail in a subsection on 2D-RT scanning.

Mitral Valve Prolapse

Mitral valve prolapse can be diagnosed readily by recognition of abrupt posterior motion of the posterior mitral leaflet (Fig. 7-4). Posterior motion of the posterior

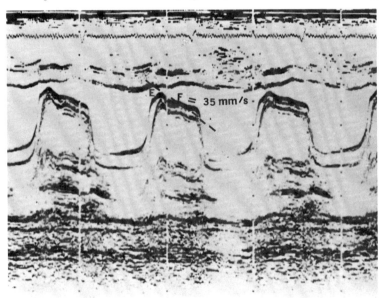

Figure 7-3. Mitral stenosis (position 2). There is diminished excursion of the mitral valve between points E and F. The E to F slope measures 35 mm per sec, which is markedly below normal. Although the severity of mitral stenosis does not correlate well with the E to F slope, an E to F slope less than 35 mm per sec is highly suggestive of mitral stenosis.

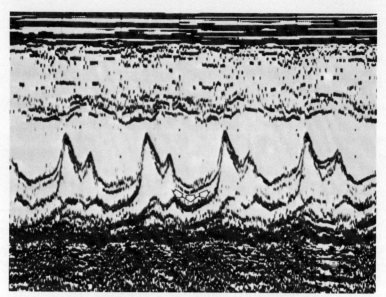

Figure 7-4. Mitral valve prolapse (position 2). The posterior leaflet of the mitral valve is noted to bulge posteriorly during systole, creating a hammock-like motion (*open arrows*).

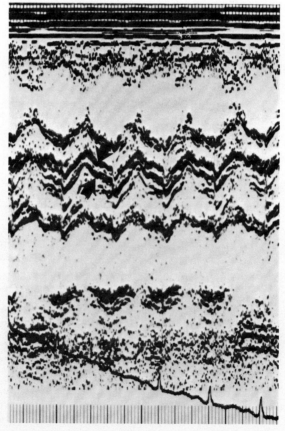

Figure 7-5. Aortic stenosis (position 1). The echoes emanating from the aortic valve are increased, and the aortic valve opening is diminished (*arrows*). These features suggest the presence of hemodynamically significant aortic stenosis.

mitral leaflet during systole greater than 3 mm is indicative of significant mitral valve prolapse. Mitral valve prolapse is a component of Barlow syndrome. It is detected clinically by a characteristic systolic click murmur. Since there are a significant number of asymptomatic patients who have evidence of Barlow syndrome, the clinical implication of this disorder is unsettled. However, if these patients have a murmur, it is usually suggested that they receive prophylactic antibiotics prior to a surgical procedure, since they are subject to an increased risk of subacute bacterial endocarditis.

PERICARDIAL EFFUSION

M-mode echocardiography is the most sensitive and accurate means for diagnosing pericardial effusion. It is difficult to quantitate the exact amount of pericardial effusion, because the distribution of fluid may not be uniform. As little as 50 cc of excess pericardial fluid can be detected. Pericardial effusion is recognized as a sonolucent band between the epicardium and pericardium that disappears as the beam is directed toward the left atrium (Fig. 7-6). Pericardial effusions can usually be differentiated from pleural effusions, since pericardial

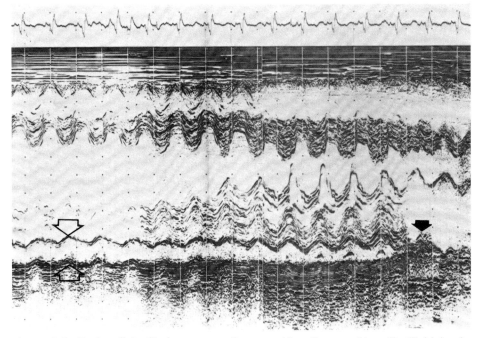

Figure 7-6. Pericardial effusion (sweep from position 2 to position 1). Fluid in the pericardium is depicted as a sonolucent band (*open arrows*) between the pericardium and the pleura and lung. Since the lung contains air, it is depicted as an echogenic interface. Fluid in the pericardial space is confirmed by the apparent lack of fluid as the transducer is aimed toward the left atrium near the origin of the pericardial sac (*solid arrow*).

fluid does not extend posterior to the left atrium. A similar pattern can be encountered, in rare instances, in patients with a thick pericardium or an unusual amount of pericardial fat around the heart.

IDIOPATHIC HYPERTROPHIC SUBAORTIC STENOSIS (IHSS)

IHSS can be diagnosed from M-mode echocardiograms (Fig. 7-7). Sonography can also be used for serial examination of these patients to evaluate response to therapy. Although not always present, the features of IHSS that can be observed either singly or in combination include an increased interventricular septum to posterior wall thickness ratio (over 1.3:1), a hypodynamic septum associated with a hyperdynamic posterior wall, failure of the septum to thicken during systole, systolic anterior motion (SAM) of the anterior mitral leaflet, narrowing of the left ventricular outflow tract during systole, diminished diastolic mitral valve slope and midsystolic closure of the aortic valve. Asymmetric septal hypertrophy may be seen in normal newborns and can simulate this condition.

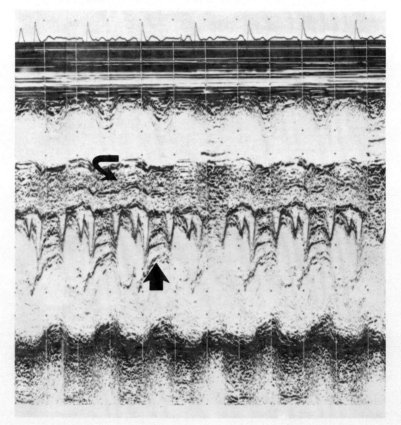

Figure 7-7. Idiopathic hypertrophic subaortic stenosis (IHSS) (position 2). The interventricular septum is abnormally thick (*curved arrow*), and there is anterior motion of the mitral valve leaflet during systole (*large arrow*). These two features are commonly encountered in this condition.

LEFT ATRIAL MYXOMA

Left atrial myxoma can be identified by the M-mode echocardiogram when the aortic valve and left atrium are visualized (Fig. 7-8). The reflections arising from this tumor appear as a cluster of echoes within the left atrium during systole and usually prolapse into the left ventricle through the mitral valve during diastole. This pattern can occasionally be simulated in scans using an improperly adjusted gain setting so that numerous artifactual echoes or "noise" are recorded. Echoes emanating from a left atrial myxoma can be differentiated from artifactual echoes created by an excessively high gain setting, because echoes from left atrial myxomas are most prominent when the beam is oriented toward the left atrium.

OTHER CARDIAC DISORDERS

In general, regurgitant lesions are difficult to diagnose by M-mode echocardiography but can be suggested by certain sonographic signs. Indirect signs, such as dilatation of the left ventricle or flattening or serration of the normally sharp echo from the anterior leaflet of the mitral valve, can occur as the result of a regurgitant jet of aortic blood striking this leaflet during diastole (Fig. 7-10). M-mode echocardiography can also be used to evaluate the function of prosthetic valves. Some prosthetic valves have characteristic M-mode patterns, and their function can be estimated by their M-mode patterns. It may be difficult to

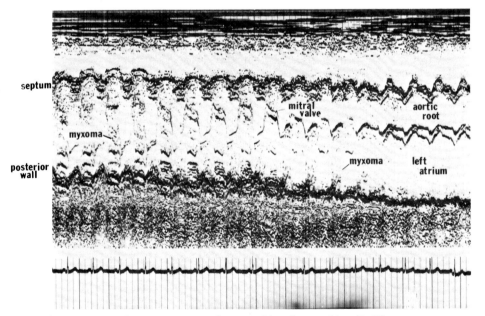

Figure 7-8. Left atrial myxoma (sweep from position 2 to position 1). The tumor appears as a cluster of echoes prolapsing into the left ventricle during diastole. (Courtesy of Rosemarie Robertson, M.D., Vanderbilt University School of Medicine, Nashville, Tenn.)

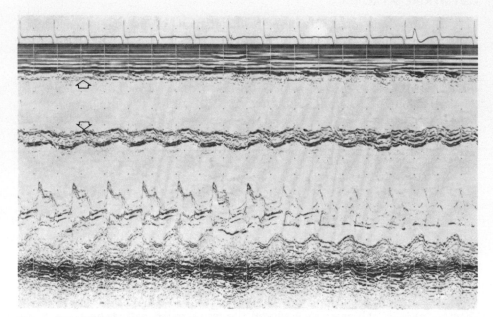

Figure 7-9. Right ventricular enlargement secondary to an atrial septal defect (position 2). The right ventricle is enlarged (*open arrows*) as the result of an atrial septal defect. Since the specific anatomical defect is rarely depicted by M-mode echocardiography, indirect signs of anatomical and functional defects, such as right ventricular enlargement, may suggest the presence of such a lesion.

diagnose valvular vegetations by M-mode echo because of the fuzziness of normal valvular echoes even in normal patients. However, vegetations can occasionally be recognized because of unusually thick and irregular valvular echoes.

TWO-DIMENSIONAL REAL-TIME SCANNING (2D-RT)

There are several types of imaging devices that display the cardiac structures by real-time sonography. These include the mechanical sector scanner and phased array scanner described in detail in Chapter 1. The linear array real-time scanner uses a transducer consisting of several smaller transducers synchronized so that the image is displayed and erased quickly, giving the illusion of dynamic imaging. The mechanical sector scanner transducer head is mechanically moved at a rapid rate in imaging the various cardiac structures. At present, mechanical sector scans and phased array systems appear to afford the best resolution of cardiac structures. In the phased array system, multiple transducers are excited at specific time interval sequences and are electronically steered to converge as a wave front at certain points. The beam is fan-shaped and is aimed in a specific direction, as in M-mode echocardiography.

The advantages of 2D-RT scanning include the ability to see anatomical structures in two dimensions as they move. The structures visualized by this scanning

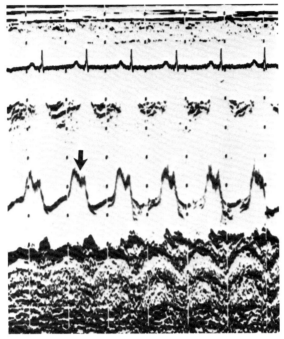

Figure 7-10. Aortic regurgitation with mitral valve flutter (position 2). The echo motion of the anterior leaflet of the mitral valve appears to oscillate (*arrow*) due to regurgitant blood from the aortic valve. The serrated appearance of the mitral valve echo in aortic regurgitation simulates the "shaggy" appearance observed with valvular vegetations.

system are limited by bony structures of the chest wall. Although the precise role of 2D-RT in cardiac diagnosis is yet to be determined, it has certain present applications and several potential applications that are discussed here (9).

IMPORTANT 2D-RT ECHOCARDIOGRAPHIC LANDMARKS AND SCANNING TECHNIQUE

Two-dimensional real-time scans are not limited to imaging the heart from the parasternal approach but allow evaluation through several acoustical windows, from the subxiphoid, apical, and suprasternal portals. Table 7-2 lists the various views, as well as the structures that are imaged from these views, that are used in echocardiography. The utility of the various views for visualizing certain cardiac structures is summarized in Table 7-2.

APPLICATIONS OF 2D-RT

Ventricular Shape, Size, and Motion

Although M-mode imaging can be used for the assessment of ventricular motion, it is limited because of the small imaging area. Since 2D-RT has the dynamic

Table 7-2. Transducer Positions in 2D-RT and Cardiac Structures Imaged (5)

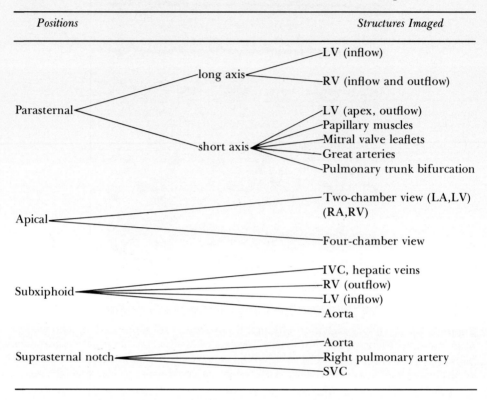

Positions	Structures Imaged
Parasternal — long axis	LV (inflow)
	RV (inflow and outflow)
Parasternal — short axis	LV (apex, outflow)
	Papillary muscles
	Mitral valve leaflets
	Great arteries
	Pulmonary trunk bifurcation
Apical	Two-chamber view (LA,LV) (RA,RV)
	Four-chamber view
Subxiphoid	IVC, hepatic veins
	RV (outflow)
	LV (inflow)
	Aorta
Suprasternal notch	Aorta
	Right pulmonary artery
	SVC

ability to image the heart wall, it can be used to establish the motion, shape, and size of the right and left ventricles (Fig. 7-11).

Changes in the shape of the left ventricle during the cardiac cycle can be portrayed by 2D-RT scanning. Areas of diminished wall excursion can be grossly identified. Focal bulging of the normally smooth wall of the left ventricle can be identified as a sign of a ventricular aneurysm (Fig. 7-12).

A major advantage of 2D-RT over M-mode echo is that 2D-RT dynamically images important structures of the right side of the heart. The tricuspid valve appears as a biconcave echogenic interface that changes configuration with the cardiac cycle. The pulmonary valve has a similar appearance but is located anterior and medial to the tricuspid valve.

Complex Congenital Heart Disease

Two-dimensional real-time scans have been used for the evaluation of complex congenital heart disorders (1,8). The ability to visualize the heart at various angles in real-time may render the functional components of congenital heart disease more apparent than they would be if imaged by M-mode echocardiography. The real-time scans are particularly helpful in the diagnosis of congenital anomalies that have a functional as well as an anatomical component, such as the malpositioned tricuspid valve in Ebstein's anomaly or the cardiac cushion defects

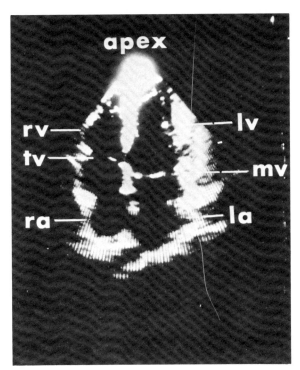

Figure 7-11. Static image taken from real-time examination of a normal heart (apical view). The right ventricle (rv), tricuspid valve (tv), right atrium (ra), left ventricle (lv), mitral valve (mv), and left atrium (la) are demonstrated. (Courtesy of Rosemarie Robertson, M.D., Vanderbilt University School of Medicine, Nashville, Tenn.)

seen with atrioventricular canal. Small atrial septal defects of the ostium primum type can be identified as an abnormal opening between the two atria by 2D-RT.

Quantifying Abnormal Valvular Motion

Although 2D-RT can be used to identify abnormal valvular motion, routine M-mode echocardiography remains the best screening procedure for assessing the presence or absence of abnormal valvular motion. Real-time scanning has an advantage over M-mode echocardiography in that the orifice size, which is a better determinant of the hemodynamic significance of a stenosis than its excursion, is readily depicted by 2D-RT. This principle is illustrated in the evaluation of the aortic valvular excursion. As stated previously, the size of the aortic valve opening as depicted by M-mode echocardiography is highly dependent upon the flow through the valve. However, the orifice size, which can be accurately determined by 2D-RT, correlates well with the physiologic gradient across an aortic valve (7).

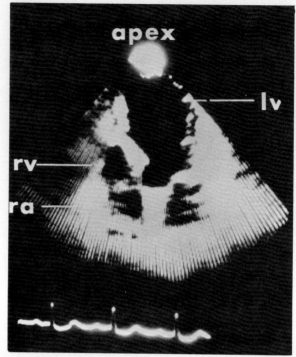

Figure 7-12. Static image obtained during real-time examination of ventricular aneurysm (apical view). There is aneurysmal dilatation of the left ventricle (lv), appearing as a focal bulge of this cardiac chamber. (Courtesy of Rosemarie Robertson, M.D., Vanderbilt University School of Medicine, Nashville, Tenn.)

SUMMARY

M-mode echocardiography is particularly useful in the evaluation of valvular disorders and pericardial effusion. 2D-RT has the advantage of dynamically portraying anatomical defects in the heart as well as displaying valvular orifice size which is a more accurate indicator of the hemodynamic significance of a valvular disorder.

REFERENCES

General

1. Feigenbaum, H.: *Echocardiography*. Second ed. Philadelphia: Lea and Febiger, 1976.

M-Mode Applications

2. Feigenbaum, H.: *Echocardiography*. Second ed. Philadelphia: Lea and Febiger, 1976.
3. Kotler, M., Segal, B., Mintg, G., Pury, W.: Pitfalls and limitations of M-mode echocardiography. *Am. Heart J.* 94 (2):227–249, 1977.

2D-RT Applications

4. Feigenbaum, H.: *Echocardiography*. Second ed. Philadelphia: Lea and Febiger, 1976.

5. Tajik, A., Seward, J., Hagler, D., Mair, D., Lie, J.: Two-dimensional real-time ultrasonic imaging of the heart and great vessels: Technique, image orientation, structure identification, and validation. *Mayo Clin. Proc.* 53 (5):271–306, 1978.

6. Lieppe, W., Scallion, R., Behar, V., Kisslo, J.: Two-dimensional echocardiographic findings in atrial septal defect. *Circulation* 56 (3):447–456, 1977.

7. Weyman, A., Feigenbaum, H., Henwith, R., Girod, D., Dillion, J.: Cross-sectional echocardiographic assessment of the severity of aortic stenosis in children. *Circulation* 55 (5):773–778, 1977.

8. Matsumato, M., Matsuo, H., Nagata, S., Hamanaha, Y., Fugita, T., Kawashima, Y., Nimiura, J., Ave, H.: Visualization of Ebstein's anomaly of tricuspid valve by two-dimensional and standard echocardiography. *Circulation* 53 (1):69–79, 1976.

9. Kisslo, J., von Ramm, O., Thurstone, F.: Cardiac imaging using a phased array ultrasound system. II. Clinical technique and applications. *Circulation* 53 (2):262–267, 1976.

8
Miscellaneous and Future Applications

OPHTHALMOLOGIC SONOGRAPHY

One of the first clinical uses of ultrasonic imaging was for the location of non-metallic foreign bodies in the eye. Since its initial use in the 1950s, sonographic imaging has been used extensively for evaluation of intra- and extraocular disorders. The aqueous humour of the eye affords good propagation of the ultrasound beam, permitting use of 10- and 15-MHz high-frequency transducers. Consequently, the resolution of ophthalmologic scanning ranges from approximately 0.2 to 0.3 mm.

There are several types of scanning devices for ophthalmologic sonography, including contact real-time B-mode scanners, water-bath scanners, and A-mode devices for estimation of axial length of the eye. The technique and indications for each of these types of scanners will be discussed separately. The most common indications for ophthalmologic sonography include:

1. Contact real-time B-mode scanning
   a. Location of nonmetallic intraorbital foreign bodies
   b. Identification of intraocular masses
   c. Diagnosis of retinal detachment
   d. Evaluation for vitreous hemorrhage
2. Water-bath scanning
   a. Evaluation of the anterior chamber
3. A-mode scanning
   a. Axial length measurement

Radiographic imaging is frequently used in combination with ultrasound studies for detection of foreign bodies in the eye. In addition, CT scanning can delineate retro-orbital fat and muscles well, but in general does not provide the same resolution of intraorbital structures as ultrasonic imaging.

Contact Real-Time B-Mode Scanning

In real-time studies a transducer is placed on the closed eyelid after gel has been applied to the surface as a couplant. The head of the transducer is approximately 4 cm wide and curved to conform to the configuration of the globe. Within the transducer housing, a smaller transducer of 10-MHz frequency is connected to a motor and sectored in a 50-degree arc. This type of imaging device affords a real-time image of the eye. During the examination, the patients are requested to move their eyes from lateral to medial and superiorly to inferiorly so that the greatest surface of the eye can be visualized.

The initial echogenic interface arises from the lens. The vitreous humor distal to the lens is sonolucent (Fig. 8-1). The retina and sclera are the most distal echogenic interfaces visualized. Because the placement of the transducer on the eyelid causes distortion of the near field, a water bath scanner is needed for evaluation of anterior chamber structures.

Intraorbital foreign bodies appear as echogenic interfaces that persist even at low gain. Occasionally, foreign bodies will produce such strong echoes as to cause reverberation artifacts distal to their interface. Metallic foreign bodies demonstrate complete posterior acoustical shadowing.

Tumors of the choroid are the most common intraocular tumors, and malignant melanoma is the most common of this group. Tumors of this kind appear

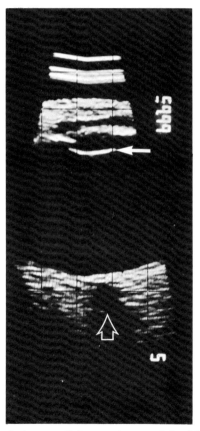

Figure 8-1. Normal B-mode image of the eye (transaxial, white-on-black image). This image of the eye was obtained with a B-mode ophthalmologic scanner. The transducer was placed on the closed eyelid and aimed axially toward the optic nerve. With this technique, the lens (*solid arrow*) and optic nerve (*open arrow*) are demonstrated. Because the aqueous humor is primarily fluid, it appears echo-free. Since ultrasound is attenuated by the optic nerve, this structure appears as an area of acoustical shadowing distal to the retina (*open arrow*). (Courtesy of Cathy Correia, R.D.M.S., St. Joseph's Hospital, Tampa, Fla.)

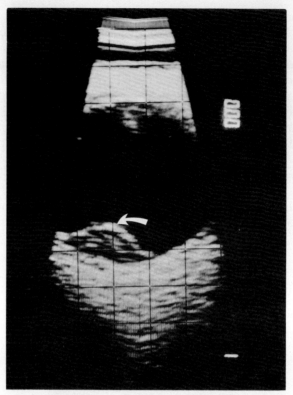

Figure 8-2A. Ocular malignant melanoma (transaxial B-mode scan). There is an echogenic mass that appears to elevate the retina (*curved arrow*). The mass is echogenic, thus distinguishing it from a retinal detachment. (Courtesy of Cathy Correia, R.D.M.S., St. Joseph's Hospital, Tampa, Fla.)

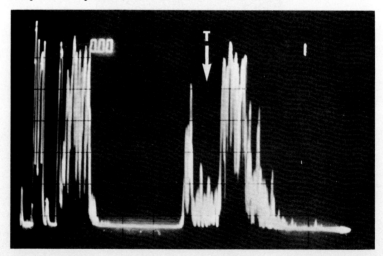

Figure 8-2B. A-mode trace through same tumor (T). This A-mode trace reveals that the tumor is echogenic, with the internal echoes appearing to decrease in amplitude due to attenuation by the solid mass. This tumor was found to represent malignant melanoma. (Courtesy of Cathy Correia, R.D.M.S., St. Joseph's Hospital, Tampa, Fla.)

as dome-shaped echogenic masses with their base on the choroid surface (Figs. 8-2A,B). The tumors may assume a mushroom shape if pedunculated. Other tumors within the eye include metastases that usually absorb much of the initial ultrasonic beam and produce high, irregular echo heights on A-mode tracings that are usually 80% of the scleral echo height. Tumors of the posterior chamber may also cause retinal detachment that can be demonstrated by sonography.

Retinal detachment is easily demonstrated by sonography and produces an echogenic interface separated from the retina but attached at the origin of the optic nerve (Fig. 8-3). Retinal detachments are thought to be produced by traction on the retina with subsequent accumulation of vitreous humor behind the retina that causes extension of a retinal detachment. In real-time scanning, detached retinal tissue can be differentiated from echoes emanating from vitreous hemorrhage by the fact that retinal detachment moves as a wavy line, whereas the echoes in vitreous hemorrhage are seen as unstructured movement within the globe.

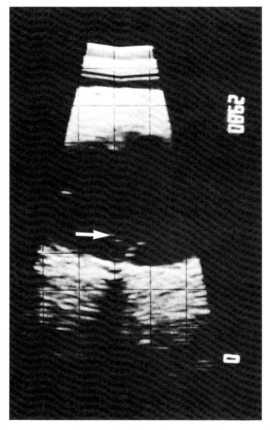

Figure 8-3. Retinal detachment (transaxial B-mode scan). There is a V-shaped interface arising from the retina in the region of the optic nerve (*arrow*). This represents a detached portion of the retina. Retinal detachments frequently reveal this configuration, for they usually retain their attachment to the retina in the region of the optic nerve. (Courtesy of Cathy Correia, R.D.M.S., St. Joseph's Hospital, Tampa, Fla.)

Water-Bath Scanning

Water-bath scanning involves placement of a plastic membrane mounted on a ring stand over the eye. The transducer is placed in the water bath and aimed toward the eye. A mechanical arm controls the movement of the transducer which makes sector scans in 2-mm intervals. The eyelids of the patient are held open by a speculum and the cornea is anesthetized.

Water-bath scanning is best used for evaluation of the structures in the anterior chamber, and scans obtained in this manner are reproducible. However, preparation time is greater than that for contact B-mode scanning, and the images do not have comparable intrinsic resolution due to the sector scanning technique.

A-Mode Scanning

A-mode determination of the axial length of the eye has become increasingly important as more intraocular lens implantations are performed. The exact determination of the axial length of the eye and its chambers is important in selecting the proper lens power for the intraocular lens. Intraocular lenses afford the least magnification of the image when compared with contact lenses substituted after cataract surgery.

The procedure for measuring the axial length of the eye begins with placing the patient in a special stand similar to that for the slit-lamp. The chin and forehead of the patient are positioned opposite the transducer. The cornea is anesthetized and the transducer brought into contact with that structure. Patients are instructed not to blink or shift their gaze during the examination.

An A-mode image is then obtained of the interfaces within the eye. First, the cornea and the anterior and posterior aspects of the lens appear as echo peaks in the A-mode tracing. The vitreous cavity is usually totally sonolucent. The most distal echoes are produced by the retina and sclera.

In order to determine whether or not the tracing corresponds to the visual axis of the eye, certain criteria for an adequate A-mode examination must be met. First, the echoes emanating from the anterior posterior aspect of the lens should be of equal height without any preceding echoes from the iris. Second, two high echo peaks should be recognized from the retina which are immediately proximal to the echo peak emanating from the sclera.

By this technique, axial length determinations are accurate and reproducible to within 0.1 mm. With these measurements, the ophthalmologist can calculate the lens power with great accuracy.

THYROID SONOGRAPHY

Sonography is useful in determining whether thyroid nodules found on radionuclide (^{99m}Tc, ^{131}I, or fluorescent) thyroid scans are cystic or solid (4). As with cysts in other parts of the body, those in and around the thyroid appear as totally sonolucent masses with well-defined margins and exhibit posterior acoustical enhancement. Diagnostic possibilities for a cystic mass include colloid cysts, thyroglossal duct cysts, and branchial cleft cysts. A wide variety of neoplasms may appear as echogenic, poorly defined thyroid masses by ultrasound study. Therefore, the sonographic pattern of a cystic mass is more specific than that of a complex or echogenic thyroid mass.

Sonographic imaging can also be used in the evaluation of other neck masses. For example, enlarged cervical nodes can be demonstrated as mildly echogenic structures that are nodular in shape.

The thyroid can be imaged by using either a contact scanning technique employing a high-frequency transducer with short internal focus (5-MHz, 3- to 6-mm focus, 6-mm diameter) or a water-bath scanner (4). In using a contact technique, the transducer is manually moved across the region of the thyroid in the transverse and longitudinal planes. Tomograms are often obtained at 0.5- cm intervals. The scanning motion should be as smooth as possible to diminish the artifacts created by uneven motion of the transducer. When a water-bath technique is used, the patient is placed in the supine position. A couplant is applied to the patient's neck and the water bath placed over the area of the thyroid. The transducer can be manually moved over the region of the thyroid while placed within the water.

A small parts ultrasound scanner has been developed for evaluation of su- perficial structures such as the thyroid. This imaging device employs a 10-MHz transducer and has resolution in the millimeter range. The transducer is sur- rounded by a water bath which is part of the transducer housing. This device has produced detailed thyroid sonograms with excellent resolution that can be used in the evaluation of superficial vessels, the abdominal viscera of neonates, and the testicles. The major limitation of the small parts scanner at present is its small field of view.

The thyroid is located on either side of the trachea, connected in the center by the isthmic portion of the gland. Vessels of the carotid sheath border the lateral aspect of the right and left lobes of the thyroid. The jugular vein and carotid artery are useful landmarks for delineating the lateral aspects of the thyroid. The jugular vein can be delineated within the carotid sheath lateral to the carotid artery because of its greater diameter and distensibility during a Valsalva maneuver. The right and left thyroid lobes may also be evaluated on longitudinal scans (Fig. 8-4). The sonographic texture of the thyroid is important to assess. It is homogeneous and moderately echogenic by comparison with the echo pattern from surrounding muscle. The sternocleidomastoid muscles appear as biconcave structures on either side of the neck beneath the skin surface.

As stated previously, cystic thyroid masses appear completely sonolucent; they are well-defined masses that have posterior acoustical enhancement. Contrary to the case with the kidney, in which cystic masses are common, only approxi- mately 20% of thyroid masses are simple cysts. Cystic masses in the thyroid include colloid cysts (Fig. 8-5) and thyroglossal duct cysts. These two entities have a similar sonographic appearance. Branchial cleft cysts are usually located in a more cephalic position than thyroid cysts but may also demonstrate a similar sonographic appearance. Most thyroid cysts spontaneously regress, but if not, sonography can be used for guided aspiration of thyroid cysts when clinically indicated.

Complex masses encountered in the thyroid include those created by ade- nomas, carcinomas, goiterous nodules, and certain colloid cysts that contain organized hemorrhage. Thus, a complex sonographic appearance is not very

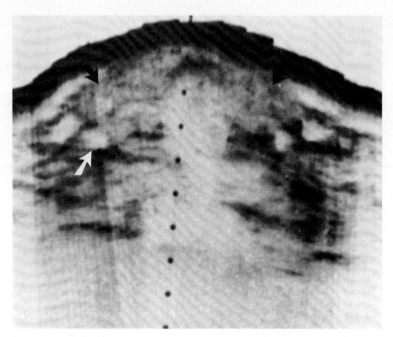

Figure 8-4. Normal thyroid (transverse, 6 cm above the sternal notch). The normal thyroid appears as a mildly echogenic structure that lies to either side of the trachea (*black arrow*). Since it contains gas, the trachea exhibits distal acoustical shadowing. The inferior medial aspect of the thyroid is delineated by the carotid artery (*white arrow*). Lateral to the carotid artery is the jugular vein, which can be distended by a Valsalva maneuver.

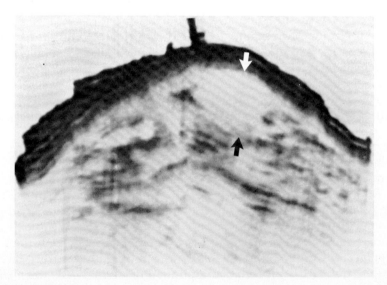

Figure 8-5. Colloid thyroid cyst (transverse, 6 cm above sternal notch). There is a sono-lucent, well-defined mass in the left lobe of the thyroid. The mass exhibits distal acoustical enhancement and smooth boundaries (*arrows*). The mass was found to represent a colloid cyst. Aspiration of benign thyroid cysts can be performed with ultrasonic guidance.

Figure 8-6. THYROID LESIONS

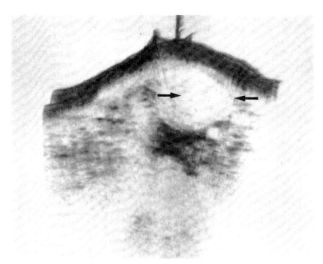

Figure 8-6A. Adenoma (transverse, 5 cm above sternal notch). This adenoma has a thick sonolucent halo around it (*arrows*). The "halo" sign is frequently seen in adenomas.

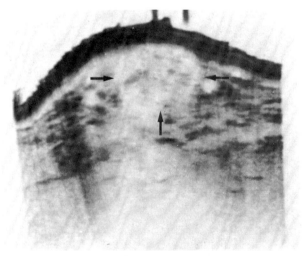

Figure 8-6B. Thyroid carcinoma (transverse, 5 cm above sternal notch). There is an irregular, moderately echogenic thyroid mass (*arrows*) that has a nonhomogeneous texture. This represented a folliculo-papillary carcinoma.

specific. However, it has been reported that a complex thyroid mass consisting of a sonolucent halo and echogenic center often represents an adenoma of the thyroid (6) (Fig. 8-6A). Solid masses that undergo cystic degeneration or that contain areas of fluid may also produce a complex echo pattern.

Echogenic masses within the thyroid may be difficult to delineate because of the similar echo pattern from the surrounding normal thyroid. However, echogenic masses have a greater likelihood of being malignant than cystic ones (Fig. 8-6B). Carcinoma should be considered as a possibility when one encounters a mass with many internal echoes, especially if it is poorly defined.

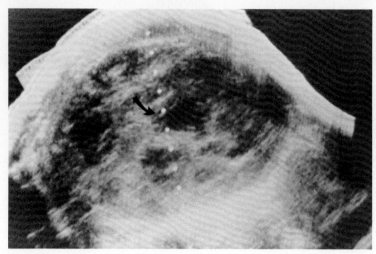

Figure 8-7. Multinodular goiter (transverse, 5 cm above sternal notch, white-on-black image). The thyroid gland is markedly enlarged, with an inhomogeneous texture. There are sonolucent areas within the thyroid, probably representing cystic degeneration within the massively enlarged gland. (Courtesy of Karen Parker, R.D.M.S.)

Sonography is less helpful in the evaluation of diffuse parenchymal disorders of the thyroid than in evaluation of specific masses. Multinodular goiter may appear as numerous nodules of variable echogenicity within the gland (Fig. 8-7). Some of these nodules may exhibit a relatively sonolucent center. The thyroid in patients with goiter is enlarged and nodular in outline. Patients with Grave's disease or thyroiditis will sometimes have a diffusely enlarged gland with an inhomogeneous echogenic texture.

PARATHYROID SONOGRAPHY

The parathyroid organs are difficult to delineate by noninvasive or invasive methods. Ultrasound studies can be used in the detection of enlargement of the parathyroids if the gland is greater than 5 mm in diameter. Delineation of the parathyroids requires meticulous sonographic technique, as well as a thorough knowledge of the anatomical structures in the area of the parathyroids.

Usually, there are four parathyroid glands, which are located in the medial-dorsal aspect of the lateral lobes of the thyroid. The individual glands are approximately 3 to 10 mm long, 2 to 6 mm wide, and 1 to 4 mm thick. The parathyroid glands are located between the medial-dorsal aspect of the lateral lobe of the thyroid and the major neurovascular bundle. These glands are in close proximity to the tracheal-esophageal groove and longus coli muscles. The superior parathyroid glands are more predictable in location than the inferior parathyroid glands. Location of the parathyroid glands may also be variable with aberrant glands located between the trachea and the thyroid as well as within the substance of the thyroid gland.

The parathyroid glands can be identified initially on transverse sonograms using a sector sweep of the tracheal-esophageal groove area on either side of the neck. Longitudinal scans are best performed with a slight medial angulation so that the beam passes through the thyroid, parathyrid region, and along the longus coli muscle. The anatomical structures around the parathyroid gland appear to be best delineated using a contact scanning technique, although the small parts scanner may also be used to delineate these structures.

Normal parathyroid glands appear as moderately echogenic, well-circumscribed structures immediately superior to the longus coli muscle and medial to the common carotid artery. Although hyperplastic glands cannot be differentiated from neoplastic glands by their sonographic appearance, enlarged glands greater than 5 mm in diameter can be detected. Pre-operative recognition of an enlarged gland contributes significantly to limiting the time necessary for identification of abnormal parathyroid glands at surgery.

CHEST SONOGRAPHY

Sonography is useful in evaluating nonspecific opacities seen on the chest radiograph (Figs. 8-8, 8-9A,B, 8-10A,B, 8-11A,B,C,D). Fluid collections can be differentiated from solid pleural and lung masses by their sonographic appearance (9,10). Loculated effusions can be distinguished from nonloculated fluid collection. In addition, many physicians have effectively employed ultrasound for guided aspiration of fluid contents within the chest; this provides a very rapid method of obtaining diagnostic specimen material.

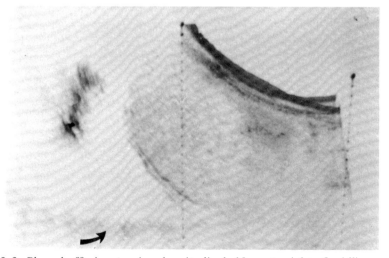

Figure 8-8. Pleural effusion (supine, longitudinal, 10 cm to right of midline, centered over xiphoid). There is a fluid collection superior to the right hemidiaphragm. Normally, the posterior aspect of the hemidiaphragm is not imaged. However, when there is fluid in the subpulmonic area, transmission through the liver to the posterior aspect of the hemidiaphragm is enhanced (*curved arrow*).

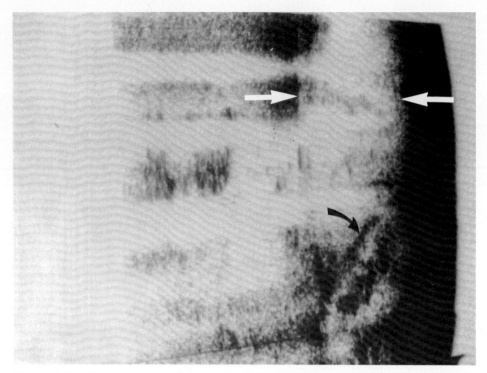

Figure 8-9A. Empyema (upright, 3 cm to right of midline). There is a sonolucent collection (*white arrows*) between the parietal and visceral pleura. Complete acoustical shadowing is seen adjacent to the ribs, which creates a "venetian blind" effect. Although this fluid collection appears to be more echogenic than benign pleural effusion, it is difficult to distinguish between a mass of inflammatory fluid and a collection of serous fluid. However, sonographic study was helpful in determining patient management in this case. It was used to localize an area of fluid that had been refractory to previous attempts at thoracentesis. The location of the pleural fluid in relation to the right kidney (*curved black arrow*) can also be demonstrated.

Since the lung normally contains air, transmission of ultrasound through this structure is minimal. However, when there is fluid or a solid mass between the chest wall and the lung, recognizable echo patterns can be produced.

In general, there is no special technique for the evaluation of opacities of the lung. The area of interest is usually scanned with a 2.25-MHz nonfocused transducer with a small diameter (about 6 mm) so that it can be placed and moved between the ribs. Sector scans in the area of interest are usually sufficient for evaluation of chest masses. Opacities that occur at the lung bases such as in pleural effusion can be examined using a sector scan with the patient supine in the longitudinal plane passing through the liver. Evaluation of the lung bases may also be performed with the patient sitting and the scans obtained along the midaxillary line.

Pleural effusions appear as sonolucent areas superior to the diaphragm. Multiloculated fluid collections are shown as sonolucent areas that have echogenic interfaces emanating from the multiple septations within the pleural effusion.

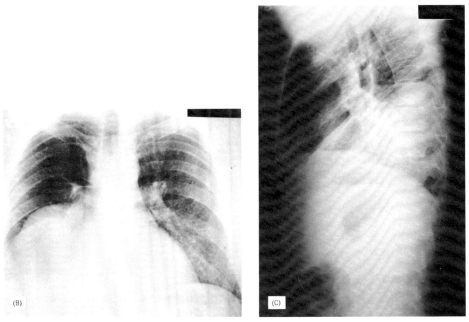

Figures 8-9B,C. Posteroanterior (B) and lateral (C) chest radiographs of same patient as in Figure 8-9A. There is a suggestion of a peripheral fluid collection in the lower right lung zone, which may be loculated. Sonography was helpful in confirming the presence of fluid posteriorly as well as serving as a guide for thoracentesis.

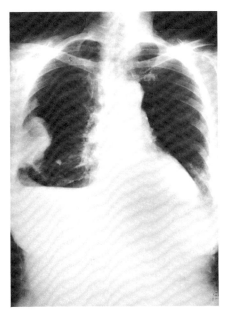

Figure 8-10A. Loculated pleural effusion. This posteroanterior chest radiograph reveals a pleural-based density along the right lateral midchest. There is also evidence of costophrenic angle blunting, suggesting that this is a loculated pleural effusion.

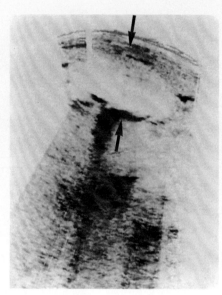

Figure 8-10B. Loculated pleural effusion (right anterior oblique limited sector scan, 2.25-MHz transducer). This limited sector scan was performed in the intercostal space. The loculated pleural effusion appears as a well-defined, lobulated sonolucent collection immediately beneath the chest wall (*arrows*).

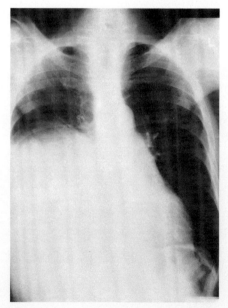

Figure 8-11A. Loculated, malignant pleural effusion. Posteroanterior chest radiograph shows the right hemidiaphragm to be obscured, suggesting a large collection of right subpulmonic fluid.

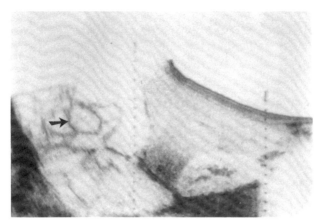

Figure 8-11B. Loculated, malignant pleural effusion (supine, 10 cm to right of midline, centered at xiphoid). Superior to the liver, there is a fluid collection that contains thin internal septations (*arrow*). This was found to represent a loculated, malignant pleural effusion. Adenocarcinoma cells were aspirated from the fluid. Loculation of pleural fluid implies malignancy. (Courtesy of R. Barry Grove, M.D.)

Loculated pleural effusions are seen in the region of the minor fissure on the right side as sonolucent collections of fluid. Solid masses that are located at the periphery of the lung or in the pleura appear as echogenic masses of variable size and shape. The signs associated with parenchymal and pleural masses may also be applied to the sonographic evaluation of solid masses of the pleura.

Artifactual echoes may be created by reverberation of intrahepatic masses and their apparent recording as an echogenic area within the thorax misdiagnosed.

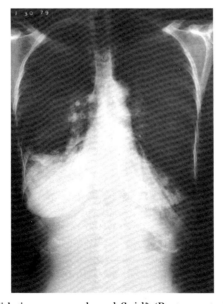

Figure 8-11C.   Consolidation versus pleural fluid? (Posteroanterior chest radiograph).

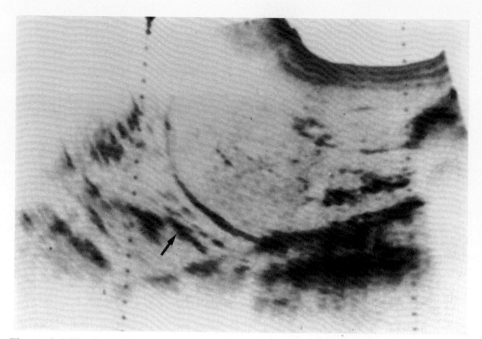

Figure 8-11D. Consolidation (longitudinal, 5 cm to right of midline). There is a solid pattern superior to the right hemidiaphragm representing consolidated lung. The branching, tubular structures represent air and mucus-filled bronchi (*arrow*), making this image a sonographic equivalent of an "air bronchogram." (Courtesy of M. Louis Weinstein, M.D.)

This phenomenon is due to multiple recording of an echogenic mass within the liver and its display as an echo interface superior to the diaphragm (10).

Flattening of the diaphragm can be assessed objectively using sonography. In patients with chronic obstructive pulmonary disease, the diaphragm is flattened, as opposed to its normally concave appearance. However, this determination must be made in a comparable state of respiration, since the configuration of the diaphragm changes during inspiration and expiration. Locating the diaphragm when there is pleural fluid above or an abscess or hematoma below can be an important clinical use of ultrasound.

BREAST SONOGRAPHY

The evaluation of breast lesions by sonography was one of the first investigations concerning the possible clinical applications of ultrasound for medical imaging (15). Recently, there has been renewed interest in the sonographic evaluation of the breast, in part generated by public concern over the possible adverse radiation effects of the more widely practiced forms of mammography. Clinical investigations are currently evaluating the clinical efficacy of ultrasound studies of breast lesions that use a scanning device specifically designed to evaluate the breast.

A method that seems to afford adequate sonographic evaluation of the breast uses a high-frequency transducer (4-MHz) that is internally focused and housed within a water bath. With this device, the patient is placed prone, with the breasts dependent and immersed in the water bath. The ultrasonic beam is directed upward toward the breasts from within the water bath. The transducers are capable of either a compound scan motion that affords acceptable spatial detail or linear simple scanning that is used to determine the attenuation values from within the breast. Transverse scans are obtained in 5-mm intervals cranial and caudal with the nipple as the reference point; 2-mm tomograms may also be obtained. The transverse scan allows display and comparison of both breasts on one image. In general, masses that are located in the center of the breast are more readily delineated than those located in the periphery because of better lateral resolution of the individual structures.

As observed with other imaging modalities of the breast, a wide range of echo patterns arise from the normal breast structures, depending primarily upon the age and parity of the patient. Sonographically, the normal glandular elements of the breast appear as a central area of mildly echogenic, relatively homogeneous tissue (Fig. 8-12). Lateral and posterior to the glandular tissue of the breast are the less echogenic supporting ligaments and fat that surrounds the breast. Intramammary ducts with diameters as small as 2 mm can be delineated as branching, tubular structures that converge toward the nipple.

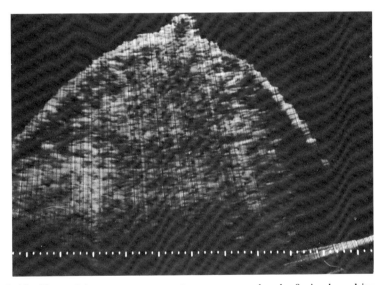

Figure 8-12. Normal breast sonogram (transverse at level of nipple, white-on-black image). Sonogram performed in a transverse manner with the breast immersed in a water bath demonstrates the normal sonographic appearance of the breast. The central portion of the breast has a mildly echogenic inhomogeneous texture arising from the mammary glands. The peripheral portions are less echogenic than the central portions and represent the ligaments and subcutaneous fat within the breast. (Courtesy of Barry Goldberg, M.D., Thomas Jefferson University, Philadelphia, Penn.)

At present, ultrasound studies are most useful in the evaluation of palpable breast masses that are thought to be cystic. As in other organs of the body, cystic lesions in the breast appear as sonolucent, well-defined masses that exhibit distal acoustical enhancement (Fig. 8-13). Even though a mass appears cystic on a breast sonogram, it may still be preferable to perform an aspiration procedure and/or biopsy of the mass. As is observed with other forms of mammary dysplasia, cystic breast lesions tend to regress after menopause.

Differentiation between benign and malignant breast masses can be inferred by ultrasound examination of the regularity of the borders of the mass. In general, benign breast masses tend to exhibit a well-defined, smooth border in relation to the surrounding tissue, whereas malignant masses demonstrate an ill-defined, irregular border. For example, most scirrhous carcinomas demonstrate an irregular border, whereas fibroadenomas are usually well circumscribed. An exception to this generalization is medullary carcinoma, which usually causes a well-defined, moderately echogenic mass. The type and quantity of calcification within a breast mass are not as apparent sonographically as on mammography studies performed by xeroradiography or conventional film emulsion radiography. As a general observation, most breast tumors are less echogenic than normal glandular tissue.

Several sonographic patterns have been observed in the various types of mammary dysplasia. Enlarged ducts greater than 2 mm in a diameter can be demonstrated by ultrasound. Sonography may be of particular use in the evaluation of a radiographically "dense" breast, for tumors in these patients may be recognized as less echogenic foci within the echogenic, dysplastic breast.

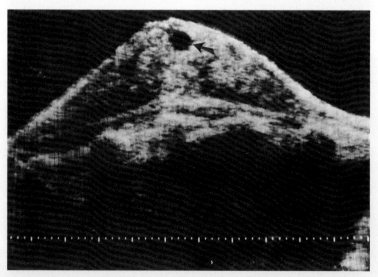

Figure 8-13. Breast cyst (transverse at level of nipple, white-on-black image). There is a well-defined, 8-mm cystic mass immediately beneath the nipple area (*arrow*). At present, sonography has its greatest application in the confirmation of breast masses that are thought to be cystic. (Courtesy of Barry Goldberg, M.D., Thomas Jefferson University, Philadelphia, Penn.)

Although at present the application of sonography for the evaluation of breast lesions is limited, this modality will probably be used more extensively as the result of further improvements in image resolution and greater clinical experience.

SONOGRAPHIC LOCALIZATION OF MASSES

As described in several sections, sonography is a useful modality for the localization and characterization of many types of masses. The ability to image a mass in several planes allows a flexible approach to the delineation of a mass for biopsy, aspiration, and radiation treatment planning. Real-time scanning provides dynamic localization of the area to be investigated.

With the recent increased use of aspiration biopsy procedures, the need for precise localization of masses has become increasingly important. Once the area of the mass is localized, its depth from the anterior skin surface and position within the body is determined. An aspiration needle is then introduced through the skin while suction is applied within the syringe. The needle is passed several times through the area of interest. The cellular material obtained is immediately sent for cytological evaluation. This method is most frequently used for the evaluation of renal and pancreatic lesions.

Sonographic localization of tumors can also be used for radiation treatment planning. The contour of the body is readily displayed when the transducer is passed over the area of interest using a high-gain setting. When a high-gain setting is used, only the "main bang" of the transducer will be displayed. The localization of a tumor relative to the skin can be established and the edges of the treatment portal marked by lifting the transducer off the patient while "writing" with the transducer.

The position of an intracavitary tandem relative to a uterine tumor is also readily depicted by pelvic sonography. The tandem appears as a curved, echogenic structure that should be symmetrically located within the uterine lumen (Fig. 8-14). The depth of the tandem from the anterior abdominal wall, its distance from the bladder and colon, and the thickness of the myometrium can be established. Perforation of the uterine wall by the tandem or improper placement can also be demonstrated (see Chapter 3).

Finally, sonography is a useful modality for assessment of the regression or growth of a mass during and after therapy.

VASCULAR SONOGRAPHY

Many of the larger arteries and veins can be delineated using gray scale techniques. With the "small parts" scanner, many of the superficial vessels can be delineated. Narrowing and vascular occlusion of the great vessels in the neck can be demonstrated using this technique.

As briefly described in the subsection on thyroid sonography, the "small parts" scanner employs a 10-MHz transducer that is encased in a water bath. This type

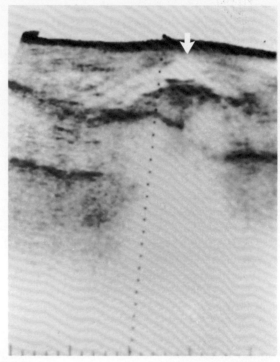

Figure 8-14. Popliteal artery aneurysm (longitudinal along course of popliteal artery). There is aneurysmal dilatation of the popliteal artery (*arrow*). These aneurysms may be difficult to demonstrate angiographically due to multiple intraluminal occlusions.

of transducer is also referred to as a water-delay type of transducer, since the incident beam passes through water before it is passed through the body. The advantages of this type of scanner are that superficial structures are readily examined and artifacts due to certain aspects of near field contact scanning are eliminated. High-frequency real-time transducers that are placed on the skin may also be used for evaluation of some of the larger superficial vessels, such as the common carotid artery.

The patency of the common carotid artery in the region of the bifurcation is readily visualized using either a high-frequency real-time transducer or the small parts scanner. Collections of atherosclerotic plaque appear as moderately echogenic areas projecting into the lumen of the vessel. Calcifications within an atherosclerotic plaque appear as a cluster of high-level echoes and can occasionally hamper delineation of the distal aspect of the vessel. Demonstration of significant narrowing of the common carotid or its branches does not, however, preclude further angiographic evaluation since data on the patency of the intracranial circulation are of primary importance in evaluating the extent of the disease. Nevertheless, sonography is useful as a screening procedure for patients who present with carotid bruits or vague symptoms of ischemia; a negative sonogram may preclude further invasive diagnostic evaluation (Fig. 8-15A).

In addition to the carotid vessels, the femoral, iliac, and popliteal arteries may be evaluated for obstruction or aneurysmal dilatation (Fig. 8-16). Evaluation of

Figure 8-15. VASCULAR SONOGRAMS

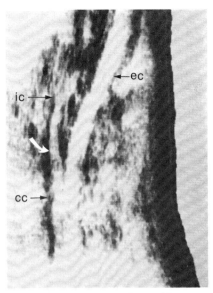

Figure 8-15A. Atherosclerotic plaque in internal carotid artery (supine, longitudinal scan along course of carotid artery). The internal (ic) and external carotid (ec) arteries can be traced from their bifurcation from the common carotid artery (cc). Narrowing at the origin of the internal carotid (ic) artery by atherosclerotic plaque is detected as echogenic, intraluminal material (*curved white arrow*). (Courtesy of Mack Williams, M.D., Cookeville General Hospital, Cookeville, Tenn.)

the renal arteries by sonography is less reliable because of their variable course and small size. In general, arteriographic evaluation is still indicated prior to surgery for an abdominal aneurysm, for extension into the renal arteries or into the iliac arteries may alter the surgical approach. Real-time or small parts scanning can also be used in the evaluation of the patency of vascular grafts in patients undergoing dialysis. Areas of aneurysmal dilatation or narrowing in the graft can be delineated.

Doppler instruments that detect flow within a vessel are frequently employed in the preoperative evaluation of areas of ischemia in the extremities (Fig. 8-15B). The data obtained by the Doppler examination of the extremity are useful

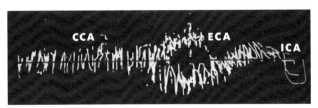

Figure 8-15B. "Dopscan" of normal arteries. This image was obtained by combining a B-scan with a Doppler device. A line is recorded where flow (Doppler signal) is present. Decreased or absent flow will be depicted as an area of diminished Doppler signal. As in B-scans of the carotid arteries, false results may be obtained when an area of calcified plaque prohibits adequate penetration of the incident beam.

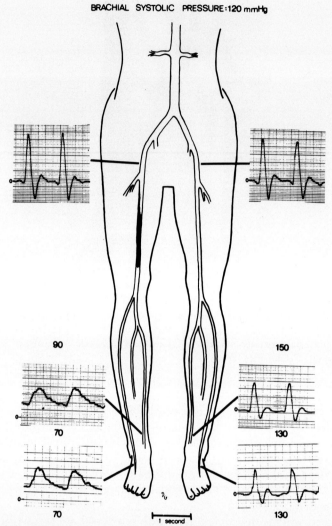

Figure 8-15C. Doppler evaluation for vascular insufficiency. Multiple Doppler tracings depicting frequency shifts caused by arterial blood flow at various regions of the lower extremity are obtained. On the side of occlusion at the level of the superficial femoral artery, the amplitude of the Doppler wave forms obtained from the dorsalis pedis and posterior tibial circulations are flattened and the systolic blood pressure is decreased. The hemodynamic significance of an occlusion can be ascertained by evaluation of the systolic blood pressure. (Courtesy of Richard Dean, M.D., Vanderbilt University School of Medicine, Nashville, Tenn.)

in determining the level at which amputation or vascular repair should be performed, as well as the relative prognosis for healing after the operation. Some scanners have the combined capability of static imaging and Doppler determinations. This correlation may reveal both the anatomic and physiologic state of a particular organ (24). Areas of occlusion can be detected by alteration of the

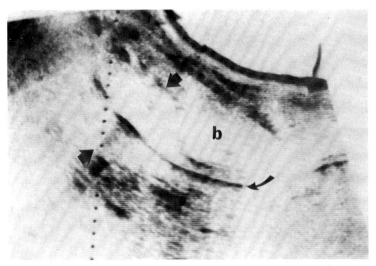

Figure 8-16. Intracavitary tandem (longitudinal, midline). The tandem appears as a curved, echogenic interface located symmetrically within the uterus (*arrow*). The tandem should be within the endometrial lumen for optimal effectiveness.

Doppler frequency shift or "wave form." The hemodynamic significance of an occlusion can be inferred by demonstration of the systolic blood pressure distal to the suspected occlusion (Fig. 8-15C). We predict that combined imaging and pulsed Doppler will be of great future clinical importance.

ORTHOPEDIC SONOGRAPHY

Because bone is highly echo-reflective, sonography has limited use in orthopedics. However, ultrasound has been employed in the evaluation of effusions around joints and in the diagnosis of a Baker's cyst. Occasionally, clotted blood can be differentiated from serous fluid around the joint, since clotted blood may emanate scattered echoes. Sonography is also helpful in evaluating soft tissue masses that are associated with bony lesions. This is commonly encountered in patients with Ewing's sarcoma. This is particularly helpful when the soft tissue extension of the lesion is not readily apparent radiographically. CT scanning can also be used to evaluate the soft tissue component of a bony lesion.

Ultrasound examination of patients with a suspected Baker's cyst is best performed with the patient prone. Longitudinal and transverse scans can be performed over the region of interest in the upper calf and popliteal fossa using a high-frequency transducer. Baker's cysts usually result from rupture of the posterior bursa and extravasation of synovial fluid into the calf muscles. A Baker's cyst appears as a complex, predominately sonolucent mass in the posterior aspect of the knee joint and may extend down into the calf area (Figs. 8-17A,B). If clotted blood is present within the cysts or if extravasation into muscle planes of the calf muscles has occurred, echoes can be seen within the mass. Since the

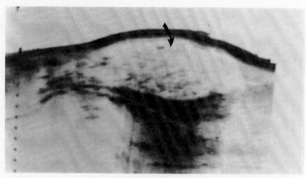

Figure 8-17A. Baker's cyst (prone, longitudinal, 2 cm to right of midline, centered over calf). There is a complex, predominantly cystic mass (*curved arrow*) in the upper thigh representing extravasated synovial fluid from a rupture of the posterior bursa of the knee in this patient with rheumatoid arthritis. Sonography is helpful in establishing this diagnosis, for the symptoms of this condition can be mimicked by thrombophlebitis. Since Baker's cysts are not true cysts, they contain echogenic components representing extravasated fluid around the muscle bundles.

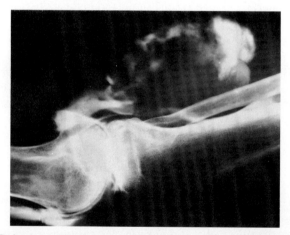

Figure 8-17B. Baker's cyst seen in Figure 8-17A (single-contrast arthrogram, lateral view). Extravasated synovial fluid forming the Baker's cyst is easily demonstrated by this single-contrast arthrogram. Sonographic study for a Baker's cyst may be the method of choice in the rare occasion when there is a history of iodine sensitivity.

symptoms produced by a Baker's cyst often mimic thrombophlebitis, ultrasound studies are clinically useful in establishing the presence of a Baker's cyst.

A similar technique can be used for evaluation of synovial effusions. As stated previously, bloody effusions can be differentiated from effusions that contain serous fluid because clotted blood is echogenic.

IMAGES FOR THE FUTURE

Over the last decade, great improvement in image resolution has resulted from extensive investigation concerning data retrieval and image processing. The addition of digital scan converters offers promise of better standardization of scanning devices as well as image interrogation through the use of pre- and postimaging processing. Automated scanning devices may also contribute to more uniform image display and have particular application in the evaluation of stationary superficial structures such as the breasts. Advances in data retrieval and image display may also allow quantification of the echo pattern of certain structures, as well as their identification through a "tissue signature." "Tissue signature" refers to recognition of a certain echo complex characteristic of the tissue of a certain organ (29). Through this method, it may be possible to convert the echo strength from any interface to a digital number. With enough samples and a sufficient repository of characteristic profiles, not only can the tissue be identified, but it is also possible to tell whether it is normal or abnormal.

Other advances in data retrieval and image display may occur with the advent of acoustical holography. With this type of display, the three-dimensional aspect of a structure can be visualized by an analysis of its interference pattern. In this method, three coherent beams of ultrasound are directed toward an object, and the changes in direction and phase of the beam are used in the reconstruction of a three-dimensional image. Because of its limited ability to penetrate structures, acoustical holography has been used in the evaluation of the extremities. By using this technique, the osseous structures as well as their tendinous attachments can be demonstrated.

As mentioned in the subsection on vascular sonography, imaging devices using both static and Doppler instrumentation can be employed for evaluation of the anatomic and physiologic state of an organ or structure. The Doppler device can detect the relative perfusion and the flow of blood through a vessel, whereas the static imaging portion of the unit can portray the anatomical region of interest.

At present, sonography can only detect morphologic abnormalities of a structure or organ system. In the future, it is anticipated that the resolution of ultrasound devices will allow evaluation of living tissue on the microscopic level. This can already be achieved by acoustical microscopy that uses frequencies in the range of 100 MHz. Very high frequencies can be used because of the thinness of the tissue being examined by this method. The resolution of acoustic microscopy now approaches that of optical microscopy (28). The information obtained by acoustic microscopy theoretically varies from that obtained using optical microscopy, since the interactions of the tissue with these two energy forms are different. However, armed with the information concerning the cellular components of an organ, it may be possible to diagnose disease at an earlier stage, before it becomes clinically manifest.

SUMMARY

We predict continued growth in utility and importance of this multifaceted discipline. Knowledge gained from this text will hopefully provide the reader with an appropriate foundation to understand the development and progress in diagnostic sonography, and to accurately assess its virtues and limitations when compared with alternative imaging modalities.

REFERENCES

Ophthalmologic Sonography

1. Bronson, N., Fisher, Y., Pickering, N., Trayner, E.: *Ophthalmologic Contact B-Mode Ultrasonography for the Clinician.* Westport: Intercontinental Publishers, 1976.
2. Coleman, D., Lizzy, F., Jack, R.: *Ultrasonography of the Eye and Orbit.* Philadelphia: Lea and Febiger, 1977.
3. Correia, C.: Use of ultrasound in ophthalmologic evaluations. *Radiol./Nucl. Med.,* October, 1978, pp. 25–34.

Thyroid Sonography

4. Chilcote, W.: Gray scale ultrasonography of the thyroid. *Radiology* 120:361–363, 1976.
5. Sackler, J., Passlaque, A., Blum, M., Amorocho, L.: A spectrum of diseases of the thyroid gland as imaged by ray scale water bath sonography. *Radiology* 125:467–472, 1977.
6. Hassani, N.: Ultrasonic investigation of solid thyroid tumors with gray scale and real time scanning: The halo sign. *Appl. Radiol.* 1977, pp. 165–180.
7. Jensen, F., Rasmussen, S. M.: The treatment of thyroid cysts by ultrasonically guided fine needle aspiration. *Acta Chic Scand.* 142:209–211, 1976.

Parathyroid Sonography

8. Sample, W., Mitchell, S., Bledsoe, R.: Parathyroid ultrasonography. *Radiology* 127:485–490, 1978.

Chest Sonography

9. Hirsch, J., Carter, S., Chikos, P., Colacurcio, C.: Ultrasonic evaluation of radiographic opacities of the chest. *Am. J. Roentgenol.* 130:1153–1156, 1978.
10. Cosgrove, D., Garburt, D., Hill, C.: Echoes across the diaphragm. *Ultrasound in Med. and Biol.* 385–392, 1978.

Breast Sonography

11. Texidor, H., Kazam, E.: Combined mammographic-sonographic evaluation of breast masses. *Am. J. Roentgenol.* 128:409–417, 1977.
12. Jellins, J., Kossoff, G., Reeve, T.: Detection and classification of liquid-filled masses in the breast by gray-scale echography. *Radiology* 125:205–212, 1977.
13. Griffins, L.: Ultrasound examination of the breast. *Med. Ultrasound* 2:13–19, 1978.
14. Baum, G.: Ultrasound mammography. *Radiology* 122:199–205, 1977.
15. Wild, J., Reid, J.: Further pilot echographic studies on the histologic structure of tumors of living intact human breast. *Am. J. Pathol.* 28:839–842, 1952.

Sonographic Localization of Masses

16. Skolnick, M., Dekker, A., Weinstein, B.: Ultrasound guided fine-needle aspiration biopsy of abdominal masses. *Gastrointest. Radiol.* 3:295–302, 1978.

Vascular Sonography

17. Corson, J., Johnson, W., LoGerfo, F., Bush, H., Menzorini, J., Kumanki, D., Nasbeth, D.: Doppler ankle systolic blood pressure—prognostic value in the venous bypass grafts of lower extremity. *Arch. Surg.* 113:932, 1978.
18. Jaques, P., Richey, W., Ely, C., Johnson, G.: Doppler ultrasonic screening prior to venography for deep venous thrombosis. *Am. J. Roentgenol.* 129:451–452, 1977.

19. Benchimol, A., Desser, K.: Clinical application of the Doppler ultrasonic flowmeter. *Am. J. Cardiol.* 29:540–545, 1972.

20. Silver, T., Washburn, R., Stanley, J., Gross, W.: Gray scale ultrasound evaluation of popliteal aneurysms. *Am. J. Roentgenol.* 129:1003–1006, 1977.

21. Gooding, G., Herzog, K., Hedgecock, M., Eisenberg, R.: B-mode ultrasonography of prosthetic vascular grafts. *Radiology* 127:763–766, 1978.

22. Kottle, S., Gonzalez, A., Macon, C., Fellner, S.: Ultrasonographic evaluation of vascular access complications. *Radiology* 129:751–754, 1978.

23. Silver, T., Washburn, R., Stanley, J., Gross, W.: Gray scale ultrasound evaluation of popliteal artery aneurysms. *Am. J. Roentgenol.* 129:1003–1006, 1977.

24. Crummy, A., Zwiebel, W., Barriga, P., Strother, C., Sackett, J., Turnipseed, W., Jarrett, F., Berkoff, H.: Doppler evaluation of extracranial cerebrovascular disease. *Am. J. Roentgenol.* 132:91–93, 1979.

Orthopedic Sonography

25. Rudikoff, J. C., Lynch, J. J., Philipps, E., Clapp, P. R.: Ultrasound diagnosis of Baker cyst. *J.A.M.A.* 235(10):1054–1055, 1976.

26. Cooperberg, P. L., Tsang, I., Truelove, L., Knickerbocker, J.: Gray scale ultrasound in the evaluation of rheumatoid arthritis of the knee. *Radiology* 126:759–763, 1978.

27. deSantos, L. A., Goldstein, H. M.: Ultrasonography in tumors arising from the spine and bony pelvis. *Am. J. Roentgenol.* 129:1061–1064, 1977.

Images for the Future

28. Quate, C.: The acoustic microscope. *Scientific American* 241(4):62–70, 1979.

29. Linzer, M., ed.: *Ultrasonic Tissue Characterization.* Washington, D.C.: National Bureau of Standards Publication No. 453, 1976.

Index